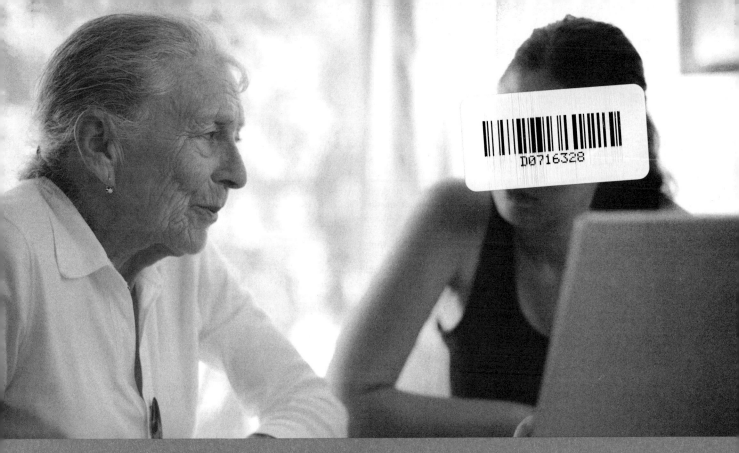

Introduction to Neurogenic Communication Disorders

M. Hunter Manasco, PhD
Department of Speech-Language Pathology
Misericordia University
Dallas, Pennsylvania

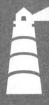

JONES & BARTLETT
LEARNING

World Headquarters
Jones & Bartlett Learning
5 Wall Street
Burlington, MA 01803
978-443-5000
info@jblearning.com
www.jblearning.com

Jones & Bartlett Learning books and products are available through most bookstores and online booksellers. To contact Jones & Bartlett Learning directly, call 800-832-0034, fax 978-443-8000, or visit our website, www.jblearning.com.

Substantial discounts on bulk quantities of Jones & Bartlett Learning publications are available to corporations, professional associations, and other qualified organizations. For details and specific discount information, contact the special sales department at Jones & Bartlett Learning via the above contact information or send an email to specialsales@jblearning.com.

Production Credits
Publisher: William Brottmiller
Senior Acquisitions Editor: Katey Birtcher
Managing Editor: Maro Gartside
Associate Editor: Teresa Reilly
Editorial Assistant: Sean Fabery
Production Editor: Amanda Clerkin
Marketing Manager: Grace Richards
Manufacturing and Inventory Control Supervisor: Amy Bacus
Composition: Publishers' Design and Production Services, Inc.
Cover Design: Michael O'Donnell

Cover Images: © Konstantin Sutyagin/ShutterStock, Inc.; (listed left to right) Courtesy of the Alzheimer's Disease Education and Referral Center, a service of the National Institute on Aging; © Lawrence Berkeley National Library/Photodisc/Thinkstock; Courtesy of the Alzheimer's Disease Education and Referral Center, a service of the National Institute on Aging; Courtesy of Dr. Giovanni Di Chiro, Neuromimaging Center, National Institute of Neurologic/National Cancer Institute
Printing and Binding: Edwards Brothers Malloy
Cover Printing: Edwards Brothers Malloy

To order this product, use ISBN: 978-1-4496-5244-9

Library of Congress Cataloging-in-Publication Data
Manasco, Hunter.
  Introduction to neurogenic communication disorders / M. Hunter Manasco.
    p. ; cm.
  Includes bibliographical references and index.
  ISBN 978-0-7637-9417-0
  I. Title.
  [DNLM: 1. Communication Disorders.   WL 340.2]
  616.85'5—dc23
                                                     2012034511

6048

Printed in the United States of America
17 16 15 14   10 9 8 7 6 5 4 3 2

Contents

CHAPTER 10   Counseling 239

Cari M. Tellis, Nicholas A. Barone, and Orlando R. Barone

Special thanks are given to all my patients, colleagues, and associates who gave their time and permission to present their clinical experiences, expertise, and personal stories in this book using the videos and written anecdotes. All personally identifying information in these components of the book has been removed or changed to protect the identities of these individuals.

M. Hunter Manasco

Preface

O the blest eyes, the happy hearts,
That see, that know the guiding thread so fine,
Along the mighty labyrinth
   —Walt Whitman from *Song of the Universal*

Only that day dawns to which we are awake.
There is more day to dawn. The sun is but a
morning star.
   —Henry David Thoreau from *Walden*

My goal for this book is to create an informal text that presents the included material in a way that is accessible to student readers while also displaying how exciting, interesting, and truly *human* this material is. If not pushed, most students fall easily into interpreting all material in a textbook as purely academic, merely facts on a page, nonemotional, and therefore not connected to real life. For the student of health science moving toward a helping profession, this is an ineffective position at best and a dangerous perception at worst. In our time of desensitization to violence, decreased face-to-face interactions, and seemingly general hardening of emotions, it is with increasing effort that the student of health science must be reminded to see, must be pushed to be attentive to the human reality of the information presented in textbooks and classrooms.

The information, conditions, and diseases discussed in this book are not simply academic problems— they are also nonacademic and emotional. It is one thing to read about and recognize intellectually that there is no effective treatment for Alzheimer's disease. It is quite another to *know* this as you view a video of a man with this disease and hear his wife explain her attempts to stall her husband's steady deterioration in cognition and describe the effects of this disease on their lives. This furthering of students' early knowledge by emphasizing the relevant effects on humanity creates more enthusiastic and more knowledgeable students who become more enthusiastic and knowledgeable professionals.

The use of clinical anecdotes in teaching health sciences has been out of style for some time, though the medical and psychological sciences have historically relied on this teaching method with good reason. I have found that by presenting academic facts *and* clinical reality, I can permanently burn into students' minds more relevant knowledge using a single 5-minute anecdote than an hour-long lecture. Hence, throughout this text I take the liberty of inserting the first person *I* to recount interesting facts, events, or anecdotes or refer readers to video clips posted on this book's website. My hope is that these additions to the text work to illustrate, inform, humanize, and reinforce the primary material for students.

I would like to remind my student readers that healthcare professionals are individuals who deal in humanity. This work can be performed humanely or inhumanely. Almost everyone has a story about themselves or a loved one being grossly misused, abused, or neglected somehow in a healthcare setting by a healthcare professional. Similarly, anyone who has spent time receiving health care also has opposite stories of being treated with extreme kindness by their healthcare workers. So, I ask my student readers openly:

> *Which of these is the more effective approach to patient care?*
>
> *Which of these experiences will you work to create in the lives of others?*

Is it surprising to think that *deliberate* kindness to others must be encouraged as a learned behavior among students and healthcare professionals? Need we look far into the past, or even beyond the present, or our own personal experiences to find instances of total abandonment of this ideal?

I encourage my students to recall a quote by the physician William Osler each time they are about to enter a hospital room or deal with a client or patient:

> Ask not what disease the person has, but rather what person the disease has.

Contributors

Nicholas A. Barone, MS
Doctoral Student
James Madison University
Harrisonburg, Virginia

Orlando R. Barone, MA
President
Barone Associates
Doylestown, Pennsylvania

Cari M. Tellis, PhD, CCC-SLP
Associate Professor
Misericordia University
Dallas, Pennsylvania

Reviewers

Features of this Text

Introduction to Neurogenic Communication Disorders incorporates a number of engaging pedagogical features to aid in the student's understanding and retention of the material.

Throughout the text, key points are explained and important information is highlighted to ensure comprehension and to aid the study of critical material. Clinical anecdotes, a colorful, engaging layout, and high-quality art coalesce in this accessible resource to enable easy reading and support the retention of important concepts. Each chapter includes bolded **Key Terms** and shaded definition boxes for student reference and review.

Broca's area The inferior, posterior region of the frontal lobe of the left hemisphere that is a specialized area of the cerebrum responsible for finding and assembling words for the appropriate expression of thought.

Wernicke's area A specialized portion of the cerebrum located at the superior marginal gyrus of the left hemisphere's temporal lobe that is responsible for interpreting and deriving meaning from the speech of others.

Central sulcus A deep groove that runs down the middle lateral surface of each cerebral hemisphere.

Lateral sulcus A deep groove that begins at the lower frontal aspect of each of the two cerebral hemispheres and travels at an upward angle, passes the central sulcus, and then terminates.

figure–ground relationships (Joseph, 1988). Visuospatial processing skills are used to piece together a jigsaw puzzle, sink a basket in a basketball game, and successfully navigate your body from place to place past and around innumerable obstacles.

The right hemisphere also plays a great role in the ability to attend to stimuli. There are various levels of attention, and the right hemisphere plays a role in regulating most kinds. Specifically, the right hemisphere specializes in the ability to keep attention on a single stimulus for an extended period of time (sustained attention) and the ability to ignore unimportant stimuli while sustaining attention on important stimuli (selective attention). An example of sustained attention is paying attention to a lecture in a classroom. If a lawn mower is running outside the classroom during the lecture, then students must actively block out the distracting sound of the lawn mower to focus on the lecture, which is an example of selective attention.

Left Cerebral Hemisphere

As mentioned, the left cerebral hemisphere has been the subject of study more than the right hemisphere has. This is mostly because the left hemisphere typically is the hemisphere that houses language. The discovery that certain locations in the left hemisphere are responsible for expressive and receptive language skills cued researchers in the late 1800s to begin examining the relationship between brain and cognition more closely.

In 1861, Paul Broca published the results of his studies indicating that the inferior, posterior region of the frontal lobe of the left hemisphere is responsible for finding and assembling words for the appropriate expression of thought. This area is now known as Broca's area (Figure 2-8). Damage to this area can produce what is known as Broca's aphasia. Individuals with this disorder usually know what they want to say but cannot find the right words.

A few years later in 1874, Carl Wernicke localized receptive language to the superior marginal gyrus of the left hemisphere's temporal lobe. This area is now known as Wernicke's area (Figure 2-8). Wernicke's area is responsible for interpreting and deriving meaning from the speech of others. Damage to this area produces a condition known as Wernicke's aphasia. Individuals with this disorder cannot comprehend the speech of others, and their own speech is often nonsensical and nonstop.

The Major Cerebral Lobes

Two important sulci are the central sulcus and the lateral sulcus (Figure 2-8). The central sulcus, also known as the fissure of Rolando or the central fissure, runs down the middle lateral surface of each cerebral hemisphere. The lateral sulcus, also known as the sylvian fissure, begins at the lower frontal aspect of each of the two cerebral hemispheres, travels at an upward angle, passes the central sulcus, and then terminates. The central and lateral sulci create important divisions among the major sections, or lobes, of the cerebrum. The lobes of the cerebrum are each named for the bones of the cranium that overlay them.

As the central sulci run down the side of each cerebral hemisphere they create a division between the

Video content is a key element of this valuable resource. Illustrative footage is included with every new print copy of *Introduction to Neurogenic Communication Disorders* on the **Companion Website** and embedded in the online, JBL eFolio edition, also available for purchase.

 Where this icon appears, visit http://go.jblearning.com/ManascoCWS to view the corresponding video.

The *Introduction to Neurogenic Communication Disorders* **Companion Website** also includes useful study activities, practice quizzes, flashcards, and more. To redeem the Access Code Card available with your new copy of the resource, or to purchase access to the website separately, visit http://go.jblearning.com/ManascoCWS.

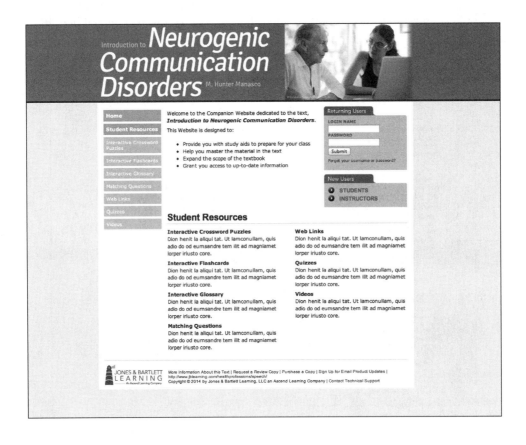

In every chapter, boxed features explore critical points further and emphasize application of clinical content. These elements enable the student to understand the experience of both the patient and the clinician:

Author's Notes provide engaging insight into key points, making abstract concepts and challenging material easily comprehensible through accessible language and examples.

Clinical Notes present illustrative anecdotes from the author's real-world experience. These illuminating case vignettes give students a window into how clinical conditions affect real people and will impact their future practice.

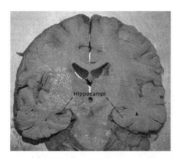

Figure 2-11   Hippocampi displayed on a coronal section of the brain.

left hemisphere (Figure 2-8). The primary auditory cortex is the section of the temporal lobes that first receives neural impulses of sound from the ears.

In the left temporal lobe, the left primary auditory cortex receives impulses of speech sounds and then passes these impulses on to Wernicke's area for processing so that, as mentioned earlier, the individual can comprehend spoken language. The right hemisphere's primary auditory cortex mostly passes impulses of environmental sounds and music to the area in the right hemisphere analogous to Wernicke's area (Bhatnagar, 2008) for the interpretation of meaning. Hence, the left hemisphere is responsible for auditory comprehension of verbal language while the right hemisphere is responsible for comprehension of the meaning of environmental sounds, such as a car starting or tree falling, as well as our appreciation of music.

Anterograde amnesia
An inability to create new memories.

Occipital lobes   The most posterior section of the cerebrum that is dedicated to receiving and processing neural impulses related to vision.

Clinical Note

Patient H.M.

The role of the hippocampus in creating new memories was brought to the attention of the medical community in the 1950s. A patient now known as H.M. was experiencing epileptic seizures to the point of being unable to work. Medications were ineffective in controlling his seizures (Scoville & Milner, 1957). Drastic action was considered to be warranted given H.M.'s severe epileptic condition. Dr. William Beecher Scoville decided to attempt a radical surgery on H.M.'s temporal lobes to relieve the patient of his seizures. Dr. Scoville removed sections of both H.M.'s temporal lobes extending into the hippocampal regions. This operation was performed in 1953 and was successful in relieving the patient of most of his seizures. However, an unexpected result of the surgery was a profound deficit in the ability to create new memories (Scoville & Milner, 1957). Although his memory of events prior to the surgery was mostly intact, Scoville and Milner (1957) report that 2 years after his surgery H.M. was still incapable of storing new information in his memory. This form of amnesia is known as **anterograde amnesia.** Scoville and Milner (1957) give some examples of the daily impact of H.M.'s memory deficit: After living in a new house for 10 months, H.M. still could not find his way around it; he would complete the same jigsaw puzzles and read the same magazines each day "without finding their contents familiar" (p. 14).

Although he possessed no conscious recollection of it, H.M. allowed a steady stream of scientists and students to study him and his memory continually throughout his life (Corkin, 2002). H.M.'s contribution to the understanding and science of memory and the brain is monumental. He also arranged for his brain to be exhumed for examination upon his death so that his case could continue to help others (Corkin, 2002). In 2008, Patient H.M., widely regarded as one of the most important individuals in the history of neuroscience, died at 82 years of age (Carey, 2008).

The occipital lobes are the most posterior of the cerebral lobes. They are located behind the parietal

Each chapter ends with useful learning and teaching tools to support student understanding, study, and review. **Main Points** are included to summarize key learning objectives and emphasize crucial concepts. **Review Questions** are designed to help students assess what they have learned and engage thoughtful consideration of the content. Finally, **References** provide a bibliography for important resources for further learning and study.

Qualified professors can also receive the full suite of **Instructor Support Resources**, including chapter PowerPoints, Test Banks, and Answer Key for Review Questions. To gain access to these valuable teaching materials, contact your Health Professions representative through www.jblearning.com.

---

apraxia of speech. However, these strategies can also be used as a stop-gap to establish funct nication until the individual with apr has regained enough speech skills for f bal communication. Compensatory s

as AAC or alternative language modalities can also

Main Points

- Motor speech disorders involve i effective manufacture, refineme sion, and execution of motor pla Motor speech disorders includ speech and the dysarthrias.
- Apraxia of speech is divided into t
  - Acquired apraxia of speech, w sult of damage to the brain
  - Developmental apraxia of sp the result of an unknown cong
- Apraxia of speech is the inability sequence (i.e., program) the ne necessary to create appropriate ments for speech.
- Apraxia of speech is the result of the motor speech programmer, v work of structures that contribut tion of motor plans for speech. Le structures such as Broca's area, th tary motor cortex, primary moto ganglia, and cerebellum are invol propriate production of motor pla
- Apraxia of speech is characterize tion errors, limited prosody, slo the visible groping about of the to mandible.
- The prosody of those with aprax usually highly affected by the de speech commonly adopted to av attempts at self-repairing speech
- The articulation errors of those v speech are inconsistent and con

---

and needs before targeting improvement of speech production.
- Restorative strategies reduce the severity of the dysarthria by restoring lost motor abilities.
- Compensatory strategies reduce the impact of the dysarthria on speech or communication while not seeking to reduce severity of the underlying neuromotor deficits.

- Speech compensatory strategies increase intelligibility of the speaker and reduce the impact of dysarthria on speech while not directly targeting the pathologic neuromotor condition producing the dysarthria.
- Nonspeech compensatory strategies entirely bypass speech production to focus on improving overall communication.

Review Questions

1. List the six major types of dysarthria.
2. Why is lesion localization important to the speech-language pathologist?
3. How do unilateral and bilateral trigeminal nerve damage affect speech differently from each another?
4. How do unilateral and bilateral facial nerve damage affect speech differently from each another?
5. How do unilateral and bilateral vagus nerve damage to the pharyngeal plexus affect speech differently from each another?
6. How do unilateral and bilateral vagus nerve damage to the extrinsic branch of the superior laryngeal nerve affect speech differently from each another?
7. How do unilateral and bilateral vagus nerve damage to the recurrent laryngeal nerve affect speech differently from each another?
8. Explain the function of the recurrent laryngeal nerve and why is it called *recurrent*.
9. How do unilateral and bilateral hypoglossal nerve damage affect speech differently from each another?
10. Why does a lesion to the UMN produce spasticity?
11. In UUMN dysarthria, explain why the lower portion of the face contralateral to the lesion is

more weakened than the upper portion of the face contralateral to the lesion.
12. In flaccid dysarthria as a result of unilateral lesion to the facial nerve, explain why this condition (in contrast to UUMN dysarthria) produces weakness equally across the entire affected side of the face.
13. What is the lesion site for ataxic dysarthria and why does a lesion at this location produce the speech qualities associated with ataxic dysarthria?
14. What are the speech characteristics of hypokinetic dysarthria?
15. What are two common profiles of mixed dysarthria and what conditions create these profiles?
16. Where in the CNS can a single small lesion create a mixed dysarthria with three dysarthrias present?
17. Strengthening exercises might be appropriate for which dysarthrias? Explain your rationale.
18. List and explain the exercise principles of strengthening exercises necessary to maximize positive impact on speech.
19. Why are relaxation techniques contraindicated for those with flaccid dysarthria? For which dysarthria(s) are relaxation techniques appropriate?
20. Give an example of a speech compensatory strategy and a nonspeech compensatory strategy.

Chapter 1

Introduction

▶ *Where this icon appears, visit http://go.jblearning.com/ManascoCWS to view the corresponding video.*

Neurogenic Communication Disorders

A **neurogenic communication disorder** is a problem with communication that arises as a result of damage to the brain or other part of the nervous system. Neurogenic communication disorders discussed in this text include the aphasias, the dysarthrias, apraxia of speech, right hemisphere disorders, dementia, as well as the myriad of deficits that can accompany these disorders and negatively affect communication in disease and trauma.

Neurogenic communication disorder A disorder of communication arising from damage to the nervous system.

The Treatment Environment

Speech-language pathologists see and treat the disorders, diseases, and deficits discussed in this book in a variety of settings. Some of these settings are as follows:

- *Skilled nursing facility.* Also known as nursing homes or long-term care facilities, skilled nursing facilities offer 24-hour care for their residents.
- *Acute care facility.* Acute care is the usually short but intensive medical care provided for severe injury or illness. The acute care facility (hospital) often has centers with professional teams that specialize in specific dangerous and severe health scenarios, such as the intensive care unit (ICU), cardiac care unit (CCU), and neonatal intensive care unit (NICU).
- *Rehabilitation facility.* Patients well enough not to require intensive acute medical attention can go to a rehabilitation facility, which provides hospital-level care for the medically stable individual while focusing on providing services such as speech-language therapy, physical therapy, and occupational therapy.
- *Outpatient rehabilitation facility.* When a patient is well enough to return home from the primary rehabilitation facility he or she might still need a great deal of therapy services. These services are often available on an outpatient basis, meaning

that the individual lives at home but returns to the rehabilitation center to take part in therapy sessions.

- *Home health care.* Often once a person leaves inpatient or outpatient rehabilitation, or when the individual's insurance does not pay for those services, the person can receive speech therapy at home.
- *Hospice care.* Hospice care is palliative care meant to manage a person's symptoms and keep the person as comfortable as possible when restoration of health is not possible. The role of the speech-language pathologist in hospice care involves ensuring that the hospice patient has a functional method of communication and swallows as safely as possible.
- *Children's hospital.* Although most of the deficits discussed in this book concern adults, many can occur, sometimes very often (such as traumatic brain injury), in the pediatric population.
- *Schools.* Children who do experience neurogenic communication disorders may never leave school and, if they do so, usually return to school to receive ongoing treatment for speech, language, and cognitive disorders from a speech-language pathologist.

Although these settings are major arenas in which speech-language pathologists treat neurogenic communication disorders, note that many other treatment settings combine characteristics of the settings mentioned. For example, neurogenic communication disorders might be treated in a long-term acute care floor in a hospital. Whereas long-term care facilities serve patients who are medically stable, the more fragile patient might require extended care in an acute facility. ▶ See the video *Rasmussen's Encephalitis, Seizures, and Hemispherectomy* for a patient description of moving through various types of facilities in recovery from brain surgery.

Speech-language pathologists usually see the disorders, diseases, and communication disorders discussed in this book in clinical settings such as medical facilities, not in schools. As a result, I often hear this question from students, "If I plan on working in schools and never working with adults, why do I need to know all this about stroke, disease, and the brain?" I am always pleased to hear this question because it gives me an opportunity to present a cautionary tale, of which there are many (see the following Author's Note).

Author's Note

Horses and Zebras

In the medical culture it is popular to say, "When you hear hoof beats, think horses, not zebras." The meaning of this charming maxim is that the most obvious diagnosis and simplest explanation for a set of symptoms are probably correct. Simply put, the horses are those patients whose symptoms are the result of the most obvious and likely diagnosis, whereas the zebras are those patients whose symptoms are the result of an unlikely and generally unexpected diagnosis.

Hence, if you are a speech-language pathologist working in the schools and a child walks into your office with a speech or language impairment, the odds are that the child is a horse and the problem is a basic developmental articulation or language disorder. Similarly, if you are a pediatrician and a child walks into your office with a low red blood cell count, it is more likely that the child is experiencing a normal variation resulting from a recent cold than it is that the child is a zebra and is one of three diagnosed cases on the continent of an extremely rare blood disorder known cryptically as Diamond Blackfan anemia—yes, this happened to my child. However, shortly after I learned the horses and zebras maxim in graduate school my father presented me with another, which goes: *It does not matter how rare if it is in your chair.*

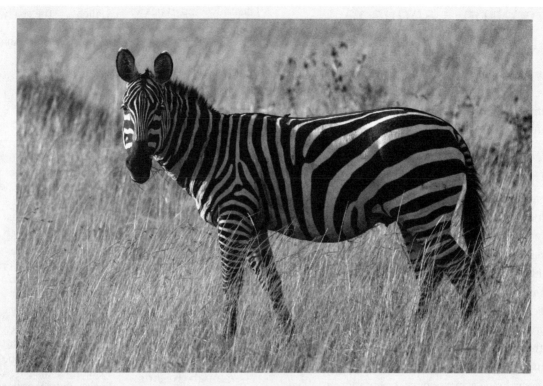

Figure 1-1
Source: © Jitendra Kumar Singh/ShutterStock, Inc.

This presents an opposite caveat from the first and emphasizes this important idea: You must be able to recognize and treat those problems in your field that are very out of the ordinary or even extraordinary.

If you work in the schools, it is true that you might not employ the brain-based knowledge you learned in college every day, but at some point a zebra will walk into your office—and probably many will come to you over the course of your career. To treat them appropriately you must have the correct knowledge.

A few years ago, a student of mine in her second year of graduate school approached me with this tale: A middle-school-aged girl had been referred to the clinic because she had been in therapy for articulation problems all her life and the problems had not improved. After a few sessions with her, my student noticed some subtle differences in the gait and muscle tone of her young client. When the student looked in this girl's mouth she was surprised to see the uvula resting on the back of the tongue, which is highly abnormal. Following her clinical judgment, the

student approached her supervisor and they referred the young girl to a neurologist for an evaluation. It turns out that just before this girl was born she had a bleed in her brain stem that lead to a mild case of flaccid cerebral palsy, which was the underlying problem affecting her speech. In short, this girl was a zebra. In the schools, a string of speech-language pathologists had seen this girl over her entire life and had failed to recognize that she was not presenting with a simple articulation disorder. If they had, her problems with speech as a result of her low muscle tone could have been more appropriately addressed.

As it was, this young girl wasted 10 years in speech therapy with speech-language pathologists who were targeting a nonexistent articulation disorder. I have also seen similar circumstances with other diseases such as multiple sclerosis and Tourette syndrome going unrecognized or being misdiagnosed in the schools for years. In short, you have to be able to recognize and treat both your horses and your zebras, no matter what setting you decide to practice in.

Cognition, Language, and Speech

Before going further, it is necessary to draw some lines in the sand. To understand the information in this book, the reader must know exactly what is meant by *cognition*, *language*, and *speech*.

Cognition

Cognition is the ability to think. Hallowell and Chapey (2008) define cognition as the ability to acquire and process knowledge about the world. The term *cognition* means slightly different things in different disciplines, but, in most settings, cognition means the ability to process thought. In the field of speech-language pathology, the specific cognitive abilities that are recognized as important to processing thought and supporting communication include arousal, attention, working memory, short-term memory, long-term memory, orientation, problem solving, inferencing, and executive function. Understanding cognition is important in speech-language pathology because many cognitive processes underlie and support appropriate and effective communication. A lack of appropriate cognitive abilities undermines the ability to communicate effectively. For instance, if a patient cannot remember what the speech-language pathologist just said, the individual will be unable to respond appropriately and communication will be impaired. Hence, the speech-language pathologist must be able to identify and treat deficits in cognition that contribute to disordered communication.

Cognition The ability to acquire and process knowledge about the world.

Arousal The level of wakefulness and the ability to respond to stimuli.

Orienting The ability to direct attention toward a stimulus.

Attention The ability to hold focus on a stimulus when aroused enough to know that the stimulus is there and using orienting skills to direct attention to the stimulus.

The following types of cognition are referred to repeatedly throughout this text:

- **Arousal**. The level of wakefulness and the ability to respond to stimuli.
- **Orienting**. The ability to direct attention toward a stimulus.
- **Attention**. In the most fundamental sense, attention is an individual's ability to hold focus on a stimulus once a person is aroused enough to know that it is there and can orient to direct his or her attention to the stimulus. However, the speech-language pathologist must be sensitive to different kinds of attention. These are presented in the following list in the hierarchical order in which speech-language pathologists usually treat them:

- **Vigilance**. The ability to stay alert to the occurrence of a possible stimulus.
- **Sustained attention**. The ability to hold attention on a single stimulus.
- **Selective attention**. The ability to hold attention on a stimulus while ignoring the presence of competing stimuli.
- **Alternating attention**. The ability to move or alternate one's attention back and forth from one stimulus to another.
- **Divided attention**. The ability to attend to one stimulus while simultaneously attending to another stimulus; also known as multitasking.

Vigilance The ability to stay alert to the occurrence of a possible stimulus.

Sustained attention The ability to hold attention on a single stimulus.

Selective attention The ability to hold attention on a stimulus while ignoring the presence of competing stimuli.

Alternating attention The ability to move or alternate attention back and forth from one stimulus to another.

Divided attention The ability to attend to one stimulus while simultaneously attending to another stimulus. Also known as multitasking.

- **Working memory.** The ability to hold a finite amount of information for immediate processing and manipulating, which is lost within a few seconds if not somehow reinforced (Parente & Herrman, 2003). In a model put forth by Baddeley (1986), working memory can be subdivided into the phonological loop responsible for retention and processing of speech and language (Martin, 1987) and the visuospatial sketchpad that is responsible for retaining visual information for active processing. In Baddeley's (1986) model, a higher-level component of working memory, the central executive, regulates the operations of the phonological loop and visuospatial sketchpad subsystems.

Working memory
The ability to hold a finite amount of information in the mind for immediate processing and manipulating.

Short-term memory
The retention of information for longer than 30 seconds to a few hours.

Long-term memory
The ability to retain information successfully for months or years.

- **Short-term memory.** There is no set and agreed upon division between short-term memory and long-term memory. Some individuals use the term *short-term memory* to refer to the ability to store information in one's memory for a period of only a few seconds or minutes (this definition of short-term memory encompasses the preceding idea of working memory) (Kempler, 2005). Others prefer to define short-term memory as the ability to store information in one's memory over hours or days. Despite the disagreement over length of time and the confusion it has created, it is clinically useful to distinguish between the memory range of a few seconds (working memory), the memory range of a few hours, and the memory range of months and years. In this book, the term *short-term memory* is used to indicate the retention of information for longer than 30 seconds up to a few hours.
- **Long-term memory.** The ability to retain information successfully over months or years.

- **Procedural memory.** The memory of sequences of actions used to complete tasks (i.e., procedures); for instance, the memory of how to brush teeth. Brushing teeth requires a series of steps that must be undertaken in the correct order for successful accomplishment of the task. However, most people brush their teeth in a completely automated and overlearned fashion. Much of procedural memory is overlearned and deployed in an entirely automatic fashion.

Procedural memory
Memory of sequences of individual actions used to achieve larger objectives.

Declarative memory
The ability to remember facts.

Episodic memory The recall of specific, recently experienced events or episodes.

Orientation The ability of individuals to know who they are, where they are, and when they are.

Problem solving The ability to find an appropriate solution to a problem.

Inferencing The ability to take previous knowledge and experience and apply it to the interpretation of the present situation. The ability to make a leap in judgment to a correct interpretation of the overall meaning.

- **Declarative memory.** The ability to remember facts.
- **Episodic memory.** Burda (2011) defines episodic memory as the recall of specific, recently experienced events (or episodes), such as a vacation.
- **Orientation.** Orientation is usually judged by person, place, and time. In other words, this is an individuals' ability to know who they are, where they are, and when they are.
- **Problem solving.** The ability to find an appropriate solution to a problem. Luria (1966) describes problem solving as the ability to pick a strategy to solve a problem, apply the strategy, and evaluate the results.
- **Inferencing.** Given details, the ability to make a leap in judgment to a correct interpretation of the overall meaning of the details.

- **Executive functions.** These are high-level cognitive systems that employ and manage other lower-level cognitive functions. Executive functions are housed within the prefrontal areas of the frontal lobes. Executive functions use cognitive functions such as attention, memory, planning, problem solving, initiating, and organizational behaviors to meet high-level goals. Brookshire (2007) states that executive functioning includes the ability to initiate purposeful behavior, the ability to plan a sequence of actions to achieve a goal, the ability to maintain behaviors meant to accomplish goals, and the ability to monitor a situation and modify behavior accordingly.

Language

Once thoughts have been formulated using cognition, if communication is desired, the brain must find the appropriate symbols that will communicate these thoughts to another person. The symbols used by people to communicate meaning are known as language. **Language** is commonly defined as a set of symbols used to communicate meaning. These symbols are most often words that are visual, as in written language; verbal, as in spoken language; or the manual signs used in signed languages. The process of symbol selection for most individuals happens automatically and below the level of awareness. For most people, the brain automatically assigns language to express meaning and automatically assigns meaning to language received.

The ability to use language to communicate is divided into receptive and expressive language abilities. Expressive language is the words people assign to ideas to express the meaning of thoughts to other people. Expressive language is usually verbal or written. Conversely, receptive language is the ability to understand language. More specifically, receptive language skills are most commonly thought of as the ability to understand spoken and written language.

Speech

Speech is simply the sounds made by the vocal and articulatory structures of the body to create verbal language. However, all sounds made by the vocal apparatus do not necessarily constitute language, just as all marks on a page do no constitute written language. Sounds can be produced nonsensically or in a way that does not communicate any meaning at all. Simply put, language is the words used to communicate and speech is the sounds made to produce those words verbally.

Interactions

It is important to keep in mind that speech is merely the verbal production of language. Deficits in language do not necessarily imply deficits in speech production. Conversely, a deficit in speech production does not imply deficits in the ability to formulate language. An individual unable to use his mouth for speech but with intact expressive language abilities might still be able to produce written or sign language to communicate.

Furthermore, a deficit in language abilities does not imply deficits in cognition. Although deficits in language and cognition often co-occur, an individual might have grossly intact cognition but devastated language abilities. This person can think clearly but cannot put those thoughts into words for communication. Conversely, an individual might display devastatingly impaired cognition and have intact language. This person can produce only disordered thoughts, but every disordered thought might be perfectly expressed and articulated because of intact speech and language abilities.

Executive functions High-level cognitive abilities used to employ other lower-level cognitive functions appropriately to meet high-level goals.

Language A set of symbols used to communicate meaning.

Speech The sounds made with the vocal and articulatory structures of the body to produce verbal language.

Changes in Speech, Language, and Cognition with Healthy Aging

Finally, consider the degree of changes to speech, language, and cognition that occur, not as a result of pathology, but as a result of normal aging. This section provides a short review of changes in speech, language, and cognition that occur with age. It is important for the student first to learn the nature of normal changes that can occur so that he or she can correctly recognize any abnormal, pathological changes. Many changes that occur for the worse in normal aging are still within the realm of *normal*. A sharp line should be drawn between the subtle and normal *decline* in abilities (often notable only in carefully controlled laboratory situations) and the immediately noticeable and incapacitating *deficits* in abilities discussed throughout the remainder of this book.

Changes in Speech with Healthy Aging

Significant physiologic changes occur in the body with age. However, in healthy aging adults these changes do not have a large negative impact on speech and voice production, which remain intact overall in most aging adults (Burda, 2011).

Changes in Cognition with Healthy Aging

Orientation

Orientation remains intact during normal aging. It is abnormal if an older adult does not know where she is, who she is, or what time of day it is.

Attention

Normally aging adults do not show changes in sustained attention (Berardi, Parasuraman, & Haxby, 2001). However, on selective attention tasks older adults perform more slowly than younger persons (Plude & Doussard-Roosevelt, 1989), indicating a greater susceptibility to distraction. Whereas divided attention skills remain normal for basic tasks, they can be compromised on higher-level or complex tasks in older adults (Simpson, Kellas, & Ferraro, 1999).

Memory

Long-term memory remains intact during normal aging. Healthy aging individuals do not forget deep-seated memories such as where they grew up or their first car. Procedural memory also shows no decline in normally aging adults, who never forget everyday procedures such as how to brush their teeth, drive their car, or wash the dishes. However, healthy aging adults can show decline in short-term memory and episodic memory (Ericsson & Kintsch, 1995; Naveh-Benjamin, Hussain, Guez, & Bar-On, 2003). This is often illustrated by older adults (or their family members) commenting on their ability to remember events from their childhood consistently but having great difficulty remembering recent events. Declarative memory and working memory also show a decline with normal aging (Craik, 2000).

Executive Functions

Older adults tend to perform more poorly on tests of executive function than do younger adults, but their use of executive function in their daily lives remains functional (Burda, 2011).

Changes in Language with Healthy Aging

As individuals age, they might experience slight delays in their processing of verbal language (Federmeier & Kutas, 2005). However, the ability to process verbal language in daily life remains functional. Also, reading might slow (Connelly, Hasher, & Zacks, 1991), but comprehension remains intact.

Evidence-based practice   The notion that therapy and evaluation procedures must be determined to be effective based on clinical opinion and/or valid and reliable research.

The most notable change in language abilities with age is a decline in word finding ability (Au et al., 1995). This most often manifests as greater difficulty with confrontational naming. Specifically, older adults often will state that they have more difficulty remembering the names of new acquaintances than they did when they were younger.

Evidence-Based Practice

Over the past decade, the field of speech-language pathology has been moving toward standard implementation of evidence-based practice. **Evidence-based practice** is the idea that therapy and evaluation techniques must be deemed effective based on clinical opinion and/or valid and reliable research. The American Speech-Language-Hearing Association (ASHA) defines evidence-based practice as the integration of "clinical expertise and expert opinion" with "scientific evidence" to provide "high-quality services" to individuals seen in therapy (American Speech-Language-Hearing Association, 2012). In other words, speech-language pathologists need to have some legitimate basis for employing the therapies used to treat individuals with speech, language, and cognitive disorders. Speech-language pathologists who do not use methods supported by evidence run the risk of not servicing their patients appropriately and damaging their professional reputations and the reputation of the profession.

The need for evidence-based practice might seem obvious, but speech-language pathology is a relatively new field of study and is very much a hybrid of many different disciplines such as education, psychology, neurology, and counseling. As such, there is no great store of past research in the field of speech-language pathology. In many cases, researchers are still struggling to understand the very nature of certain disorders, much less having built up a repository of supportive research on how to treat these disorders effectively. However, over the last 20 years researchers have made strides to build support for certain therapies.

Nevertheless, a lack of evidence-based practice or even a perceived lack can seriously affect speech-language pathologists and the populations that rely on them for rehabilitation. A powerful and recent example of this is the refusal of the U.S. Department of Defense to pay for rehabilitative cognitive therapy for soldiers returning from battle with traumatic brain injuries (the signature injury of modern U.S. warfare). These soldiers are now returning home in huge numbers after multiple deployments to the wars in Iraq and Afghanistan. To avoid paying for therapy for the cognitive deficits following these traumatic brain injuries, in 2010 the Department of Defense cited a lack of appropriate scientific evidence that cognitive therapies help individuals with brain injuries recover (Miller & Zwerdling, 2010). As a result, many U.S. soldiers and veterans still cannot get the appropriate speech-language pathology services they need to maximize their recovery after being wounded in battle.

The need for speech-language pathologists to use evidence-based practice in their clinical decision making is paramount. Therapists must constantly explore expert opinion as well as keep up with recent and valid research on the efficacy of therapy methods to ensure that they administer the highest level of care to their patients.

Main Points

- A neurogenic communication disorder is a problem with communication that arises as a result of damage to the brain or other part of the nervous system.
- Neurogenic communication disorders include the aphasias, the dysarthrias, apraxia of speech, as well as the myriad of communication problems that may arise following deficits associated with right hemisphere disorders, traumatic brain injury, and dementia.
- Speech-language pathologists treat the communicative difficulties that result from neurogenic communication disorders in a variety of settings.
- Treatment settings include skilled nursing facilities, acute care facilities, rehabilitation facilities, outpatient rehabilitation facilities, home health care, hospice care, children's hospitals, and schools.
- The aspects of neurogenic communication disorders that speech-language pathologists target in therapy include speech, language, and cognition, and the subcategories of each.
- Cognition is the ability to think, acquire, and process knowledge about the world. This is important because many cognitive processes underlie and support effective communication.
- Cognitive abilities important to the processing of thought and support of communication include arousal, attention (which includes vigilance, sustained attention, selective attention, alternating attention, and divided attention), working memory, short-term memory, long-term memory (which includes procedural memory and declarative memory), orientation, problem solving, inferencing, and executive functions.
- Language is an agreed upon set of symbols used to communicate meaning. If communication is desired, the brain must find the appropriate symbols to be produced to communicate thoughts to others.
- Language abilities are generally divided into expressive language and receptive language abilities.
- Speech is the sounds made by the vocal and articulatory structures of the body to produce verbal language. The sounds produced are used as vehicles for language to express thoughts to others.
- Deficits in speech, language, or cognition can occur separately or can co-occur, though a deficit in one area does not imply deficits in all other areas: A person can have a deficit in speech, though not in language and vice versa. However, deficits in both language and cognition do often occur. Different deficits can interact with one another and change the overall presentation of deficits in patients.
- There are degrees of change to speech, language, and cognition that occur not as a result of pathology, but as a result of normal aging. It is important to understand the nature of normal changes so that abnormal, pathological changes can then be recognized.
- Changes in healthy aging generally do not negatively affect a person's daily life. If daily life is disrupted, an abnormal change not associated with aging should be suspected.
- Healthy aging can result in varying levels of slight decline in cognition such as in selective attention, divided attention for complex tasks, short-term memory, episodic memory, declarative memory, and working memory. However, healthy older adults retain orientation, long-term memory, divided attention for basic tasks, procedural memory, and executive functions.
- Healthy aging can result in varying levels of slight decline in language abilities such as verbal language processing, reading, and word finding;

however, healthy older adults retain functional verbal processing and comprehension.

- Generally, subtle changes in speech ability and voice production do occur with normal aging, but not enough to negatively affect daily life or warrant therapy.

- Evidence-based practice is the integration of research evidence with clinical expertise and expert opinion to provide effective and high-quality services.

- Speech-language pathologists must keep their knowledge base up to date with the latest research on evidence supporting therapy methods.

Review Questions

1. What is a neurogenic communication disorder?
2. What are some examples of neurogenic communication disorders?
3. What are some settings in which a speech-language pathologist provides therapy for neurogenic communication disorders?
4. Why is it important to know and understand neurogenic communication disorders even if you never plan on working in a clinical setting?
5. Compare and contrast speech, language, and cognition.
6. What are some subcategories of cognition?
7. How might communication be compromised if a person's cognition is not intact?
8. What is a general definition of attention?
9. List and describe the individual levels of attention.
10. Compare and contrast working memory and short-term memory.
11. What are the two gross divisions of language?
12. Do deficits in one aspect of speech, language, or cognition constitute a deficit in another area of speech, language, or cognition? Why or why not?
13. What are three areas of cognition that can decline in healthy aging?
14. What are three areas of cognition that are retained in healthy aging?
15. What are three areas of language that can decline in healthy aging?
16. What are three areas of language that are retained in healthy aging?
17. Why is it important to know changes in speech, language, and cognition that are brought about by healthy aging?
18. Why is evidenced-based practice important?
19. How might speech-language pathologists know that the therapy techniques they use are evidence based?
20. What rationale did the U.S. Department of Defense present in 2010 for denying cognitive rehabilitation services for veterans and soldiers returning from wars in Iraq and Afghanistan?

References

1. American Speech-Language-Hearing Association. (2012). Introduction to evidence-based practice. Retrieved from http://www.asha.org/Members/ebp/intro/

2. Au, R., Joung, P., Nicholas, M., Obler, L., Kass, R., & Albert, M. (1995). Naming ability across the adult life span. *Aging and Cognition, 2,* 302–311.

3. Baddeley, A. (1986). *Working memory*. Oxford, England: Oxford University Press.

4. Berardi, A., Parasuraman, R., & Haxby, J. (2001). Overall vigilance and sustained attention decrements in healthy aging. *Experimental Aging Research, 27*, 19–39.

5. Brookshire, R. (2007). *Introduction to neurogenic communication disorders* (7th ed.). St. Louis, MO: Mosby-Elsevier.

6. Burda, A. (2011). *Communication and swallowing changes in healthy aging adults*. Burlington, MA: Jones & Bartlett Learning.

7. Connelly, L., Hasher, L., & Zacks, R. (1991). Age and reading: The impact of distraction. *Psychology and Aging, 6*, 533–541.

8. Craik, F. (2000). Age-related changes in human memory. In D. Park & N. Schwarz (Eds.), *Cognitive aging: A primer* (pp. 75–92). Philadelphia, PA: Psychology Press.

9. Ericsson, K., & Kintsch, W. (1995). Long term working memory. *Psychological Review, 201*, 211–245.

10. Federmeier, K., & Kutas, M. (2005). Aging in context: Age-related changes in context use during language comprehension. *Psychophysiology, 44*, 491–505.

11. Hallowell, B., Chapey, R. (2001). Introduction to language intervention strategies in adult aphasia. In R. Chapey (Ed.), *Language intervention strategies in aphasia and related neurogenic communication disorders* (4th ed.). (pp. 341–382). New York, NY; Lippincott Williams & Wilkins.

12. Kempler, D. (2005). *Neurocognitive disorders in aging*. London, England: Sage.

13. Luria, A. (1966). *Higher cortical functions in man*. New York, NY: Basic Books.

14. Martin, R. (1987). Articulatory and phonological deficits in short-term memory and their relation to syntactic processing. *Brain and Language, 32*(1), 159–192.

15. Miller, C., & Zwerdling, D. (2010 December 20). Pentagon plan won't cover brain-damage therapy. *National Public Radio*.

16. Naveh-Benjamin, M., Hussain, Z., Guez, J., & Bar-On, M. (2003). Adult age differences in episodic memory: Further support for an associative-deficit hypothesis. *Journal of Experimental Psychology: Learning, Memory, and Cognition, 29*, 826–837.

17. Parente, R., & Herrman, D. (2003). *Retraining cognition: Techniques and applications* (3rd ed.). Austin, TX: Pro-Ed.

18. Plude, D. J., & Doussard-Roosevelt, J. A. (1989). Aging, selective attention, and feature integration. *Psychology and Aging, 4*, 98–105.

19. Simpson, G., Kellas, G., & Ferraro, F. (1999). Age and the allocation of attention across the time course of word recognition. *Journal of General Psychology, 126*, 119–136.

Basic Brain Anatomy

To understand how a part of the brain is disordered by damage or disease, speech-language pathologists must first know a few facts about the anatomy of the brain in general and how a normal and healthy brain functions. Readers can use the anatomy presented here as a reference, review, and jumping off point to understanding the consequences of damage to the structures discussed. This chapter begins with the big picture and works down into the specifics of brain anatomy.

The Central Nervous System

The nervous system is divided into two major sections: the central nervous system and the peripheral nervous system. The **central nervous system** (CNS) consists of the brain and spinal cord. The **peripheral nervous system** (PNS) consists of the nerve tracts that connect the rest of the body to the central nervous system. An easy way to differentiate the CNS and the PNS is to remember that the CNS is entirely encased in bone whereas the PNS is not (**Figure 2-1**).

The Brain

The average weight of an adult human brain is about 3 pounds. That is about the weight of a single small cantaloupe or six grapefruits. If a human brain was placed on a tray, it would look like a pretty unimpressive mass of gray lumpy tissue (Luria, 1973). In fact, for most of history the brain was thought to be an utterly useless piece of flesh housed in the skull. The Egyptians believed that the heart was the seat of human intelligence, and as such, the brain was promptly removed during mummification. In his essay *On Sleep and Sleeplessness*, Aristotle argued that the brain is a complex cooling mechanism for our bodies that works primarily to help cool and condense water vapors rising in our bodies (Aristotle, republished 2011). He also established a strong argument in this same essay for why infants should not drink wine. The basis for this argument was that infants already have too much moisture in their heads. Nonetheless, thanks to advancements in the fields of science, medicine, and the birth of the fields of psychology and neurology, we

Central nervous system The brain and spinal cord.

Peripheral nervous system The nerve tracts outside of the central nervous system that work to connect the central nervous system to the rest of the body.

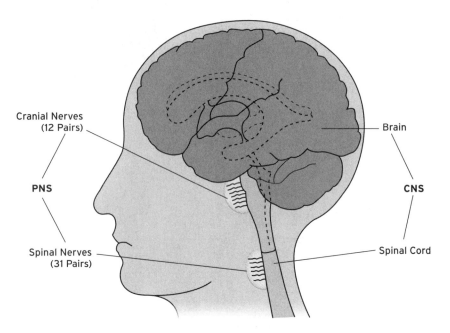

Figure 2-1   The central and peripheral nervous systems.

now know that the brain is much more than an inert mass of head stuffing. And though we know Aristotle was correct in stating that infants should not drink wine, we know that it is not because infants are born with copious amounts of head vapors. We know now that the brain is the organ that coordinates and regulates all functions and other organs in our bodies. It is the seat of consciousness, intelligence, and language.

The brain has three gross divisions, the cerebrum, the brain stem, and the cerebellum (Figure 2-2).

When asked to describe a brain, most individuals describe the cerebrum of the brain. This is the most recently evolved and most easily recognizable part of the brain. The cerebrum is the rounded gray section of the brain riddled with tiny ridges and valleys that makes so many appearances in zombie movies. The cerebrum rests on top of the brain stem. The cerebrum houses our highest and most complex cognitive functions. This is where our consciousness originates as well as our ability to do things such

Cerebrum   The rounded gray section of the brain with gyri and sulci.

Cerebral cortex   The most superficial layer of the cerebrum.

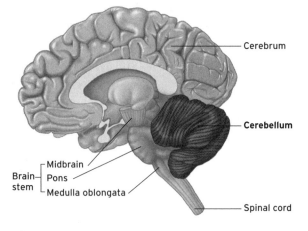

Figure 2-2   Cerebrum, brain stem, and cerebellum.

as produce language and cognition and organize body movements. The surface tissue of the cerebrum is known as the cerebral cortex. The cortex is the most superficial layer of the cerebrum (Figure 2-3).

The cerebral cortex is gray and folded and marked by various ridges and valleys. The cerebrum is folded in on itself so that more neural tissue can be packed

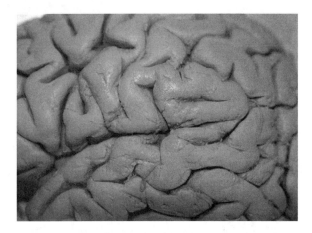

Figure 2-3   Cerebral cortex.

into a much smaller space. The gray coloration of the surface of the cerebral cortex results from the gray color of the cell bodies of the neurons and is therefore said to consist of gray matter. Gray matter is where processing and regulating of information occurs in the CNS. Gray matter is found in the cortex and some subcortical structures such as the cerebellum, thalamus, basal ganglia (to be discussed), in addition to the spinal cord. This is in contrast to white matter. The white matter of the CNS consists of the axons of neurons that are covered in a white sheath of a protein and fatty substance called myelin. Myelin insulates the axons of neurons (like a rubber sheath insulates the copper wire in electrical wiring) and allows electrical chemical impulses of the nervous system to be conducted at approximately 100 meters per second. Unmyelinated neurons are able to conduct neural impulses only at about 1 meter per second. White matter is responsible for

connecting different areas and structures of the brain to one another and enabling them to communicate.

The myelinated axons of neurons make white matter appear white and the lack of myelin makes gray matter gray. There are three primary types of white matter tracts in the CNS: association fibers, commissural fibers, and projection fibers. Association fibers are the pathways of white matter that connect different structures and areas of the brain in a single hemisphere. Commissural fibers are white matter pathways that connect analogous areas between the two cerebral hemispheres. Projection fibers are white matter tracts that project from the brain to the spinal cord and transmit motor (movement) signals from the CNS out to the PNS and sensory signals from the PNS back up through the lower CNS to be processed in the brain.

Certain diseases attack and break down the myelin sheath of white matter. These are known as demyelinating illnesses. Demyelinating illnesses degrade the potential of neurons to conduct neural impulses. This degradation of the myelin inhibits appropriate neural functioning by disrupting communication between different areas of the CNS or PNS, or both. Amyotrophic lateral sclerosis (ALS) and multiple sclerosis are two such demyelinating diseases. ▶ See the video, *Living with Multiple Sclerosis* for a discussion of this disease as well as an interview with an individual living with multiple sclerosis.

The folds on the cerebral cortex are created by small convolutions and furrows, or ridges

Gray matter
Unmyelinated neurons responsible for the processing and regulating of information within the nervous system.

White matter
Myelinated neurons responsible for the transmission of impulses from one area of the brain to another.

Myelin   An insulating layer of protein and fatty substances that forms a layer around the axons of certain neurons, which allows for the fast and effective transmission of neural impulses.

Association fibers
White matter pathways that connect different structures and areas of the brain within a single hemisphere.

Commissural fibers
White matter pathways that connect analogous areas between the two cerebral hemispheres.

Projection fibers   White matter pathways that project from the brain to the spinal cord and transmit motor (movement) signals from the CNS out to the PNS and also transmit sensory signals from the PNS back up through the lower CNS to be processed in the brain.

and valleys. The ridges are known as gyri (singular: gyrus). The valleys are known as sulci (singular: sulcus). (See the following Clinical Note on lissencephaly for a discussion of the clinical relevance of the gyri and sulci.) Deeper grooves that make more pronounced divisions in the anatomy of the brain are referred to as fissures. Knowledge of the major gyri, sulci, and fissures is important to learning about the rest of the anatomy of the brain because they are important landmarks for describing the location of many other areas and structures of the brain. The following sections on the cerebral hemispheres and the major cerebral lobes revisit the importance of these structures.

Between the surface of the brain and the skull are three anatomic layers of tissue known as the cerebral meninges. The outermost of these layers is the dura mater. The dura mater (Latin for *tough mother*) is a dense, fibrous protective layer of tissue enveloping the brain and spinal cord. Beneath the dura mater is the arachnoid mater. The arachnoid mater is a far more delicate layer of tissue than the dura mater. The arachnoid mater wraps the brain and spinal cord and plays a large role in supplying blood to the surface of the brain by the

Gyri Ridges forming the visible portion of the cerebral cortex.

Sulci Inward folds of the cerebral cortex.

Fissure A deep groove that creates major divisions in the anatomy of the brain.

Lissencephaly A group of congenital malformations that create a lack of appropriate gyri and sulci of the cortex and a consequent reduction in cortical tissue.

Cerebral meninges Three layers of tissues with various functions that encase and envelope the brain and spinal cord.

Dura mater A dense, fibrous protective layer of tissue that envelopes the brain and spinal cord. This is the superficial-most layer of the cerebral meninges.

Arachnoid mater A layer of the cerebral meninges that exists between the dura mater and the pia mater that plays a large role in supplying blood to the surface of the brain through the many blood vessels it contains.

Clinical Note

Lissencephaly

As mentioned, the human cerebrum is folded in on itself to allow far more cortical tissue to be packed into the skull. If you smoothed out the gyri and sulci of the human cortex, the surface area would be far greater than that of the inside of the skull. This system of folding allows the body to fit as much cortical tissue within the skull as possible. It is this great amount of cortex that allows for normal cognitive functioning. However, there is a group of congenital malformations categorically referred to as lissencephaly, or smooth brain syndrome, in which the brain develops in the mother's womb without these folds in the cortex (**Figure 2-4**). There are many different etiologies that account for the varying types of lissencephaly. Some etiologies are viral infection and gene mutation. Children who are born this way usually have profound neurologic impairments, feeding difficulties, and can have a very short life span. Nonetheless, lissencephaly does occur on a spectrum and the long-term medical and developmental prognosis of an affected child depends on the level of severity of the brain disorder.

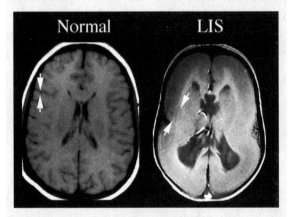

Figure 2-4 Imaging scan of a normally developed brain and cortex alongside a lissencephalic brain. Missing from the lissencephalic brain are the many folds of cortical tissue seen in the normally developing brain.

Source: Courtesy of Dr. Joseph G. Gleeson, University of California San Diego

many blood vessels that it contains. The arachnoid mater is so named because of the dense spider-web-like appearance of the blood vessels in this layer. The **pia mater** (Latin for *gentle mother*) is the innermost and most delicate meningeal layer. The pia mater closely hugs the surface of the brain and spinal cord as it rises and falls along the gyri, sulci, and fissures of the brain. Blood vessels from the arachnoid mater pass through the pia mater to nourish the surface of the brain and spinal cord. **Figure 2-5** shows the dura mater as it is being pulled back from the brain below to expose the **leptomeninges** (i.e., the arachnoid mater and the pia mater). See Figure 2-14 for an image depicting the meningeal layers.

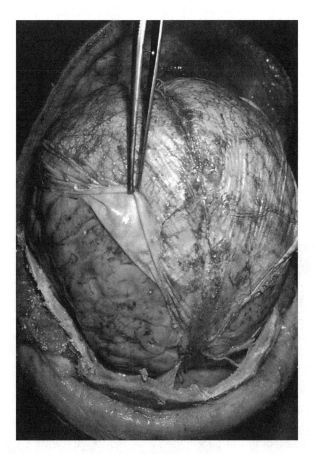

Figure 2-5 Head autopsy revealing dura mater and leptomeninges.

Courtesy of Department of Health and Human Services, Centers for Disease Control and Prevention. Dr. Edwin P. Ewing, Jr.

The Cerebral Hemispheres

Observable on the surface of the brain is a deep groove running front to back. This groove is known as the **longitudinal fissure** and it runs the length of the brain and divides the brain into left and right halves. These halves are known as the left and right cerebral hemispheres (**Figure 2-6**).

Generally speaking, each cerebral hemisphere is responsible for different cognitive and motor functions. For instance, the right hemisphere is responsible for movement of the left side of the body and processing sensory information coming up to the brain from the left side of the body. The left hemisphere is responsible for moving the right side of the body and processing sensory information coming up to the brain from the right side of the body.

Although the hemispheres are often spoken of as discrete and separate units that operate independently, it is a false and outdated assumption that each hemisphere performs its own functions in isolation without input from the other. The two hemispheres work in tandem and communicate with one another by a mass of white matter tracts known as the **corpus callosum**. The corpus callosum is located between the cerebral hemispheres and is found deep within the longitudinal fissure, at its very base. The corpus callosum houses the largest white matter pathways responsible for connecting the left and right hemispheres. See the following Clinical Notes on split-brain syndrome.

Pia mater The innermost and most delicate layer of the cerebral meninges that hugs the surface of the brain and spinal cord closely as it rises and falls along the gyri, sulci, and fissures of the brain.

Leptomeninges The thin layers of the meninges including the arachnoid mater and the pia mater.

Longitudinal fissure A deep groove running front to back along the brain that divides the brain into the right and left cerebral hemispheres.

Corpus callosum A mass of white matter tracts located at the base of the longitudinal fissure that connects the analogous areas between the two hemispheres.

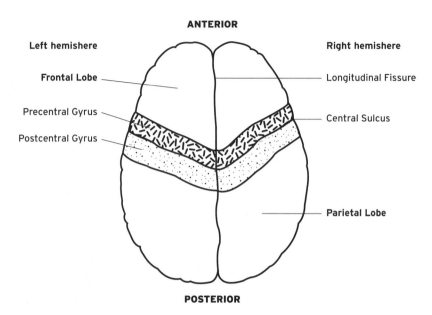

Figure 2-6 A superior view of the cerebral hemispheres.

See the *Split Brain Demonstration* video for a live demonstration.

Typically, the left cerebral hemisphere is the hemisphere that houses most language abilities. Also, most individuals are right handed. This creates the situation where the language-dominant hemisphere (most often the left hemisphere) also controls a person's writing hand (most often the right hand). More often than not, the right cerebral hemisphere is not the language-dominant hemisphere. Even in left-handed individuals the left hemisphere usually

Clinical Note

Split-Brain Syndrome

All brains operate using electricity. Electrical chemical impulses are how our brains communicate with themselves and our bodies. However, it is possible to have too much electricity generated in the brain. A seizure is a result of an excess and pathologic amount of electricity in the brain. Seizures can be very dangerous and can create severe and permanent damage to the brain and even death. The most common group of seizure disorders are categorized as forms of epilepsy. In some very severe forms of epilepsy, seizure activity is so threatening to an individual's brain that it is deemed necessary to perform a surgery on the two cerebral hemispheres by cutting the corpus callosum. This surgery, known as a corpus commisurotomy, decreases seizures but results in what is known as split-brain syndrome. Individuals with split-brain syndrome have cerebral hemispheres that are unable to communicate with one another. This makes perception sometimes difficult and creates motor problems as well. With the modernization and perfection of this surgery in the 1960s and 1970s, scientists were able to study the functioning and abilities of the individual cerebral hemispheres in isolation from one another.

Clinical Note

Split-Brain Demonstration

Find a friend and try this little experiment to demonstrate to yourself the value of communication between your right and left cerebral hemispheres. You need a friend and a shoe with laces.

To begin, take the shoe in your own hands, close your eyes, and tie the laces with your eyes closed. Probably this isn't a difficult task for you. Your brain can draw on years of motor memory developed by the thousands of times you have tied your shoes. As you are tying the shoe, your left cerebral hemisphere is controlling your right hand and your right cerebral hemisphere is controlling your left hand. Your hands probably move dexterously together as if they know exactly what the other is doing, even though you have your eyes closed. In fact, each hand does know what the other is doing because your left and right cerebral hemispheres are communicating with each other by the corpus callosum and telling each other what the other is doing with each hand.

Now, sit side by side with your friend. The two of you should be shoulder to shoulder. One of you lace your arm under the arm of the other (**Figure 2-7**) so that each of you has one hand that will attempt to work together with the other to tie the shoe. Now there is a left and a right hand each controlled by a separate cerebral hemisphere. This is almost just like when you tied your shoe yourself but with an important difference. The difference is that when you were by yourself, the two cerebral hemispheres controlling the hands were connected. With your friend, the two cerebral hemispheres controlling the hands are not connected at all and, therefore, cannot communicate with one another (you are not allowed to talk to your friend or open your eyes as you do this experiment). Therefore, one hemisphere does not know what the other hemisphere's hand is doing.

In this side-by-side position where each of you contribute the use of one hand, hold the untied shoe, both of you close your eyes, and attempt to tie the shoe. Probably you'll find it far more difficult than when you attempted this task by yourself. Why is this? It is because each hand does not know exactly what the other is going to do and when. Individuals with split-brain syndrome face these motoric problems on all tasks requiring more than one side of the body.

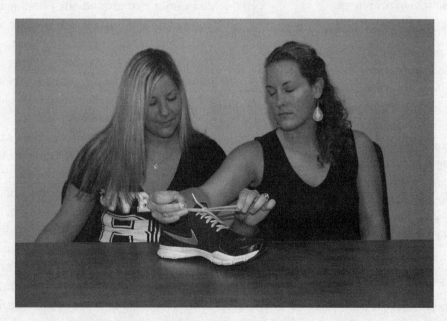

Figure 2-7   **Split-brain demonstration.**

houses language or a greater part of it. Although certainly not always the case, in the rest of this book, unless otherwise stated, it is assumed for the sake of brevity that the term *left hemisphere* is synonymous with *language-dominant hemisphere* and *right hemisphere* is synonymous with *nondominant hemisphere for language*.

Right Cerebral Hemisphere

If the brain was neglected as an important organ for most of known history, then the right hemisphere has suffered almost the same fate since the inception of serious study of the brain. For most of the history of neuroscience, the right hemisphere was deemed most insignificant and such terms as *silent*, *minor*, *unconscious*, or *subordinate* were almost universally applied when describing the right hemisphere. Only in the last 20 to 30 years (really beginning with the split-brain studies of the 1960s and 1970s) has the scientific community come to acknowledge the right hemisphere as a truly significant structure in cognition and language. In fact, damage to the right hemisphere produces some of the most bizarre and noteworthy deficits in neurology.

As it is understood now, the right hemisphere plays some very important roles in communication. Communication not only involves language but facial expressions, body language, gestures, and prosody of speech. It is these nonlinguistic aspects of communication that the right hemisphere specializes in. The right hemisphere deals heavily in the perception of emotion by processing these nonlinguistic components of communication. The appropriate processing of nonlinguistic aspects of communication can facilitate effective communication and mutual understanding between speakers, whereas a failure to process nonlinguistic information appropriately can completely derail efforts at communication.

In regard to speech, the right hemisphere is responsible for our perception of prosody. **Prosody** is the changes in tone and intensity we use when we speak that allow us to give the words we say an emotional component. Usually most of the emotional content of speech (the mood and emotional state of the person) is conveyed in prosody. For instance, when a person is angry, a listener often does not really need to hear the actual words said to know that the speaker is angry. The listener will probably be able to detect anger in the speaker's prosody, their tone of voice. Or when a person produces a verbal insult, a listener can tell the utterance is meant to be an insult even if they don't understand the language or have never heard the insult. Another example is of two people arguing in a closed room. Listeners in adjacent rooms might hear the muffled sound of these two people arguing. Even though the listeners might not hear the actual words spoken, they cannot mistake the angry tone of the voices as two people having a pleasant conversation. The right hemisphere allows people to perceive emotions through interpretation of prosody.

> **Prosody**   The changes in pitch, stress, timbre, cadence, and tempo a person uses to infuse utterances with emotional content.

The ability to comprehend the information embedded within prosody and other nonlinguistic signals during communication is especially important in social interactions because, often, the words that a person says do not reflect the true intent of the utterance. For example, when a person says, "It is a beautiful day" accompanied by a pleasant smile, she probably is communicating that it is, in fact, a beautiful day. However, by using a sarcastic tone, furrowing her brows, and snarling her upper lip, she can use the words "It is a beautiful day" to communicate very effectively that she does not believe that the day is beautiful in any way, shape, or form. The right hemisphere enables listeners to know that the literal interpretation of a person's words does not always accurately reflect the thoughts the speaker intends (or does not intend) to communicate. Due to the loss of these abilities, individuals with right hemisphere damage tend to be very concrete in their comprehension of language. For example, if asked to explain the phrase "She is warm-hearted," an individual with right hemisphere damage might state that the person in question has a heart temperature that is much higher than most other people's hearts.

Processing and recognizing faces and facial expressions are also right hemisphere responsibilities. A loss of the ability to perceive and recognize faces often follows damage to the right occipital area (Luria, 1973). Difficulty with the visual processing of the faces of others is known as **prosopagnosia**. In severe cases, individuals with lesions in the occipital area of the right hemisphere might have difficulty recognizing the faces of their loved ones or even their own face. In less severe cases, they might simply be unable to interpret facial expressions appropriately. Their understanding of the communicative intent of others can be affected by this.

The right hemisphere is responsible not only for comprehending emotion in speech and on faces, but also for producing appropriate prosody and facial expression to convey emotion. Individuals who have damage to the right cerebral hemisphere can often appear expressionless and sound monotone and emotionless to listeners. Hence, listeners might not be able to perceive that a person with right hemisphere damage is in a highly agitated state or experiencing some other strong emotion as it is occurring because of these deficits. Clinically, this can make the treatment of cognitive deficits in individuals with right hemisphere damage difficult as the speech-language pathologist may have no idea of the frustration or enthusiasm level of the patient.

The right hemisphere is also responsible for processing melody and rhythm in music. Individuals who have experienced right hemisphere damage can display **amusia**, or the loss of the ability to recognize and interpret music (Luria, 1973). Amusia can also affect the ability of the person to produce music as well as hear and interpret it correctly.

The right hemisphere also is largely responsible for the perception of environmental sounds. Damage to certain areas in the right hemisphere might result in a lack of ability to discern the meaning of non-speech sounds that occur in the environment such as a door slamming, a car driving by, or a bird singing (Joseph, 1988). This can happen in the absence of any difficulty interpreting speech sounds. See the following discussion on the temporal lobe for more specific information regarding this function of the right hemisphere.

Also significant is that the right hemisphere has a role in processing the **macrostructure**, or gestalt. **Macrostructure processing** is the ability to effectively piece together many smaller details (microstructure) to arrive at the correct perception of the big picture (the macrostructure). An example of macrostructure processing is being able to perceive four wheels, doors, trunk, hood, and headlights and from that being able to perceive that the object is a car. Individuals with deficits of macrostructure processing tend to perseverate on details and cannot piece together the details and perceive the whole. Therefore, individuals with right hemisphere lesions are often known as being unable *to see the forest for the trees.*

> **Prosopagnosia** A neurologic deficit in the specific ability to cognitively process sensory information regarding the faces of others for the purposes of recognition.
>
> **Amusia** An acquired deficit in the ability to interpret and recognize music.
>
> **Macrostructure** The bigger picture composed of many details. Also known as the gestalt.
>
> **Macrostructure processing** The ability to generate a correct perception of macrostructure.
>
> **Visuospatial processing** The ability to understand visual information, visual representations, and spatial relationships among objects.

The spatial component of math skills as well as **visuospatial processing** is also a primary responsibility of the right hemisphere. Examples of some specific visuospatial skills are perception of depth, distance, and shape; localizing targets in space; and identifying

Broca's area The inferior, posterior region of the frontal lobe of the left hemisphere that is a specialized area of the cerebrum responsible for finding and assembling words for the appropriate expression of thought.

Wernicke's area A specialized portion of the cerebrum located at the superior marginal gyrus of the left hemisphere's temporal lobe that is responsible for interpreting and deriving meaning from the speech of others.

Central sulcus A deep groove that runs down the middle lateral surface of each cerebral hemisphere.

Lateral sulcus A deep groove that begins at the lower frontal aspect of each of the two cerebral hemispheres and travels at an upward angle, passes the central sulcus, and then terminates.

figure–ground relationships (Joseph, 1988). Visuospatial processing skills are used to piece together a jigsaw puzzle, sink a basket in a basketball game, and successfully navigate your body from place to place past and around innumerable obstacles.

The right hemisphere also plays a great role in the ability to attend to stimuli. There are various levels of attention, and the right hemisphere plays a role in regulating most kinds. Specifically, the right hemisphere specializes in the ability to keep attention on a single stimulus for an extended period of time (sustained attention) and the ability to ignore unimportant stimuli while sustaining attention on important stimuli (selective attention). An example of sustained attention is paying attention to a lecture in a classroom. If a lawn mower is running outside the classroom during the lecture, then students must actively block out the distracting sound of the lawn mower to focus on the lecture, which is an example of selective attention.

Left Cerebral Hemisphere

As mentioned, the left cerebral hemisphere has been the subject of study more than the right hemisphere has. This is mostly because the left hemisphere typically is the hemisphere that houses language. The discovery that certain locations in the left hemisphere

are responsible for expressive and receptive language skills cued researchers in the late 1800s to begin examining the relationship between brain and cognition more closely.

In 1861, Paul Broca published the results of his studies indicating that the inferior, posterior region of the frontal lobe of the left hemisphere is responsible for finding and assembling words for the appropriate expression of thought. This area is now known as **Broca's area** (**Figure 2-8**). Damage to this area can produce what is known as Broca's aphasia. Individuals with this disorder usually know what they want to say but cannot find the right words.

A few years later in 1874, Carl Wernicke localized receptive language to the superior marginal gyrus of the left hemisphere's temporal lobe. This area is now known as **Wernicke's area** (Figure 2-8). Wernicke's area is responsible for interpreting and deriving meaning from the speech of others. Damage to this area produces a condition known as Wernicke's aphasia. Individuals with this disorder cannot comprehend the speech of others, and their own speech is often nonsensical and nonstop.

The Major Cerebral Lobes

Two important sulci are the **central sulcus** and the **lateral sulcus** (Figure 2-8). The central sulcus, also known as the fissure of Rolando or the central fissure, runs down the middle lateral surface of each cerebral hemisphere. The lateral sulcus, also known as the sylvian fissure, begins at the lower frontal aspect of each of the two cerebral hemispheres, travels at an upward angle, passes the central sulcus, and then terminates. The central and lateral sulci create important divisions among the major sections, or lobes, of the cerebrum. The lobes of the cerebrum are each named for the bones of the cranium that overlay them.

As the central sulci run down the side of each cerebral hemisphere they create a division between the

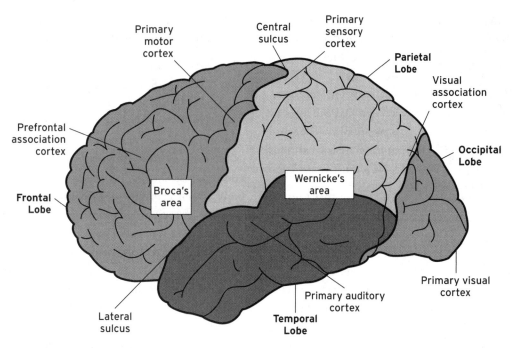

Figure 2-8 External surface of the left cerebral hemisphere.

frontal lobes and the parietal lobes (Figure 2-8). The lateral sulci create a division between the temporal lobes and the above frontal and parietal lobes (Figure 2-8). These are both unlike the longitudinal fissure, which divides the brain into right and left cerebral hemispheres.

Each cerebral lobe houses different major functions of the brain and specializes in certain functions.

The left **frontal lobe** (Figure 2-8) houses expressive language in Broca's area in the inferior and posterior sections. The frontal lobes also play a large role in motor movement. All voluntary movement originates in the anterior portion of the brain (i.e., the frontal lobes). The frontal lobes house cortical areas responsible for the initiation and construction of plans for motor movement such as the **primary motor cortex**, which is also known as the motor strip (Figure 2-8). The primary motor cortex is located on the most posterior gyrus of the frontal lobe, just in front of the central sulcus. The primary

motor cortex is responsible for issuing motor plans for volitional movement. More surface area of the cortex within the primary motor cortex is devoted to body parts that are capable of producing delicate or fine motor movements, including the face, lips, mouth, and hands. Less cortical tissue in the primary motor cortex is dedicated to the control of body parts that execute only gross motor functions. The knee, for instance, has less surface area dedicated to its control within the primary motor cortex than does the mouth or hands. The spatial representation of

Frontal lobes The most anterior sections of the cerebral hemispheres that are delineated posteriorly by the central sulcus and inferiorly by the lateral sulcus and that houses expressive language and deals heavily in motor movement.

Primary motor cortex A strip of tissue oriented vertically along the last gyrus of each frontal lobe that plays a large role in voluntary motor movement.

Motor homunculus   A visual illustration of the amount of cortical tissue dedicated to the movement of each body part within the primary motor cortex.

Parietal lobes   A section of the cerebrum located posterior to the frontal lobes and anterior to the occipital lobes that is largely responsible for receiving and processing sensory information concerning the body.

Primary sensory cortex   A section of cortex along the first gyrus of the parietal lobes dedicated to receiving and processing sensory information.

Proprioception   An individual's sense of where their extremeties and their body is in space.

Sensory homunculus   A visual illustration of the amount of cortical tissue within the primary sensory cortex dedicated to processing sensory information from each body part.

Frontal lobotomy   A procedure of damaging or removing tissue from the prefrontal area of the frontal lobes for the supposed remediation of psychological problems.

Temporal lobe   A section of the cerebrum located inferior to the parietal lobes that is largely responsible for memory and processing of auditory stimuli.

the amount of space in the brain dedicated to the movement of each body part is represented by an illustration known as the **motor homunculus**. The word homunculus is Latin for *little man* (**Figure 2-9**).

The left primary motor cortex is responsible for issuing motor movements for speech. Damage at or near Broca's area, near the base of the left primary motor cortex, disrupts the brain's ability to execute appropriate motor plans for speech. This condition is known as apraxia of speech.

The frontal lobes, specifically the prefrontal regions (the very front of the frontal lobes), also store personality and some memory. Damage to the prefrontal regions of the frontal lobes can produce changes in personality ranging from mild to drastic. Examples of these changes include a sudden lack of social inhibitions leading to inappropriate sexual advances or physical/verbal aggression, or impulsivity. However, less obvious changes in personality can also take place, such as changes in food

and clothing preferences. See the following Clinical Notes on Phineas Gage and frontal lobotomies.

The **parietal lobes** are located behind the frontal lobes (Figure 2-8) and are responsible for receiving and processing sensory information concerning the body. The first gyrus of the parietal lobes house the **primary sensory cortex** (Figure 2-8), also known as the sensory strip. This section of cortex receives and processes tactile information coming from the body as well as proprioceptive information. The left primary sensory cortex receives sensory information from the right side of the body, and the right primary sensory cortex receives sensory information from the left side of the body. **Proprioception** is an individual's sense of where their extremities and their body is in space. For instance, when an individual closes his eyes and extends his arms in front of himself, he can feel his arms out there and knows exactly where they are in space, despite having his eyes closed.

More cortical tissue within the primary sensory cortex is dedicated to body parts that have higher numbers of sensory receptors than those that have fewer. For instance, the mouth and lips are very sensitive to touch and to temperature. Accordingly, very large sections of the primary sensory cortex are dedicated to receiving and processing sensory information coming from the mouth and lips. In contrast, the skin on the back has far fewer sensory receptors and therefore has very little representation in the primary sensory cortex. As in the primary motor cortex, the topographical arrangement of cortical tissue representing the associated body parts creates an arrangement that is referred to as the sensory homunculus. On the **sensory homunculus**, body parts that have the most cortical tissue dedicated to processing their sensory information are represented as being larger than those body parts that have little cortical tissue dedicated to processing their tactile and proprioceptive information (Figure 2-9). Extending the previous example, the mouth and lips on the sensory homunculus are quite large, while the trunk of the sensory homunculus is very small.

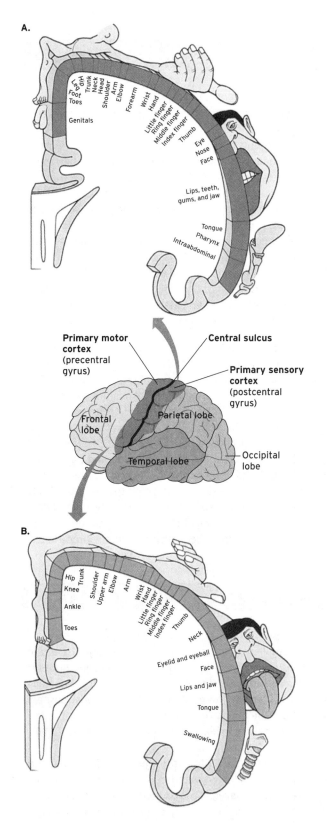

A.

Leg
Hip
Trunk
Neck
Head
Shoulder
Arm
Elbow
Forearm
Wrist
Hand
Little finger
Ring finger
Middle finger
Index finger
Thumb
Eye
Nose
Face
Foot
Toes
Genitals
Lips, teeth, gums, and jaw
Tongue
Pharynx
Intraabdominal

Primary motor cortex
(precentral gyrus)

Central sulcus

Primary sensory cortex
(postcentral gyrus)

Frontal lobe

Parietal lobe

Temporal lobe

Occipital lobe

B.

Hip
Trunk
Knee
Shoulder
Upper arm
Elbow
Arm
Wrist
Hand
Little finger
Ring finger
Middle finger
Index finger
Thumb
Neck
Ankle
Toes
Eyelid and eyeball
Face
Lips and jaw
Tongue
Swallowing

Figure 2-9 A. Sensory homunculus. B. Motor homunculus.

Clinical Note

Frontal Lobotomy

In the 1940s and 1950s, the frontal lobotomy, a procedure of damaging or removing tissue from the prefrontal area of the frontal lobes for the supposed remediation of psychological problems, was at its height. This procedure was popularized in the United States by Dr. Walter Freeman, whose name is closely associated with the procedure though use of the frontal lobotomy was widespread (Acharya, 2004).

The frontal lobotomy began as a surgical procedure to treat those with profound schizophrenia. At this point, the frontal lobotomy was still considered a highly experimental procedure (Kucharski, 1984). Freeman and most other medical professionals of the time initially used the frontal lobotomy as only a last-resort treatment. However, Freeman eventually came to believe that once psychological problems got to a certain level of severity, patients became unresponsive to other treatments. Following this belief, he shifted his position to using the frontal lobotomy as a more general treatment to be applied earlier to a range of problems including depression, criminality, schizophrenia, alcoholism, obsessive-compulsive disorder, and hysteria among others (Acharya, 2004; Kucharski, 1984).

To perform this treatment as often and as efficiently as necessary to meet his new criteria, Freeman abandoned the surgical suite, the surgical team, and general anesthesia. In his office, he began knocking his patients out with electroshock (electric currents to the brain) and inserting ice picks through the orbital process of their skull behind their eyes and moving the ice picks back and forth in a lateral (side-to-side) fashion, effectively damaging the prefrontal areas of the frontal lobes. Thousands and thousands of individuals were lobotomized in this manner during the 1940s and 1950s in assembly-line-like procedures. Eventually, Freeman abandoned the use of ice picks, which occasionally broke off in the skulls of his patients, and had custom instruments made that were far stronger than the average ice pick.

Despite grossly inconsistent results from the procedure, varying from improvement of conditions to extreme worsening of conditions and severe side effects, Freeman continued advocating for the procedure well after pharmaceutical treatments in the mid-1950s had been developed to target the same psychological conditions (Acharya, 2004). The frontal lobotomy was a product of its time and part of the scientific zeitgeist of the 1940s and 1950s. In retrospect, it is seen as being accepted too enthusiastically and blindly as an effective procedure by not only the scientific community but the popular culture at large willing to subject their loved ones to the procedure.

Clinical Note

Phineas Gage

Perhaps the most famous case documenting personality change following damage to the frontal lobes is that of Phineas Gage. Mr. Gage was a railway construction worker who lived in the mid-1800s. He was known to those around him to be moderate in his habits and possessing self-restraint and was rarely known to be profane (MacMillan, 2000). In 1848, while Mr. Gage was packing explosive powder into a hole to clear away rock for a railway, the explosives ignited unexpectedly and blew the metal tamping rod he was using beneath his cheekbone up through the frontal lobes of his brain and out through the top of his skull (Figure 2-10). This injury damaged both his frontal lobes and took out his left eye. It is generally accepted that he might not have lost consciousness from the injury. He is said to have sat upright in the cart that drove him to see a doctor (MacMillan, 2000).

Despite the severity of the injury, Mr. Gage lived and had generally recovered after 3 months (MacMillan, 2000). However, it was noted by friends and relatives that his personality changed dramatically after his accident. He was reported to have become very uninhibited and had difficulties not indulging in all his desires. He also had significant memory loss. His employers found that he could no longer complete his previous duties in railway construction. Years after

his death his skull was exhumed and it was determined that the areas of Mr. Gage's brain that were damaged by the metal rod were within the frontal cortex, parts of the brain responsible for inhibiting socially inappropriate behavior.

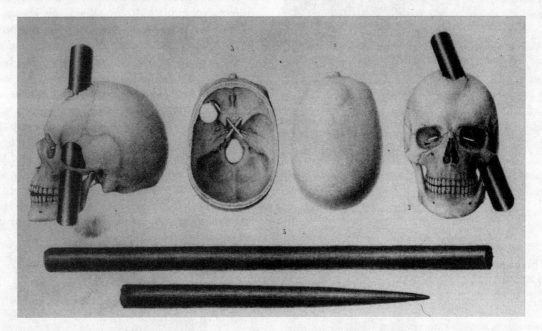

Figure 2-10 Phineas Gage.
Source: © National Library of Medicine.

The **temporal lobes** are located inferior to the posterior portion of the frontal lobes and inferior to the anterior portion of the parietal lobes (Figure 2-8). The temporal lobes house more memory than any other cerebral lobes. Most of the memory ability of the temporal lobes can be attributed to the hippocampi (plural). **Hippocampus** (singular) is Latin for *seahorse*. The hippocampi are located within the inferior and medial section of the temporal lobe where the cortex curls up into itself (**Figure 2-11**).

The hippocampi of the temporal lobes are so named because of their curled shape, which early anatomists thought resembled a *seahorse*. The hippocampal region takes new experiences and turns them into memories that can be stored and accessed later.

Individuals who have damage to the hippocampal regions in both temporal lobes display severe to profound deficits in short-term memory because they cannot create new memories (Scoville & Milner, 1957), and long-term memory abilities might be destroyed as well. See the following Clinical Note about Patient H.M.

Hippocampus A region of the temporal lobe responsible for storing and creating memories. (Plural: hippocampi.)

Primary auditory cortex A region of cortex located within the temporal lobes responsible for receiving and processing neural impulses related to sound.

The **primary auditory cortex** is located on the superior temporal gyrus, anterior to Wernicke's area in the

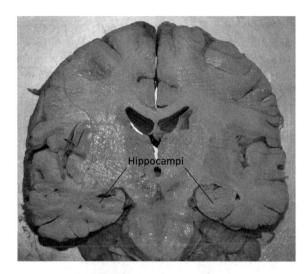

Figure 2-11 Hippocampi displayed on a coronal section of the brain.

left hemisphere (Figure 2-8). The primary auditory cortex is the section of the temporal lobes that first receives neural impulses of sound from the ears.

In the left temporal lobe, the left primary auditory cortex receives impulses of speech sounds and then passes these impulses on to Wernicke's area for processing so that, as mentioned earlier, the individual can comprehend spoken language. The right hemisphere's primary auditory cortex mostly passes impulses of environmental sounds and music to the area in the right hemisphere analogous to Wernicke's area (Bhatnagar, 2008) for the interpretation of meaning. Hence, the left hemisphere is responsible for auditory comprehension of verbal language while the right hemisphere is responsible for comprehension of the meaning of environmental sounds, such as a car starting or tree falling, as well as our appreciation of music.

Anterograde amnesia An inability to create new memories.

Occipital lobes The most posterior section of the cerebrum that is dedicated to receiving and processing neural impulses related to vision.

The **occipital lobes** are the most posterior of the cerebral lobes. They are located behind the parietal

Primary visual cortex
The posterior-most section of the occipital lobes dedicated to receiving neural impulses of vision from the eyes.

and temporal lobes (Figure 2-8). The occipital lobes are concerned mostly with vision. The occipital lobes house the **primary visual cortex** (Figure 2-8), which receives visual information from the eyes. The primary visual cortex is located on the most posterior section of each occipital lobe. The right and left divisions of the primary visual cortex receive and process information from the contralateral visual field.

Just anterior to the primary visual cortex is the **visual association cortex** (Figure 2-8). This is the section of the brain that processes and interprets visual information received from the primary visual cortex allowing for appropriate visual perception (i.e., the visual association cortex allows people to make sense with the brain of what they are seeing with their eyes). This area performs much the same function for vision that Wernicke's area performs for spoken language. Just as a lesion at Wernicke's area creates a condition (an aphasia) in which the person might be able to hear spoken words but cannot deduce the meaning of the sounds, bilateral lesions at the visual association cortices often create a condition known as visual agnosia in which a person can see but cannot comprehend what she is seeing.

Subcortical Structures

Beneath the cortex is the **subcortex**, its name literally meaning *below the cortex*. Unlike the cortex, which is responsible for very high-level reasoning and cognitive abilities, the subcortex is responsible for performing functions that are more automatic and usually beneath the level of our awareness. Examples of subcortical functions are refining and monitoring motor plans, regulating automatic life-sustaining body functions such as heartbeat as well as automatic breathing, coordinating functions of

the digestive system, and regulating level of arousal (this includes the sleep–wake cycle). The following subsections discuss four primary structures of the subcortex: the brain stem, cerebellum, thalamus, and basal ganglia.

The Brain Stem

In evolutionary terms, the **brain stem** is the oldest part of the brain. As a species, we were sleeping, breathing, and mating long before we were enjoying Shakespeare or learning the Pythagorean theorem. Higher levels of cognition came only with the more recent evolution of the huge cerebrum that sits on top of our brain stems.

Visual association cortex   A section of cortex within the occipital-parietal region responsible for processing and interpreting visual information received from the primary visual cortex.

Subcortex   The portion of the brain located beneath the cortex that deals less in reasoning abilities and higher-level cognition and more in autonomic, life-sustaining functions.

Brain stem   A subcortical structure that connects the spinal cord to the rest of the brain and houses many structures involved in autonomic functions.

Medulla   The superior-most section of the spinal cord that connects the spinal cord to the pons and is the site of decussation of a large portion of the motor tracts descending through the brain stem.

In a basic sense, the brain stem is the structure that connects the spinal cord to the brain. There are three main divisions of the brain stem. From top to bottom these are the midbrain, the pons, and the medulla (**Figure 2-12**). The **medulla** is the superior-most section of the spinal cord that connects the spinal cord to the pons. The medulla is the place where many of the motor fibers that transmit impulses of motor movement cross over or decussate to the other side of the body (**Figure 2-13**).

Because of the decussation of these motor fibers, the left side of the body is controlled by the right cerebral hemisphere and vice versa. Because of the decussation of these fibers, a lesion to the

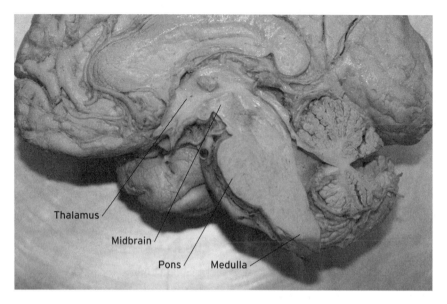

Figure 2-12 Sections of brain stem shown in midsaggital section.

descending motor tracts above the medulla creates a hemiplegia (one-sided paralysis) or a hemiparesis (one-sided weakness) on the side of the body contralateral (opposite) the lesion. If a lesion occurs below the level of decussation (such as within the spinal cord), the resulting hemiplegia or hemiparesis is on the side of the body ipsilateral (same) to the lesion.

Hemiplegia A unilateral spastic paralysis of the body.

Hemiparesis A unilateral spastic weakness of the body.

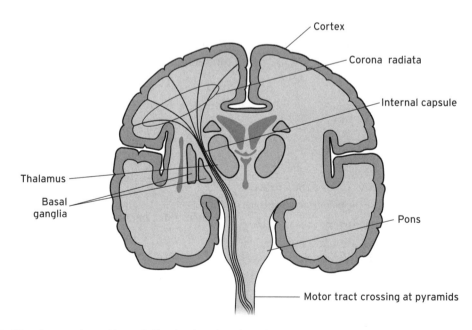

Figure 2-13 Coronal section of the brain showing decussation of descending motor tracts at the level of the medulla.

Pons   The middle and slightly bulbous portion of the brain stem that provides an attachment between the cerebellum (not cerebrum) and the rest of the CNS.

Midbrain   The superior-most section of the brain stem that houses the substantia nigra.

Substantia nigra   A structure located within the midbrain responsible for the production of the neurotransmitter dopamine.

Reticular formation   A series of nuclei stretching among the midbrain, pons, and medulla that regulates arousal, respiration, and blood pressure.

Located above the medulla is the pons (Figure 2-12). The **pons** is a slightly bulbous portion of the brain stem that provides an attachment between the cerebellum (not cerebrum) and rest of the CNS. The pons also connects the medulla below to the midbrain above.

The superior-most section of the brain stem is the **midbrain** (Figure 2-12). The midbrain houses the substantia nigra. The **substantia nigra** is where the brain produces a neurotransmitter known as dopamine. When the substantia nigra fails to produce enough dopamine, the symptoms of Parkinson's disease begin to arise.

Stretching between the midbrain, pons, and medulla is a series of nuclei called the reticular formation or the reticular activating system. The **reticular formation** regulates arousal (i.e., level of wakefulness), respiration, and blood pressure (Seikel, King, & Drumright, 2010).

The Cerebellum

Hanging off the back of the brain stem under the occipital lobes is the cerebellum (**Figure 2-15**). The **cerebellum** is known as the *little brain* because of its resemblance to the cerebral hemispheres. The cerebellum resembles the cerebral hemispheres because it also is divided into right and left hemispheres (**Figure 2-14**), each with a tightly packed and folded gray matter layer superficial to white matter coursing below. These are the cerebellar hemispheres. Students must be sure not to confuse the cerebellar hemispheres with the cerebral hemispheres.

When cut through at midline in a saggital (front to back) fashion, the distinctive plant-like shape of the white matter fibers of the cerebellar hemispheres is apparent (Figure 2-15). This plant-shaped

Cerebellum   A subcortical structure hanging off the back of the pons and under the occipital lobes that is known as an error control device for body movement and ensures that body movements are smoothly coordinated and as error free as possible.

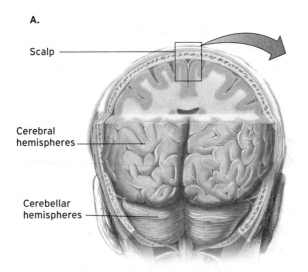

A.

Scalp

Cerebral hemispheres

Cerebellar hemispheres

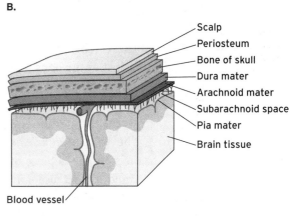

B.

Scalp
Periosteum
Bone of skull
Dura mater
Arachnoid mater
Subarachnoid space
Pia mater
Brain tissue

Blood vessel

Figure 2-14   **A. The cerebellar and cerebral hemispheres. B. The meningeal layers.**

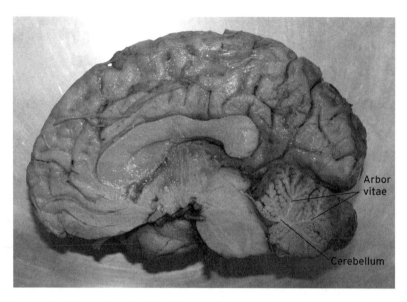

Figure 2-15 The cerebellum attached to the pons.

structure is known as the **arbor vitae** (Latin for *tree of life*). The right and left cerebellar hemispheres are connected to each other at midline by the unpaired vermis. The **vermis** is the midline gray matter that connects the cerebellar hemispheres and receives somatosensory information about the body through projections coursing through the pons.

The cerebellum is attached to the pons and communicates with the rest of the CNS by the cerebellar **peduncles**. The word *peduncle* is used primarily to refer to the stalk that a piece of fruit hangs from. The word is used here because early anatomists perceived that the cerebellum resembled a piece of fruit hanging off the pons under the cerebrum. In order from top to bottom, there are three cerebellar peduncles: the superior, middle, and inferior cerebellar peduncles.

Arbor vitae The distinctive plantlike shape of the fibers of the cerebellar hemispheres evident upon dissection and some imaging studies.

Vermis The midline gray matter that connects the two cerebellar hemispheres and receives somatosensory information about the body through projections coursing through the pons.

Peduncles Attachments between the cerebellum and the pons.

The cerebellum is known as an error control device for body movement. It makes sure that body movements are smoothly coordinated and error free. After motor plans are assembled in the primary motor cortex they are sent to the cerebellum to be checked for errors. The cerebellum monitors the intended movements of the motor plan and compares those plans with what the body is actually doing (Duffy, 2005). If there are any discrepancies between the motor plan and the body's execution of the motor plan, which are errors, the cerebellum makes corrections in the body's movements to match the motor plan to avoid the error. It does this by altering force, timing, and sequencing of muscle contractions (Diener & Dichgans, 1992). Although this discussion makes this process sound like it occurs in a step-by-step manner, the monitoring of the body's appropriate execution of motor plans by the cerebellum is an ongoing activity that continues in time as body movements continue.

Each cerebellar hemisphere receives and monitors motor plans from the contralateral cerebral hemisphere (Duffy, 2005). This means that motor signals from the left cerebral hemisphere are checked for errors in the right cerebellar hemisphere and motor signals from the right cerebral hemisphere are checked for errors in the left cerebellar hemisphere. Because of this arrangement each cerebellar hemisphere is

Thalamus A subcortical structure that rests on top of the brain stem beneath the cerebrum and functions as a relay station for neural impulses of sensation (excluding olfaction).

Basal ganglia A group of subcortical structures located deep within the cerebral hemispheres on either side of the thalamus that works to regulate body movement.

Spinal cord A bundle of white matter tracts and gray matter housed within the bony vertebral column that enables afferent (sensory) impulses coming from the body to be transmitted to brain and efferent (motor) impulses from the brain to be transmitted to the body.

responsible for monitoring movement occurring on the ipsilateral side of the body (Duffy, 2005).

The more rapid and precise a body movement is, the greater the likelihood that an error in the execution of motor plans will occur and the harder the cerebellum will work to minimize that risk. For example, as a professional pianist performs a complicated piece, the cerebellum works much harder to monitor for errors the motor plans of finger movements than it does if the pianist simply waved her arm in the air. A far more common activity that also requires a great deal of rapidity and precision in motor execution and that is used by almost everyone every single day is speech. Because the act of producing smoothly articulated speech requires a great deal of cerebellar input, difficulties in articulation can be a first indicator of cerebellar pathology. Pathology of the cerebellum often produces a speech problem known as ataxic dysarthria.

The Thalamus

The **thalamus** sits on top of the brain stem and under the cerebral hemispheres (Figure 2-12, Figure 2-13). This is a perfect location for the thalamus because the thalamus is responsible for taking sensory signals from one part of the nervous system and directing them to another part of the nervous system. The tag line associated with the thalamus is that it is a *relay station*. Specifically, all afferent (sensory) information (excluding olfaction) passes through the thalamus before arriving at the correct portion of the cerebral cortex for processing. For example, the optic nerve from the eyes passes through the thalamus on its way to the occipital lobes. Afferent impulses of proprioception and taction coming up from the body pass up the spinal cord, through the brain stem, and through the thalamus to the primary sensory cortex in the parietal lobes. The thalamus also takes the motor plans that the cerebellum has checked for errors and sends those motor plans to the appropriate places for execution (Duffy, 2005).

The Basal Ganglia

The term *ganglia* refers to a collection of nerve cells. The **basal ganglia** is a group of subcortical structures located deep within the cerebral hemispheres on either side of the thalamus (Figure 2-13). The structures of the basal ganglia include the caudate nucleus, the putamen, and the globus pallidus (Duffy, 2005). These structures have complex circuitry and interconnections among themselves and other portions of the CNS. The basal ganglia and its connections and circuitry are far from being perfectly understood. Nonetheless, it is clear that the basal ganglia play a strong role in motor movement. Lesions to the basal ganglia create problems with initiation of movement, muscle tone, and extra movements. These are all the symptoms of Parkinson's disease, which is created by dysfunction of the basal ganglia. Parkinson's disease occurs when the substantia nigra fails to produce dopamine, which the basal ganglia requires to operate properly.

The Spinal Cord

The **spinal cord** is a bundle of white matter tracts and gray matter housed within the bony vertebral column. It allows afferent (sensory) impulses coming from the body to be transmitted to brain and efferent (motor) impulses from the brain to be transmitted to the body.

The spinal cord originates superiorly at the medulla. The spinal cord then passes inferiorly through the vertebral column until it narrows at a section known as the conus medullaris. The spinal cord terminates inferiorly at the **conus medullaris** in the lumbar region of the lower back. Below the level of the conus medullaris the spinal cord breaks up into loose strands of spinal nerves called the **cauda equina**, or *horse's tail*, so named because of the resemblance of the loose strands of nerves to the hairs of a horse's tail (Figure 2-16).

Conus medullaris
Conical point of inferior termination of the spinal cord in the lumbar region of the lower back.

Cauda equina The loose strands of spinal nerves that separate from the inferior termination of the spinal cord.

In a cross section or transverse cut of the spinal cord, a gray butterfly or H shape appears in the middle (Figure 2-17). The grayness of the butterfly shape stands out in contrast to the whiteness of the surrounding tissue. This gray tissue is spinal nerve matter and can be thought of as the location where the spinal nerves enter and leave the spinal cord. The topmost wings of the butterfly shape are known as the dorsal horns. The nerve cells of the dorsal horns deliver the sensory (afferent) information from the spinal nerves to the surrounding white matter tracts to be transmitted to the brain. The bottom wings of the butterfly shape are known as the ventral horns. The nerve cells of the ventral horns deliver motor

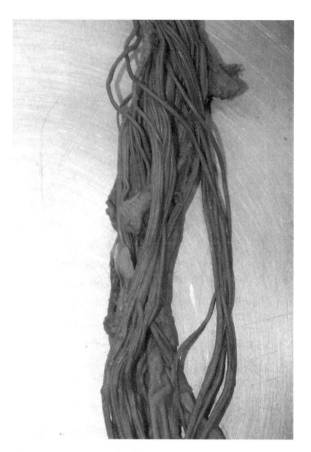

Figure 2-16 Cauda equina of the spinal cord.

(efferent) information from the associated white matter tracts in the spinal cord to the spinal nerves to be delivered to the organs and muscles. In the usual orientation of the spinal cord within the vertebral column the dorsal horns point posteriorly while the ventral horns point anteriorly.

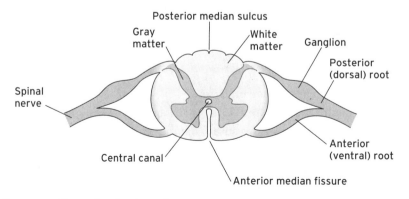

Figure 2-17 Cross section of spinal cord.

In addition to being a major highway between the brain and body for afferent and efferent signals, the spinal cord is also involved in basic reflexes. A **reflex** is the production of a physical movement that occurs automatically in response to a stimulus and is initiated below the level of awareness. Perhaps the most salient example of a reflex is the pain withdrawal reflex. Accidentally laying a hand on a hot stove produces this reflex: When a person's hand touches the hot surface, he pulls his hand away from the stove very quickly. In fact, he begins pulling the hand away before he realized his hand was being burned or that he was even in pain. In other words, the rest of this person's CNS does not wait for the cerebral cortex (which is the portion of the CNS farthest away from the burning hand) to realize the hand is burning before deciding to get it off the hot stove. This is a survival mechanism that allows people to react much faster than they would be able to if they had to wait for the sensation of pain to travel all the way up to the cerebral cortex, which is the farthest section of the CNS from the extremities.

Reflex   The production of a physical movement that occurs automatically in response to a stimulus and is initiated below the level of awareness.

Stretch reflex   A contraction of a muscle in response to a passive stretching of a muscle spindle within a muscle. This reflex enables the body to correct any unintended changes in body position in a timely manner without waiting for input from the cerebral cortex as well as keep appropriate tone in the muscles.

One very important reflex of concern to speech-language pathologists is the **stretch reflex**. The most well known example of this is the kick a leg makes unintentionally after the knee is tapped, the patellar reflex. When a doctor taps an individual's knee, she is momentarily stretching a muscle in the person's leg. A sensory receptor in that muscle called a muscle spindle is stretched as well and sends an afferent signal to the spinal cord indicating that the muscle has moved. The spinal cord receives this signal and recognizes that the leg muscle has been moved and yet no instructions came down from the brain telling that muscle in the leg to do so. The spinal cord knows that it is problematic for a body part to be moving with no commands from the brain to do so.

The spinal cord here is a mediator between the body and the brain. The spinal cord monitors the motor plans for the muscles as they come down from the brain, and then it sends those motor plans out along the cranial and spinal nerves to the muscles for execution. When a muscle behaves in a way contradictory to the motor plans sent down from the brain, the spinal cord is the first to know. It is problematic for survival if a person's muscles or body parts are not where the brain wants them to be and doing what the brain has told them to do. In evolutionary terms, this could mean the difference between a narrow escape with a saber-tooth tiger or a saber-tooth tiger tearing off an arm. Fortunately, the spinal cord doesn't wait for information concerning this discrepancy to travel all the way up to the cerebral cortex and rise to the level of conscious awareness. It recognizes the situation as an emergency and takes immediate action without consulting the brain.

Now back to the knee. When a muscle is lengthened passively, as when a doctor tests the patellar reflex, the spinal cord recognizes the discrepancy between the motor plans sent by the brain and the afferent signal coming from the muscle informing the spinal cord that the muscle has moved out of place (i.e., the spinal cord recognizes that no signal came from the brain telling the muscle that just moved to move). The spinal cord then originates and sends its own efferent (motor) signal out to the muscle to correct the situation and contract the muscle into its original and intended position. This contraction causes the leg to kick in response to the tap on the knee. In short, before the brain realizes there is a problem the spinal cord steps in and tells the offending muscle or body part to get to where it is supposed to be to correct the situation.

Normally, the stretch reflex is a good thing. In healthy individuals, the stretch reflex allows their bodies to correct any unintended changes in body position in a timely manner without waiting for input from the cerebral cortex as well as keeps appropriate tone in the muscles. However, the stretch reflex can be problematic when it becomes hyperactive. In some clinical scenarios, the spinal cord overapplies the stretch reflex and uses this hyperactive stretch reflex to create hypertonia in affected musculature which, combined with the weakness discussed previously, inhibits the individual's ability to move the affected body parts. This overactive stretch reflex also resists passive muscle movement. In these cases, a person's muscles might tighten, accomplish volitional movement with difficulty, and be resistant to movement when the clinician attempts to passively move the affected limbs or musculature. This resistance to passive movement brought about by an overactive stretch reflex is a big part of producing spasticity in musculature.

Spasticity is a combination of hypertonia (overtightness of muscles) and the resistance to passive movement caused by a hyperactive stretch reflex that makes movement of a body part difficult (i.e., it creates a spastic weakness). A clinical example is spastic cerebral palsy. Spastic cerebral palsy is the most common form of cerebral palsy and can be mild, affecting only a single extremity, or severe enough to affect an individual's entire body. If an individual's laryngeal, oral, or thoracic musculature is spastic, then the ability to move those structures is weakened, which can affect production of speech. This communication disorder is termed spastic dysarthria and occurs as a result of bilateral damage to motor tracts within the CNS usually by stroke.

> **Spasticity** A combination of hypertonia and the resistance to passive movement caused by a hyperactive stretch reflex that makes movement of a body part difficult.

Blood Supply to the Brain

Although the average human brain is only about 2% of total body weight, the brain consumes between 20% and 25% of the total amount of oxygen and glucose used by the body. In other words, up to a fourth of the body's oxygen and energy supplies is used to power this single organ. Any interruption of blood flow to the brain, such a stroke, has immediate and possibly dire consequences. To keep up the supply of blood to the brain necessary to meet these massive requirements the body must get blood first from the heart to the head.

The two pairs of large arteries whose function it is to deliver blood superiorly to the brain to be distributed throughout the brain by other arteries are the internal carotid arteries and the vertebral arteries. The paired right and left **internal carotid arteries** course superiorly from the thorax in the anterior portion of the neck (**Figure 2-18**). The pulse in the neck is felt by palpating the internal carotid. The internal carotid arteries course through the neck to the base of the brain to link with the **circle of Willis**. Once the internal carotid arteries reach the circle of Willis, the paired left and right anterior cerebral arteries and middle cerebral arteries branch off from the internal carotids (**Figure 2-19**). The **anterior cerebral arteries** course anteriorly to supply blood to the frontal and parietal lobes, basal ganglia, and corpus callosum (Seikel et al., 2010). The **middle cerebral arteries** course laterally to supply blood flow to Broca's area, Wernicke's

> **Internal carotid arteries** Paired arteries that course superiorly from the thorax within the anterior portion of the neck to the base of the brain to link with the circle of Willis.
>
> **Circle of Willis** A series of anastomoses that connects the internal carotid and vertebral/basilar system, acts to ensure equal blood flow to all areas of the brain, and acts as a safety valve if an occlusion occurs within the circle of Willis or below the circle of Willis.
>
> **Anterior cerebral arteries** Paired arteries that originate from the internal carotid arteries at the circle of Willis and course anteriorly to supply blood to the frontal and parietal lobes, basal ganglia, and corpus callosum.
>
> **Middle cerebral arteries** Paired arteries that originate from the internal carotid arteries at the circle of Willis and course laterally to supply blood flow to Broca's area, Wernicke's area, the temporal lobes, and the primary motor cortex.

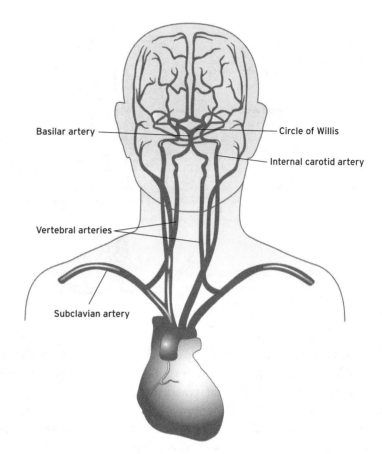

Figure 2-18   Major arteries supplying blood flow to the brain.

Vertebral arteries
Paired arteries that course superiorly through the cervical vertebrae of the spinal column in the posterior aspect of the neck and come together to form the basilar artery at the pons.

Basilar artery   A single unpaired artery that joins the circle of Willis posteriorly and branches into the paired posterior cerebral arteries.

Posterior cerebral artery   Paired arteries that branch off the basilar artery at the circle of Willis to course posteriorly and deliver blood to the occipital lobes, cerebellum, and the inferior temporal lobes.

Anastomosis   A connection between blood vessels. (Plural: anastomoses.)

Anterior communicating artery   An unpaired anastomosis between the right and left anterior cerebral arteries that forms the anterior portion of the circle of Willis.

Posterior communicating arteries   Paired anastomoses coursing from the left posterior cerebral artery to the left middle cerebral artery and also coursing from the right posterior cerebral artery to the right middle cerebral artery.

area, the temporal lobes, and the primary motor cortex.

Meanwhile, the paired right and left **vertebral arteries** course superiorly through the cervical vertebrae of the spinal column in the posterior aspect of the neck (Figure 2-18). The vertebral arteries come together to form the basilar artery at the pons. The **basilar artery** then proceeds to join to the posterior section of the circle of Willis (Figure 2-19). Once the basilar artery reaches the circle of Willis, it branches into the **posterior cerebral arteries** (Figure 2-19), which delivers blood to the occipital lobes, cerebellum, and the inferior temporal lobes (Seikel et al., 2010).

The circle of Willis is a set of **anastomoses** (i.e., connections between arteries) between the anterior, middle, and posterior cerebral arteries that together form a circle at the base of the brain. The **anterior communicating artery** connects the left and right anterior cerebral arteries. The **posterior communicating arteries** link the posterior cerebral arteries to the middle cerebral arteries.

The circle of Willis is highly important because by connecting the internal carotid and vertebral/basilar systems it acts to ensure equal blood flow to all areas of the brain and acts as a safety valve if an occlusion

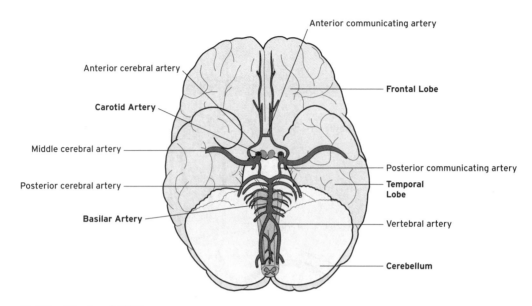

Figure 2-19 Circle of Willis.

(i.e., a clot) occurs within the circle of Willis or below the circle of Willis. For instance, if there is a sudden reduction in blood flow from the left internal carotid artery, blood can course through communicating arteries from the basilar and right internal carotid arteries to sustain blood flow to those areas of the brain dependent on the internal carotid artery for blood supply. In this way, brain tissue can be saved from oxygen deprivation and tissue death.

The Peripheral Nervous System

The PNS is composed of the nerves that connect the CNS to the rest of the body. These nerves can be thought of as wires that connect at one end to a muscle, organ, or gland and at the other end to the brain, brain stem, or the spinal cord.

Efferent signals from the brain travel along the PNS to reach the muscles to command them to move. Examples of efferent information sent from the CNS are commands to muscles to contract or relax to move a body part or to make the heart beat as well as commands regulating body metabolism.

Afferent signals originating with the body are transmitted along the PNS on their way back to the CNS for processing. Afferent information is analyzed and interpreted by the CNS in the cerebrum. For example, the sensory information about the way an individual feels following striking his thumb with a hammer is transmitted along the nerves of the PNS to the CNS where that afferent signal is processed and understood as pain.

The two primary divisions of the PNS are the cranial nerves and spinal nerves.

The Spinal Nerves

As their name implies, **spinal nerves** are associated with the spinal cord. Whereas the cranial nerves contribute to control of the head and neck, the spinal nerves contribute to control of the rest of the body. The spinal cord and spinal nerves are associated with movement and control of the trunk of the body and the arms and legs. There are 31 pairs of spinal nerves. Each spinal nerve arises within the gray matter of the spinal cord and then courses out from

Spinal nerves Nerves that course between the spinal cord and the body.

between the 33 individual bones of the vertebral column (the vertebrae) to innervate the body (Figure 2-17). Each spinal nerve connects the spinal cord to a muscle, organ, or gland of the body.

Most spinal nerves do not play a direct role in speech. However, the **phrenic nerve** innervates the diaphragm. The **diaphragm** is the muscle that is primarily responsible for the inspiration of air into the lungs. Of course, respiration is necessary to life, but it also is essential for the production of phonation for speech.

The Cranial Nerves

As their name implies, the **cranial nerves** are associated with the cranium. The cranium is the bony part of the skull that encases and protects the brain. The cranial nerves connect muscles and structures of the head, face, and neck to the CNS. There are 12 cranial nerves. Each of the cranial nerves is a paired nerve, meaning that there is one for the right side of the body and an analogous one for the left side of the body.

Thorough knowledge of the function and location of the cranial nerves is a powerful diagnostic tool for the speech-language pathologist. Based on the presence of certain speech, voice, or swallowing difficulties, a speech-language pathologist often can discern the presence of pathology in the PNS and, using knowledge of the function of the cranial nerves, can determine with which nerve(s) the problem originates.

The cranial nerves are numbered by roman numerals in the order that they synapse, or connect, to the CNS from superior to inferior. The olfactory nerve is numbered I because, from superior to inferior, it is the first cranial nerve to synapse with the CNS. In contrast, the hypoglossal nerve is XII because the other 11 cranial nerves attach to the portions of the brain and brain stem above it.

The cranial nerves are all either motor nerves, sensory nerves, or mixed sensory-motor. Cranial nerves that are motor in nature carry only efferent impulses from the CNS out to the body. Those that are sensory in nature transmit only afferent impulses from the body back to the CNS. The cranial nerves that function both as sensory and motor nerves relay both efferent and afferent information between the CNS and the body. See **Table 2-1** for a complete listing of the cranial nerves and their function.

Although all the cranial nerves are very important to know, this book focuses on those whose function is important for communication. The cranial nerves that are most directly important to speech are trigeminal V, facial VII, glossopharyngeal IX, vagus X, accessory XI, and hypoglossal XII.

The Trigeminal V

The fifth cranial nerve, the trigeminal, is one of the largest cranial nerves and one of the most important cranial nerves for speech (see **Figure 2-20**.) It is a mixed motor and sensory nerve. The trigeminal emerges from the pons and splits into three primary branches: the **ophthalmic branch**, the **maxillary branch**, and the **mandibular branch** (Seikel et al., 2010). The ophthalmic branch is sensory in nature

Phrenic nerve A spinal nerve that provides innervation to the diaphragm.

Diaphragm The primary muscle of inspiration.

Cranial nerves Nerves that course between the brain stem and the head/neck/face and are either motor/efferent, sensory/afferent, or mixed sensory-motor in function.

Ophthalmic branch A branch of the trigeminal nerve that is sensory in nature and transmits afferent information from the upper face, forehead, and scalp to the central nervous system.

Maxillary branch A branch of the trigeminal nerve that is sensory in nature and is responsible for transmitting afferent information from the teeth, upper lip, buccal and nasal cavities, as well as the sides of the face to the CNS.

Mandibular branch A branch of the trigeminal nerve with both sensory and motor functions. The afferent portion of this nerve carries sensory information from the lower teeth, lower gums, bottom lip, as well as somatic information from portions of the tongue. The efferent component innervates muscles of mastication.

Table 2-1 Cranial Nerves

Roman Numeral	Cranial Nerve	Origin	Type	Function
I	Olfactory	Cerebral hemispheres	Sensory	Smell
II	Optic	Thalamus	Sensory	Vision
III	Oculomotor	Midbrain	Motor	Movement of the eyes
IV	Trochlear	Midbrain	Motor	Movement of the eyes
V	Trigeminal*	Pons	Sensory	Somatic sensation from face, lips, jaw
			Motor	Movement of the mandible
VI	Abducens	Pons	Motor	Movement of the eyes
VII	Facial*	Pons	Sensory	Gustation (taste) from the anterior two-thirds of the tongue
			Motor	Movement of the lips and face
VIII	Cochleovestibular	Pons, medulla	Sensory	Hearing and balancing
IX	Glossopharyngeal*	Medulla	Sensory	Gustation (taste) from the posterior one-third of the tongue
			Motor	Movement of superior portion of pharynx
X	Vagus*	Medulla	Sensory	Sensation from larynx, pharynx, abdominal viscera
			Motor	Movement of the larynx, pharynx, velum
XI	Accessory*	Medulla, spinal cord	Motor	Movement of the muscles of shoulder and neck (trapezius)
				Assisting vagus on movement of the larynx, pharynx, and velum
XII	Hypoglossal*	Medulla	Motor	Movement of the tongue

* Necessary for speech production.

and transmits afferent information from the upper face, forehead, and scalp to the CNS (Figure 2-20). The maxillary branch is also a sensory nerve and is responsible for transmitting afferent information from the teeth, upper lip, buccal and nasal cavities, as well as the sides of the face to the CNS (Figure 2-20). In contrast, the mandibular branch has both sensory and motor functions. The afferent portion of this nerve carries sensory information from the lower teeth, lower gums, and bottom lip and somatic information from portions of the tongue (Figure 2-20). The efferent component of the mandibular branch of the trigeminal nerve innervates muscles of mastication. ▶ For an interview with an individual regarding pathology of the trigeminal refer to the video *Trigeminal Neuralgia*.

The Facial Nerve VII

The seventh cranial nerve, the facial, is a mixed sensory-motor nerve. The facial nerve emerges from the inferior pons. The primary motor function of the facial nerve is to provide motor innervation to the muscles of the face. The primary sensory function of the facial nerve is to transmit afferent information concerning taste from the anterior two-thirds of the tongue to the CNS (Gertz, 2007).

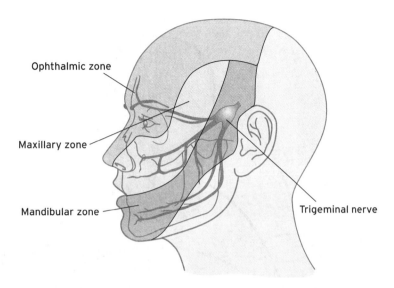

Ophthalmic zone

Maxillary zone

Mandibular zone

Trigeminal nerve

Figure 2-20 Areas of the face and scalp innervated by the Mandibular, Maxillary, and Opthalmic branches of the trigeminal nerve.

The facial nerve has four branches. From superior to inferior these are the temporal branch, the zygomatic branch, the buccal branch, and the mandibular branch. A distinctive feature of the facial nerve is that the temporal and zygomatic branches, which innervate the muscles of the upper face, receive plans of volitional motor movement for the upper face from the contralateral *as well as* the ipsilateral cerebral hemispheres (Figure 2-21). When one side of a paired nerve (the right or the left) receives motor plans from both the right and left cerebral hemispheres, it is termed **bilateral innervation**.

In contrast, the inferior branches of the facial nerve, the buccal and the mandibular branches, which innervate the muscles of the lower face, are unilaterally innervated. **Unilateral innervation** of a nerve indicates that the nerve receives motor plans from only the contralateral cerebral hemisphere. More simply: The muscles of each side of the upper face receive motor plans from both the right cerebral hemisphere and the left cerebral hemisphere (Figure 2-21). So, when an individual moves one side of her upper face and forehead, those motor plans come from both cerebral hemispheres. However, the muscles of either side

of the lower face receive motor plans only from the contralateral cerebral hemisphere (Figure 2-21). Therefore, when an individual twitches the right side of her mouth, that motor plan comes only from the left cerebral hemisphere.

Other cranial nerves besides the facial nerve are also bilaterally innervated, though sometimes inconsistently between individuals. The facial nerve presents a unique opportunity to learn unilateral and bilateral innervation because the superior branches receive bilateral innervation whereas the inferiorly located branches receive only unilateral innervation.

There is a **protective redundancy** in bilateral innervation. With bilateral innervation, a lack of motor

Bilateral innervation An innervation pattern that occurs when one side of a paired nerve (the right or the left) receives motor plans from both the right and left cerebral hemispheres.

Unilateral innervation An innervation pattern that occurs when a nerve receives motor plans from only the contralateral cerebral hemisphere.

Protective redundancy When the body duplicates systems to protect proper functioning.

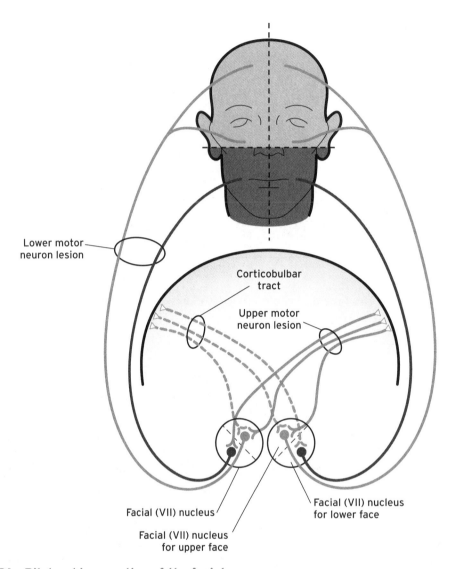

Figure 2-21 Bilateral innervation of the facial nerve.

plans coming from one cerebral hemisphere does not completely incapacitate a body part if that body part can still receive motor plans from the opposite hemisphere. So, why is this important? Take the phrenic nerve, which innervates the diaphragm, for example. The diaphragm is the primary muscle for respiration and the phrenic nerve, which supplies motor commands to the diaphragm, is bilaterally innervated. If the phrenic nerve was not bilaterally innervated, then damage to one cerebral hemisphere

would incapacitate the entire contralateral half of the diaphragm. However, due to the protective redundancy of bilateral innervation, an individual can suffer damage to a cerebral hemisphere and still retain some function in the contralateral portion of the diaphragm. Because moving the diaphragm is important to sustaining life, the significance of bilateral innervation becomes evident. Figure 2-21 shows an illustration of the bilateral innervation of the superior portions of the facial nerve.

Glossopharyngeal IX

The ninth cranial nerve, the glossopharyngeal, has both sensory and motor functions. The primary sensory function of the glossopharyngeal is transmitting taste from the posterior one-third of the tongue and also from a portion of the soft palate. The motor function of the glossopharyngeal nerve is to deliver efferent signals to the superior muscles of the pharynx, which are involved in swallowing, as well as to the parotid gland, which produces saliva (Gertz, 2007).

Vagus X

The 10th and largest cranial nerve, the vagus, is perhaps the most important cranial nerve for the speech-language pathologist. The vagus is a long and complex nerve with both sensory and motor functions. The vagus exits the medulla and travels inferiorly to innervate the muscles of the soft palate, pharynx, and larynx. **Figure 2-22** is an illustration of the sections of the vagus.

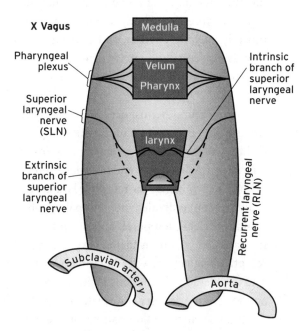

Figure 2-22   Sections of the vagus nerve.

Upon leaving the medulla, the first branch of the vagus innervating a structure important for speech is the pharyngeal plexus. This branch of the vagus innervates most of the muscles of the inferior pharynx as well as most of the muscles of the velum. The muscles of the inferior pharynx are responsible for pharyngeal constriction, which is used during swallowing, while the muscles of the velum are important for sealing off the nasal cavity for production of nonnasal phonemes and also for avoiding nasal regurgitation during swallowing.

Continuing inferiorly, the second branch of the vagus important for speech is the superior laryngeal branch, or the superior laryngeal nerve (SLN). The SLN has an intrinsic and an extrinsic branch. The intrinsic branch of the SLN is sensory in nature and responsible for transmitting sensory information from the inside of the larynx to the CNS. The extrinsic portion of the SLN is responsible for innervating the cricothyroid muscle (the primary tensor of the vocal folds).

The vagus then courses and passes inferiorly into the thorax. The right vagus nerve passes under the right subclavian artery within the right side of the thorax. The left vagus passes under the arch of aorta of the heart within the left side of the thorax. Both of these branches then immediately change course and pass superiorly back, *recurring*, into the neck and to the larynx to innervate all the remaining intrinsic muscles of the larynx (those muscles responsible for adduction and abduction of the vocal folds). These branches of the vagus are known appropriately as the recurrent laryngeal nerve (RLN).

Accessory XI

The 11th cranial nerve, the accessory, is an efferent nerve and as such is only motor in function. The accessory nerve has a spinal component responsible for innervating muscles of the shoulders such as the trapezius, but also has a cranial component. The cranial component of the accessory nerve and the functional differences between it and the vagus nerve are poorly understood. The cranial component of the accessory nerve works alongside the vagus (as an accessory). The spinal component of the accessory nerve innervates some of the muscles of the shoulders.

Hypoglossal XII

The 12th and last cranial nerve is the hypoglossal. The hypoglossal nerve exits the brain stem at a more inferior location off the medulla than any other cranial nerve. The hypoglossal nerve is motor in nature. The primary role of the hypoglossal nerve is to innervate all the intrinsic muscles of the tongue and most of the extrinsic muscles of the tongue. The intrinsic muscles of the tongue are the muscles that comprise the actual body of the tongue and are responsible for the more fine motor movements of the tongue involved in articulation. The extrinsic muscles of the tongue are those muscles responsible for gross movements of the tongue, such as the extension and retraction of the tongue. These gross motor movements of the tongue are more likely to be used during mastication and swallowing than during speech.

Main Points

- The nervous system is divided into the central nervous system (CNS), which is made up of the brain and spinal cord, and the peripheral nervous system (PNS), which is made up of the cranial nerves and spinal nerves.
- The brain is grossly composed of the cerebrum, brain stem, and cerebellum.
- The surface of the cerebrum is the cerebral cortex and is composed of folded tissue that creates gyri and sulci. These folds of cortical tissue enable more neural tissue to be packed into a smaller space.
- The brain is made up of gray and white matter. Gray matter lacks myelin, a fatty substance used to facilitate the conduction of electrical impulses along tracts of white matter. Gray matter is responsible for processing information. White matter is responsible for transmitting information. White matter is made up of three types of fibers. These include association fibers, commissural fibers, and projection fibers.
- The cerebrum is divided into right and left cerebral hemispheres by the longitudinal fissure.

- The right and left cerebral hemispheres are connected by a thick band of commissural fibers called the corpus callosum.
- The right cerebral hemisphere is responsible for the interpretation of nonlinguistic stimuli such as facial expressions, body language, gestures, prosody, melody, rhythm, and environmental sounds; understanding macrostructure; visuospatial processing; and attention (sustained and selective).
- The left cerebral hemisphere is primarily responsible for expressive and receptive language abilities. Broca's area is primarily responsible for expressive language, and Wernicke's area is primarily responsible for receptive language.
- The cerebrum is divided into four paired lobes: frontal, parietal, temporal, and occipital. The frontal lobes' functions include expressive and receptive language, as well as motor movements. The parietal lobes' functions include receiving and processing sensory information regarding the body such as taction and proprioception. The temporal lobes' functions include memory

as well as receiving and processing auditory information through the primary auditory cortices. Last, the occipital lobes' functions include receiving afferent signals of vision as well as processing visual information.

- The frontal and parietal lobes are divided by the central sulci, which run laterally down the side of each cerebral hemisphere in a vertical fashion. The frontal and parietal lobes are divided from the temporal lobes by the lateral sulci, which run anteriorly to posteriorly at an upward angle through each cerebral hemisphere.

- Structures of the subcortex are the brain stem, cerebellum, thalamus, and basal ganglia. The subcortex is responsible for less volitional and more automatic/visceral functions such as heartbeat, breathing, and sleep–wake cycles.

- The brain stem is composed of (from superior to inferior) the midbrain, pons, and medulla. The brain stem connects the spinal cord to the brain.

- The cerebellum is made up of two hemispheres connected by the vermis at midline. The cerebellum is attached to the pons by the inferior, medial, and superior peduncles. The cerebellum is as an error control device and works to create smoothly coordinated and errorless body movements.

- The thalamus rests on top of the brain stem and is the relay station for afferent signals.

- The basal ganglia is made up of the caudate nucleus, putamen, and globus pallidus and is responsible for regulation of motor movement, muscle tone, and inhibition of extraneous movements.

- The spinal cord, which begins at the medulla, narrows and terminates at the conus medullaris and divides into in loose strands of nerves. The spinal cord transmits afferent information from the PNS to the brain and transmits efferent information from the brain to the PNS. The spinal cord is also responsible for originating the stretch reflex, which can become hyperactive in

certain pathologic situations, such as damage to the motor pathways within the CNS, and result in spasticity.

- The brain consumes 25% of all oxygen and glucose brought into the body.

- The internal carotid arteries and the basilar artery transmit blood from the thorax to the brain.

- The anterior cerebral arteries, middle cerebral arteries, and posterior arteries transmit blood out to certain portions of the brain.

- The anterior communicating artery and the posterior communicating arteries link up the internal carotid system with the vertebral/basilar system to form the circle of Willis. The circle of Willis acts as a safety valve to protect the brain from a lack of blood supply.

- The 31 paired spinal nerves connect the spinal cord to muscles, organs, and glands that usually do not play a direct role in speech production. However, the phrenic nerve is a spinal nerve that innervates the diaphragm, the muscle primarily responsible for inspiration of air into the lungs.

- The 12 paired cranial nerves connect the muscles and structures of the head, face, and neck to the CNS and function as sensory, motor, or both sensory and motor nerves. Important cranial nerves for speech include the trigeminal (V), facial (VII), glossopharyngeal (IX), vagus (X), accessory (XI), and hypoglossal (XII).

- The trigeminal (V) nerve is a paired sensory-motor nerve that transmits sensory information from the upper and lower face to the CNS and transmits motor information from the CNS to the muscles of the mandible. The trigeminal is divided into ophthalmic, maxillary, and mandibular branches.

- The facial (VII) nerve is a paired sensory-motor nerve that provides motor to the face and sensation (taste) from the anterior two-thirds of the tongue and is divided into the temporal and zygomatic branches, which are bilaterally inner-vated, and the buccal and mandibular branches, which are unilaterally innervated.

- The glossopharyngeal (IX) nerve is a paired sensory-motor nerve that provides sensory information to the posterior one-third of the tongue and motor information to the pharynx for swallowing.
- The vagus (X) nerve is a paired sensory-motor nerve that provides motor information to the soft palate, pharynx, and larynx and sensory information from the pharynx, larynx, and viscera through its many branches, including the pharyngeal plexus, superior laryngeal nerve (intrinsic and extrinsic branches), and recurrent laryngeal nerve.
- The accessory (XI) nerve is a paired motor-only nerve whose cranial portion works alongside the vagus for innervation of the larynx, pharynx, and velum and whose spinal portion in-nervates some of the muscles of the shoulders.
- The hypoglossal (XII) nerve is a paired motor nerve that innervates the intrinsic and extrinsic muscles of the tongue.

Review Questions

1. Describe the two major sections of the nervous system, including each section's anatomy and functions.
2. What three gross structures constitute the brain?
3. What are the ridges and valleys of the cerebral cortex called and why are they there?
4. What is myelin? What is the function of myelin and what type of neurons have myelin?
5. Which fissure separates the left and right cere-bral hemispheres? What major band of commis-sural fibers connects the right and left cerebral hemispheres?
6. List five functions of the right hemisphere.
7. List two functions of the left hemisphere.
8. Name the four lobes of the cerebral hemispheres and describe the function and any important areas of each lobe that enable those functions to occur.
9. Which sulci run laterally and divide the frontal and temporal lobes? Which sulci run superiorly to inferiorly and divide the frontal and parietal lobes?
10. List three structures of the subcortex and iden-tify the main functions of those structures.

11. List the three sections of the brain stem and de-scribe functions of each.
12. What structures of the cerebellum attach it to the pons and the CNS?
13. What is the location and primary function of the thalamus?
14. Describe the function of the basal ganglia.
15. Why is the circle of Willis an important structure?
16. Describe the location, anatomy, and role of the spinal cord.
17. Describe how a healthy stretch reflex occurs and describe how a hyperactive stretch reflex contributes to spasticity.
18. In your opinion, which cranial nerve is the most important for speech production and why?
19. What are the six most important cranial nerves that are central to the production of speech?
20. What is bilateral innervation? What is unilat-eral innervation? Why is bilateral innervation a good thing?

References

1. Acharya, H. (2004). The rise and fall of the frontal lobotomy. *Proceedings of the 13th Annual History of Medicine Days*.

2. Aristotle. (2011). *On sleep and sleeplessness* (I. Beare, Trans.). Amazon Digital Services.

3. Bhatnagar, S. (2008). Neuroscience for the Study of Communicative Disorders. Philadelphia, PA: Wolters Kluwer/Lippincott Williams & Wilkins.

4. Carey, B. (2008). H.M., an unforgettable amnesiac, dies at 82. *New York Times*. http://www.nytimes.com/2008/12/05/us/05hm.html?pagewanted=al&_rmoc.semityn.www

5. Corkin, S. (2002). What's new with the patient H.M.? *Nature Reviews: Neuroscience, 3*, 153–160.

6. Diener, H., & Dichgans, J. (1992). Pathophysiology of cerebellar ataxia. *Movement Disorders, 7*(2), 95–109.

7. Duffy. J. (2005). *Motor speech disorders: Substrates, differential diagnosis, and management* (2nd ed.). St. Louis, MO: Mosby.

8. Gertz, S. (2007). *Liebman's neuroanatomy made easy and understandable* (7th ed.). Austin, TX: Pro-Ed.

9. Joseph, R. (1988). The right cerebral hemisphere: Emotion, music visual-spatial skills, body-image, dreams, and awareness. *Journal of Clinical Psychology, 44*(5), 630–673.

10. Kucharski, A. (1984). History of frontal lobotomy in the United States, 1935–1955. *Neurosurgery, 14*(6), 765–772.

11. Luria, A. (1973). *The working brain: An introduction to neuropsychology*. New York, NY: Basic Books.

12. MacMillan, M. (2000). Restoring Phineas Gage: A 150th retrospective. *Journal of the History of the Neurosciences, 9*(1), 46–66.

13. Scoville, W. B., & Milner, B. (1957). Loss of recent memory after bilateral hippocampal lesions. *Journal of Neurology, Neurosurgery, and Psychiatry, 20*(11), 11–21.

14. Seikel, J., King, D., & Drumright, D. (2010). *Anatomy and physiology for speech, language, and hearing* (4th ed.). Clifton Park, NY: Delmar Cengage.

Chapter 3

Acute Etiologies of Neurogenic Communication Disorders

▶ *Where this icon appears, visit http://go.jblearning.com/ManascoCWS to view the corresponding video.*

Whereas degenerative disorders are diseases that result from a systemic breakdown or destruction of structures within the peripheral or central nervous systems, usually from unknown or partially known mechanisms, acute etiologies include acute or traumatic events such as stroke, traumatic brain injury, seizure, tumor, surgical trauma, and infection.

> **Etiology** The underlying cause of a symptom or deficit.
>
> **Idiopathic** To be of unknown origin.

Clinicians use the term **etiology** to refer to the underlying cause of a symptom or deficit. Neurogenic communication disorders vary greatly in their etiologies. The most common etiologies of neurogenic communication disorders in the general population are stroke, traumatic brain injury, surgical trauma, and degenerative diseases. However, infectious disease and other conditions can also produce deficits in speech, cognition, and language. It is not uncommon for individuals with neurogenic communication disorders to have an unknown etiology of their deficits or symptoms. If an etiology is unknown or obscure, it is said to be **idiopathic**.

The etiologies mentioned in this chapter produce damage to the central and/or peripheral nervous system. How this damage to the nervous system manifests in deficits in communication, cognition, and behavior is determined by the site of the damage as well as the severity of the damage. Often, the site and severity of damage to the nervous system are intimately associated with the etiology. For instance, certain diseases attack specific parts of the nervous system.

It is important for speech-language pathology students to secure a basic understanding of stroke. Strokes are an overwhelmingly common condition encountered in the adult and aging populations. Before tackling the communication disorders that a stroke can produce, students must understand the physiologic mechanisms behind this etiology and be able to recognize the early warning signs of stroke so that medical help can be acquired for the patient before permanent damage to the brain occurs.

Stroke: Cerebrovascular Accident

A stroke is the result of blood flow to a part of the brain being interrupted by a clot or a hemorrhage. Medical professionals refer to stroke as a cerebrovascular accident or, simply, CVA. Speech-language pathologists who work in hospitals and other medical settings inevitably work with many individuals who have had a stroke. Strokes can produce damage to any area of the brain or brain stem and, therefore, can create most any type of neurogenic communication disorder or cognitive deficit.

Cerebrovascular accident A stroke. An interruption of blood flow to or within the brain that permanently destroys brain tissue or causes a temporary cessation of function.

Stroke is the third leading cause of death in the United States behind heart disease and cancer (American Heart Association [AHA], 2010; Bonita, 1992). Stroke is a leading cause of hospital admission and long-term disability (AHA, 2010; Bonita, 1992). It has been estimated that every 40 seconds someone in the United States has a stroke and every 4 minutes someone dies of a stroke (AHA, 2010). Although the actual percentage of individuals experiencing communication difficulties following stroke is unknown, studies show that the presence of aphasia alone among individuals who have had strokes can be as high as 41.2% (Guyomard et al., 2009). Also, more women tend to die of stroke than men (AHA, 2010). Known factors that contribute to the likelihood of experiencing a stroke are a history of tobacco use (which doubles a person's risk for stroke), physical inactivity, atrial fibrillation, and high blood pressure (Rosamond et al., 2008).

Specifically, a stroke is when brain tissue is either permanently destroyed or temporarily ceases to function as a result of decreased or absent blood supply to the affected area. When brain tissue is permanently destroyed, the body reabsorbs the dead cells and an empty space is left on the cortex or within the brain where the tissue once was.

During a stroke, a primary source of damage to brain tissue is from the loss of oxygen supply resulting from a lack of blood supply, which transports oxygen-rich blood to the brain. The complete lack of oxygen supply to tissue is a condition known as anoxia. The partial loss of oxygen supply to tissue is hypoxia. Typically, the brain can go 6 to 8 minutes without oxygen before anoxia begins to cause permanent cell death within the brain. It is therefore extremely important to be able to recognize quickly when an individual is experiencing a stroke so that appropriate medical care can be acquired.

Stroke A lesion in the brain that occurs when brain tissue is either permanently destroyed or temporarily ceases to function as a result of a lack of blood flow or a disturbance of blood supply to the affected area.

Anoxia A condition of being completely without oxygen; an extreme lack of oxygen to brain tissue.

Hypoxia A condition in which the body lacks appropriate oxygen supply.

Ischemia Blockage of or restriction in a blood vessel.

Hemorrhage Bleeding of an open blood vessel.

There are two main forms of stroke: ischemic and hemorrhagic. The term ischemia means a blockage of or restriction in a blood vessel. The term *hemorrhagic* is derived from the word hemorrhage, which means to bleed. The majority of strokes are ischemic in nature. Typically, strokes can produce immediate deficits in cognition and language as well as weakness and difficulty seeing, hearing, and balancing.

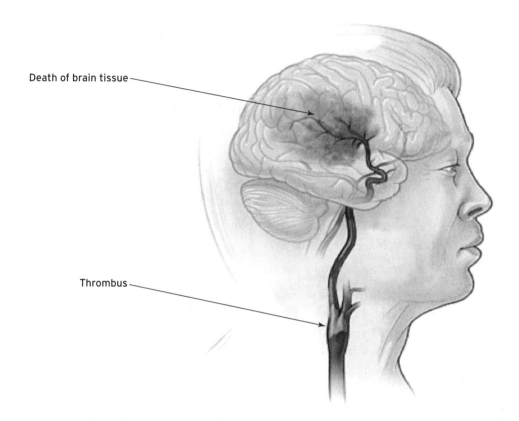

Death of brain tissue

Thrombus

Figure 3-1 Thrombus reducing bloodflow to the brain.

Ischemic Stroke

An **ischemic stroke** occurs when a blood vessel supplying bloodflow to the brain becomes occluded (**Figure 3-1**). An occlusion in a blood vessel deprives brain tissue of the blood supply necessary for survival of the tissue. Symptoms of ischemic stroke typically develop over minutes or hours. Early warning signs or symptoms of an ischemic stroke include "loss of strength or sensation on one side of the body, problems with speech and language, or changes in vision or balance" (AHA, 2007, p. 1). See the videos *Brain Stem Stroke* and *Recovering from Stroke and Nonfluent Aphasia* for descriptions of the onset of ischemic strokes.

There are three main forms of ischemic stroke. The first is a thrombotic stroke. A **thrombus** is an occlusion that forms slowly in an artery. A **thrombotic stroke** occurs when a thrombus interrupts blood flow to the brain, resulting in a stroke. A thrombus usually is the result of atherosclerosis. **Atherosclerosis** is a condition in which a person has a buildup of fatty materials such as cholesterol in the blood and this material accumulates

Ischemic stroke A cerebrovascular accident that occurs as a result of a blood vessel becoming occluded or blocked.

Thrombus A site of occlusion of a blood vessel usually the result of slow accumulation of fatty materials such as cholesterol on the walls of the artery.

Thrombotic stroke A cerebrovascular accident that occurs when a thrombus forms and interrupts blood flow to the brain.

Atherosclerosis A condition in which a person has a buildup of fatty materials such as cholesterol in the blood and this material accumulates slowly on the walls of the arteries, narrowing the arteries and possibly restricting blood flow.

slowly over time on the walls of arteries, narrowing them and possibly restricting blood flow.

A mass, such as a blood clot, that originates in the body and travels through the vascular system is known as an embolus. An embolic stroke occurs when an embolus, formed elsewhere in the body, travels to the brain and lodges in a blood vessel, restricting or cutting off blood circulation within the brain. A piece of a thrombus can become an embolus (a thrombo-embolus) if, for instance, a piece of thrombus breaks off of an arterial wall and travels elsewhere within the brain to lodge and create an occlusion within a blood vessel.

The third type of ischemic stroke is the transient ischemic attack, known in the medical community simply as TIA and commonly as a mini stroke. A TIA is a small ischemia within the brain that resolves within 24 hours. An individual experiencing a TIA can present with mild motor and cognitive deficits that go away when the blood clot causing the ischemia is successfully broken down by the body, resolving the occlusion. Transient ischemic attacks usually do not cause permanent deficits or life-threatening health issues. However, TIAs are usually warning signs of a larger, more destructive stroke to come. Although a single TIA usually does not cause lasting deficits, multiple reoccurring TIAs can, over time, cause significant cognitive and language deficits, possibly creating what is known as vascular dementia.

When an ischemic stroke occurs, the portion of brain tissue that is immediately deprived of the necessary level of blood flow to survive dies within an hour.

Embolus A mass within the blood stream that is carried through the vascular system by the forces of circulation.

Embolic stroke When an embolus lodges within a blood vessel and restricts or cuts off blood circulation to the brain.

Thrombo-embolus When a piece of a thrombus breaks off and travels through the circulatory system, thereby becoming an embolus.

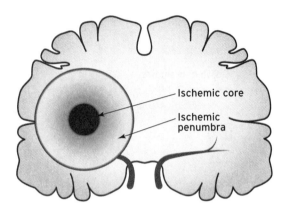

Figure 3-2 Ischemic core and penumbra.

This area of dead tissue is referred to as the ischemic core. The ischemic core, also known as the infarct, is the location of the focal damage within the brain following ischemia (Figure 3-2). The death of cells, or tissue necrosis, within the core is irreversible. However, circumscribing the ischemic core is the ischemic penumbra (Figure 3-2). The ischemic penumbra is the area of tissue that, although it has lost the appropriate level of blood supply to function, still receives enough collateral blood flow from other vessels to stay alive. The penumbra is important because, whereas the core has experienced permanent tissue damage, the tissue within the penumbra can often be salvaged with prompt and appropriate medical treatment. This means that with timely medical intervention the brain tissue within the penumbra can be saved. Saving the penumbra improves the short-term and long-term prognoses for the patient (Sallustio, Diomedi,

Transient ischemic attack A small ischemia within the brain that resolves itself within 24 hours.

Ischemic core The location of the focal damage of tissue within the brain following ischemia. Also known as the infarct.

Tissue necrosis The death of body tissue.

Ischemic penumbra An area of tissue within the brain surrounding the ischemic core that has lost the appropriate level of blood supply to function but that is still receiving enough collateral blood flow from other vessels to stay alive.

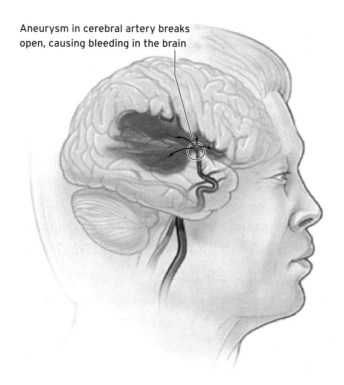

Aneurysm in cerebral artery breaks open, causing bleeding in the brain

Figure 3-3 Hemorrhagic stroke.

Centonze, & Stanzione, 2007). Damage within the ischemic penumbra can typically be reversed within 2 to 4 hours of onset of ischemia.

Hemorrhagic Stroke

A **hemorrhagic stroke** is when a blood vessel within the brain ruptures (hemorrhages). (See **Figure 3-3**.) About 13% of strokes are hemorrhagic (AHA, 2010). These strokes usually occur in individuals with high blood pressure and often during periods of high physical activity. By far the most significant risk factor associated with hemorrhagic stroke is high blood pressure, also known as **hypertension**.

> **Hemorrhagic stroke** A cerebrovascular accident that occurs when a blood vessel within the brain ruptures.

Alcohol abuse and the presence of relatives who have experienced hemorrhagic strokes also increase a person's risk. Typically, hemorrhagic strokes require immediate surgery to repair the broken blood vessel and to stop the bleeding. Individuals who experience a hemorrhagic stroke usually have less chance of survival than those who experience an ischemic stroke. However, individuals who do survive a hemorrhagic stroke often have fewer enduring deficits than those who experience ischemic strokes.

There are two primary kinds of hemorrhagic stroke, the subarachnoid hemorrhage and the intracerebral hemorrhage. A **subarachnoid hemorrhage** is a bleed that occurs between the surface of the cerebrum and the skull. Specifically, the hemorrhage occurs in an area known as the subarachnoid space that exists between the arachnoid mater and the pia mater, which

> **Hypertension** High blood pressure.
>
> **Subarachnoid hemorrhage** A hemorrhagic stroke that occurs when a blood vessel between the arachnoid mater and the pia mater ruptures.

Intracerebral hemorrhage A hemorrhage that occurs within the brain, often of traumatic origin.

Intracranial pressure The level of pressure within the skull and therefore the amount of pressure that is exerted on the brain and the amount of pressure the heart must pump against for blood to reach the brain.

overlay and protect the cerebrum. An **intracerebral hemorrhage** occurs when a blood vessel bursts within the brain itself.

Unlike symptoms of ischemic stroke, which can develop relatively slowly over minutes or hours, the onset of symptoms of a hemorrhagic stroke is sudden and definite. A hemorrhagic stroke is usually announced by a sudden and very severe headache, which might be associated with nausea and vomiting (AHA, 2007). Those who experience these headaches say they fall like a clap of thunder, hence their name thunderclap headaches. Although a sudden headache is considered typical of a hemorrhagic stroke, at times it can indicate an ischemic stroke.

Three primary and very dangerous mechanisms of damage to the brain are associated with hemorrhagic strokes. The first is, like ischemic stroke, when blood supply to a portion of the brain is interrupted. Unlike ischemic stroke, where blood flow simply stops because of an occlusion of a blood vessel, in hemorrhagic stroke the blood is diverted out of the burst or broken blood vessel and pours into the brain. Therefore, the second mechanism of damage following a hemorrhagic stroke is blood spilling outside of the circulatory system into the brain tissue where it does not belong, which damages the surrounding tissue that comes into contact with the blood. Finally, the continued release of blood into the brain or between the surface of the brain and the cranium increases intracranial pressure. **Intracranial pressure** is the level of pressure within the skull and thus the level of pressure to which the brain is exposed. Heightened levels of intracranial pressure create a very inhospitable environment for the brain. Increased intracranial pressure makes it increasingly difficult for the heart to pump blood to the brain and can quickly lead to death if not promptly treated. Many individuals have survived stroke, surgery, and worse only to die a few hours later as a result of heightened levels of intracranial pressure.

Aneurysm

An **aneurysm** is an abnormal stretching and ballooning of the wall of a blood vessel (Figure 3-4). An aneurysm can result from disease or hereditary factors that weaken the wall of an artery. Hypertension (high blood pressure) and atherosclerosis also can contribute by placing above-normal amounts of pressure on artery walls. Symptoms of a cerebral aneurysm are severe headache, nausea, vomiting, blurred vision or sensitivity to light, seizures, or loss of consciousness. However, there might be no symptoms at all until

Aneurysm An abnormal stretching and ballooning of the wall of a blood vessel.

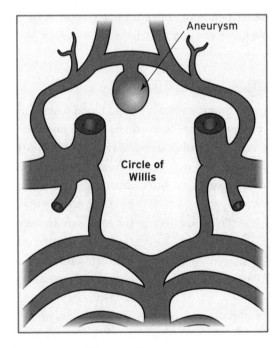

Figure 3-4 Aneurysm.

the aneurysm ruptures. Once a cerebral aneurysm ruptures it becomes a hemorrhagic stroke with a sudden and rapid spilling of blood into the brain. Aneurysms of the brain commonly occur within the circle of Willis (Figure 3-4). Ruptured aneurysms tend to be deadly and most of those who survive have some form of permanent disability.

Traumatic brain injury Damage to the brain that is the result of an external and forceful event.

Traumatic Brain Injury

A **traumatic brain injury** (TBI) is when serious and life-threatening damage to the brain occurs as the result of an external and forceful event. This definition of TBI rules out damage to the brain as a result of disease, stroke, seizure, or surgery. Usual causes of traumatic brain injury are falls, motor vehicle and traffic accidents, being struck by an object, and violent assaults (Faul, Xu, Wald, & Coronado, 2010). The immediate impact of a TBI can range from a mild concussion to coma or death. It is estimated that about 1.4 million individuals experience a TBI each year in the United States (Faul et al., 2010).

Deficits in language and cognition following TBI are many, complex, and varied and are typically a function of which areas of the brain were damaged and to what extent. Speech-language pathologists see and treat individuals with TBI for speech, language, cognition, and swallowing disorders. The hospital-based speech-language pathologist usually begins therapy for these disorders before long-term rehabilitation efforts begin. In a best-case scenario, speech-language pathologists work with an individual with TBI from shortly after his or her admittance to the hospital all the way to the point when the individual begins returning to his or her previous life at home, work, or school. However, many of those with TBI do not make such a complete recovery and continue to live out their lives in various debilitated conditions such as coma or vegetative state.

For children with TBI, rehabilitation eventually culminates (hopefully) in the release of the child from the hospital. At this point, responsibility for continued rehabilitation of the child is passed from the in-hospital speech-language pathologist to the speech-language pathologist in the child's school. Also, because TBI is very common in children ages 4 years and younger, school-based speech-language pathologists must be familiar with TBI treatment.

Brain Tumors

A **brain tumor** is an abnormal growth of cells in the brain (Figure 3-5). Also known as a **neoplasm**, a tumor serves no purpose to the body. A **primary tumor** of the brain is a tumor that originates within the brain and has not spread from a tumor elsewhere in the body. A **secondary tumor**, or a **metastatic tumor** of the brain, is a cancerous tumor that spread from another part of the body to the brain. In 2009, there were an estimated 12,920 cases of brain cancer in the United States (American Cancer Society, 2009). Brain tumors are composed of the types of cellular tissue from which they originally arise. A tumor that arises within the brain is composed of abnormal growths of certain brain cells. The names given to brain tumors reflect the type of cell the tumor is composed of. For instance, cells called oligodendrocytes are myelin-producing cells in the brain

Brain tumor An abnormal growth of cells in the brain.

Neoplasm A brain tumor. An abnormal growth of cells in the brain that serves no purpose to the body.

Primary tumor A tumor that does not originate from another tumor.

Secondary tumor A cancerous tumor that spread from another part of the body. Also known as a metastatic tumor.

Metastatic tumor A cancerous tumor that spread from a primary tumor to grow in another part of the body. Also known as a secondary tumor.

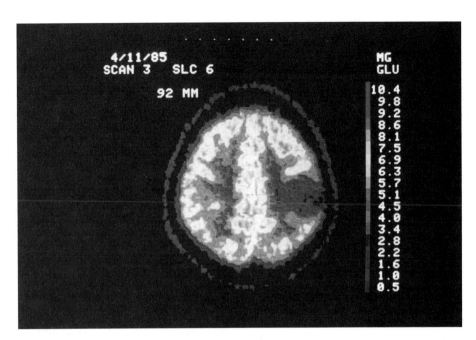

Figure 3-5   **A PET (positron emission tomography) scan of a 17-year-old girl with a longstanding history of epilepsy, who has a brain tumor (the large dark spot on the right side of the image).**

Source: Courtesy of Dr. Giovanni Di Chiro, Neuroimaging Center, National institute of Neurologic/National Cancer Institute.

(Baumann & Pham-Dinh, 2001). A tumor arising from oligodendrocytes is termed an oligodendroglioma.

Brain tumors can be either benign or malignant. Medical doctors remove a small piece of the tumor's tissue to determine if the tumor is benign or malignant. The minor surgery to remove a piece of tissue for testing is a biopsy. A malignant brain tumor is brain cancer. Brain cancer is life threatening and can grow quickly and spread throughout the body. Brain cancer is often treated with surgical removal of the tumor followed by radiation therapy. These treatments pose their own dangers to the brain. Damage to the brain usually occurs as a result of the surgical process of cutting into the brain to remove a tumor. Radiation therapy destroys the targeted cancerous tissue in an attempt to kill a malignant tumor and cancer cells left in the area of the tumor after surgical removal. However, radiation therapy destroys healthy and cancerous cells indiscriminately; therefore, it can also damage the brain or surrounding structures. If radiation therapy is not carefully targeting the tumor, healthy tissue cells exposed to the radiation will die.

Unlike a malignant tumor, a benign brain tumor cannot spread to other parts of the body. Although the word *benign* implies a lack of possible harm, benign tumors can be quite dangerous and problematic as well. For example, even a benign tumor can grow uncontrollably within the brain, crushing an otherwise healthy brain against the skull and damaging the healthy brain tissue. When a tumor displaces or crushes areas of the brain, possibly causing

Oligodendroglioma   A brain tumor arising from oligodendrocytes, which are myelin-producing cells within the brain.

Biopsy   Surgery to remove a piece of tissue for diagnostic purposes.

Malignant brain tumor   Brain cancer.

Brain cancer   A malignant tumor of the brain or one located centrally within the spinal cord.

Benign brain tumor   A tumor within the brain that cannot spread to other parts of the body.

Mass effect   The displacement effect or crushing force on nearby tissues that a tumor exerts.

Surgical trauma   The collateral damage to the tissues of the body that occurs during the process of surgery.

symptoms, it is said to be creating a **mass effect**. As mentioned previously, surgical intervention to remove a benign tumor can itself be damaging to the brain and can produce even more complications and deficits than the tumor itself, though the individual's life is preserved.

Brain tumors can produce focal damage within the brain as a stroke might, but usually present with different symptoms. Deficits produced by a tumor depend on the area of the brain the tumor affects and to what degree. However, headache is a common symptom. Whereas symptoms of stroke occur somewhat suddenly, symptoms of tumor occur and worsen gradually over longer periods of time as the tumor grows.

Surgical Trauma

Surgery is performed on a person's brain for various reasons. Surgery on the brain is often performed to remove a tumor or repair a hemorrhagic stroke. Surgery on the brain is never lightly considered and is usually undertaken only in very serious or life-threatening circumstances. Brain surgery often results in surgical trauma. **Surgical trauma** is the collateral damage to the delicate tissues of the brain that occurs during the process of achieving the objective of the surgery. Surgical trauma is often a necessary consequence of removing a tumor or repairing a bleed to save the patient's life. Unfortunately, once these individuals are medically stable, a speech-language pathologist might need to evaluate and treat them for acquired language, cognitive, speech, or swallowing deficits. Medical professionals must also try to manage the secondary risks of brain surgery: seizures, additional cerebrovascular accidents, acquired in-

fections, and increased intracranial pressure. ▶ See the *Surgical Trauma to the Vagus* video for a discussion of related material.

Infection

Many infections are capable of damaging the central nervous system (CNS) and the peripheral nervous system (PNS). Infections can be viral, fungal, bacterial, or parasitic. The impact an infection has on cognition, language, or motor movement (i.e., speech and swallowing) depends on the site of the infection, the nature of the infection, and the extent of damage created by the infection. Some infections might affect only the CNS and create alterations and deficits in cognition and language. Others affect only the PNS, affecting motor control of the body, which affects speech. Some infections affect both the CNS and PNS. The diseases addressed in the following subsections, selected for their clinical as well as historical and educational significance, are but a few that involve the human nervous system.

Encephalitis

Encephalitis is a general term indicating an acute infection and/or inflammation of the brain or spinal cord. There are many different forms of encephalitis. Generally, encephalitis is caused by a viral or bacterial infection of the brain or spinal cord. The

Encephalitis   A general term that refers to an acute infection and/or inflammation of the brain or spinal cord.

symptoms often reflect the type as well as location of the infection. Symptoms often include headaches, fevers, confusion, and seizures.

A particularly interesting form of encephalitis that made its way into public awareness is encephalitis lethargica. In the early part of the 20th century, there was an epidemic of this disease. This outbreak of encephalitis lethargica occurred alongside and was possibly the result of a simultaneous influenza epidemic

(Mortimer, 2009). Known as the sleepy sickness in the 1910s and 1920s, first signs of the disease are a fever accompanied by a low level of arousal or sleep state. Eventually, this disease leads to muscle rigidity and weakness, disturbances in initiating movement, and cardiac and respiratory abnormalities. Encephalitis lethargica is fatal in approximately one-third of its victims. It causes inflammation and damage to subcortical structures that are responsible for autonomic processes such as the sleep/wake cycle, heart rate, breathing rate, and the control of movement. Specifically, these structures are the midbrain, basal ganglia, and substantia nigra (Anderson, Vilensky, & Duvoisin, 2009). Survivors of this disease usually display distinctly Parkinsonian features as a result of the damage to their subcortical structures. These symptoms can include difficulty initiating and controlling volitional movement as well as inhibiting nonvolitional movement.

Encephalitis lethargica was virtually forgotten by modern medicine until the publication of *Awakenings* by Oliver Sacks in which he details his administration of the then-experimental drug levadopa (L-Dopa) during the 1960s to survivors of the 1920s encephalitis lethargica epidemic. Sacks (1990) wrote of the survivors of the 1920s epidemic who were still living and had been placed, years earlier, in a long-term care hospital where he worked. He described these patients as being alive, yet not fully awake, and unable to move or speak. The patients displayed an extreme form of Parkinsonism resulting from the damage the disease wrought in their subcortices. Although no large-scale outbreaks of encephalitis lethargica have occurred since the 1920s, sporadic cases are still regularly diagnosed and reported (Anderson et al., 2009).

A rare and idiopathic form of encephalitis is Rasmussen's encephalitis. Rasmussen's is a fast-moving encephalitis characterized by T cells of the immune system attacking and causing inflammation in either the right or left cerebral hemisphere. As a result of this inflammation, the presenting symptom of Rasmussen's encephalitis is seizure activity that creates a unilateral tremor in an extremity contralateral to the affected cerebral hemisphere. Individuals with Rasmussen's encephalitis progress over the course of months into seizures that grow more severe as more of the diseased cerebral hemisphere is affected. Treatment is medical to control seizure activity, but seizures ultimately grow so debilitating and life threatening that individuals with this disease must undergo surgery to remove large portions of the affected cerebral hemisphere or even the entire cerebral hemisphere. This surgery is known as a hemispherectomy. Hemispherectomy is most often performed to remove large tumors existing in a single cerebral hemisphere or to control intractable seizure activity, as in conditions such as Rasmussen's encephalitis. ▶ See the video *Rasmussen's Encephalitis, Seizures, and Hemispherectomy* for an interview with an individual who underwent a hemispherectomy for the remediation of Rasmussen's encephalitis.

HIV/AIDS

Human immunodeficiency virus (HIV) is the virus that leads to AIDS **(acquired immune deficiency syndrome).** HIV/AIDS can be transmitted through sexual contact, through blood, or from an infected mother to her child. HIV slowly weakens the immune system until another pathogen overtakes the individual's body, leading to death. HIV/AIDS is a pandemic, and no known cure for the disease exists. In 2007, the World Health Organization (WHO) estimated that there were 32.2 million people infected with HIV (UNAIDS, 2007). That same year, the World Health Organization estimated that 2.1 million people died of AIDS (Joint United Nations Programme on HIV/

> **Human immunodeficiency virus (HIV)** The virus that leads to AIDS (acquired immune deficiency syndrome).
>
> **Acquired immune deficiency syndrome (AIDS)** The final stage of HIV disease characterized by severe damage and impairment of the immune system.

AIDS [UNAIDS] & World Health Organization [WHO], 2007), including 330,000 children.

AIDS is known to cause neurologic changes and deficits. Neurologic symptoms can occur before an individual knows he or she is infected (Singer, Valdes-Sueiras, Commins, & Levine, 2010). However, until recently, individuals with AIDS often did not live long enough for these cognitive and motor deficits to be a concern. With the advent of more effective medical treatments in the form of combinations of medicines known as drug cocktails, individuals with HIV are living long enough to experience these neurologic symptoms, often referred to as **neuoroAIDS** or HIV/AIDS dementia (Gendelman, Grant, Everall, Lipton, & Swindells, 2005) and more recently as HIV-associated neurocognitive disorder (HAND) (Singer et al., 2010). The term **HIV/AIDS dementia** is applied only if neurocognitive deficits are severe enough to affect the individual's daily life. The most common neurocognitive changes seen in AIDS include impairments in ability to learn new information, loss of gross and fine motor abilities including gait disturbances, reduced attention abilities, slowness in processing information, disfluent speech, and impaired recall (Gendelman et al., 2005; Singer et al., 2010). Although language is often unaffected, mild language deficits and severe deficits in functional use of language in individuals with HIV/AIDS dementia have also been reported (McCabe, Sheard, & Code, 2008).

neuroAIDS Neurological changes as a result of HIV/AIDS that create cognitive deficits and dementia. Also known as HIV/AIDS dementia and HIV-associated neurocognitive disorder (HAND).

Creutzfeldt-Jakob Disease

In the 1920s, Hans Creutzfeldt and Alfons Jakob documented a degenerative and fatal brain disease. This illness came to be known as Creutzfeldt-Jakob disease and has genetic as well as infectious etiologies (Praveen, Sinha, Chandrasekhar, Vijayan, & Taly,

2006). It is currently believed that most cases are produced by a type of infectious pathogen known as a prion. A **prion** is a small infectious protein with its own genetic coding. Although debatable, it is commonly believed that the prion disease known in animals as mad cow disease produces a variant of Creutzfeldt-Jakob disease in humans.

HIV/AIDS dementia Cognitive changes as a result of HIV/AIDS that are severe enough to affect an individual's activities of daily living.

Prion A small infectious protein with its own genetic coding that attacks structures within the central or peripheral nervous system.

Myoclonus An involuntary rapid twitching of a muscle or group of muscles.

Creutzfeldt-Jakob disease attacks the central nervous system, currently has no known cure, and is usually fatal within a year of onset of symptoms. General symptoms of this disease include dementia with rapid onset and involuntary movement disturbances called myoclonus. **Myoclonus** is the involuntary rapid twitching of a muscle or group of muscles.

Praveen and colleagues (2006) document the dementia symptoms of a 69-year-old woman with Creutzfeldt-Jakob disease as including behavioral abnormalities, emotional volatility in the form of inappropriate anger or crying, and "irrelevant talk" (p. 418). One month later, this woman developed slurred speech, gait abnormalities, and "excessive sleepiness" (p. 418). She later developed myoclonus in her limbs and became bedbound.

Creutzfeldt-Jakob disease has also been noted to cause akinetic mutism (Gozke, Erdal, & Unal, 2008), which is an inability to speak as a result of being unable to move. Saigusa and colleagues (2008) document a case of bilateral paralysis of the vocal folds in a case of Creutzfeldt-Jakob disease. Certain Alzheimer-like neuropathologic changes are present in the brain tissue of those affected by Creutzfeldt-Jakob disease. One of these is the occurrence of amyloid plaques (**Figure 3-6**).

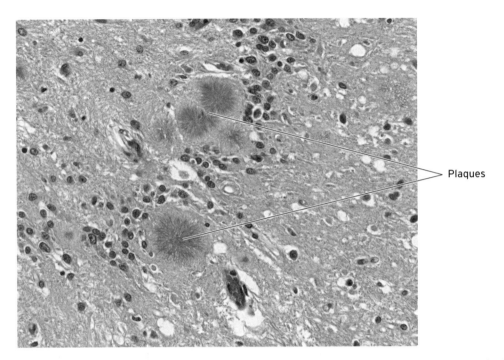

Figure 3-6 Stained photomicrograph of brain tissue displaying amyloid plaques created by variant Creutzfeldt-Jakob disease.

Source: Courtesy of Teresa Hammett, Department of Health and Human Services Centers for Disease Control and Prevention.

Syphilis

Syphilis is a sexually transmitted disease that is highly treatable with the antibiotic penicillin and is curable. This disease is caused by corkscrew-shaped bacteria called spirochetes. The spirochete that causes syphilis is *Treponema pallidum* (**Figure 3-7**). Syphilis infection initially causes an open sore at the site of initial infection. Symptoms then progress to include ulcers, rashes, fevers, and headaches. If left untreated, symptoms become more severe, progressing to anemia, liver and heart disease, as well as disease of the nervous system.

A specific variation of syphilis that affects the nervous system is **neurosyphilis**. Neurosyphilis usually occurs years after an individual is initially infected and treated for a primary infection of syphilis. However, infiltration of the CNS by syphilis can begin as early as a few days or weeks following infection (Ho & Lukehart, 2011). Neurosyphilis can present with an array of neurologic signs and symptoms including meningitis, headache, stiff neck, changes in vision or visual abnormalities, facial weakness, cognitive deficits, motor problems, and involvement of individual cranial nerves (Ho & Lukehart, 2011; Jacob et al., 2005). Intensive penicillin therapy is used to treat neurosyphilis. The earlier the treatment is provided, the better the prognosis for recovery.

Simultaneous infection of both syphilis and HIV is high among individuals with syphilis (Ho & Lukehart, 2011). This is because syphilis causes open sores on or around the genitalia. HIV, also a sexually transmitted disease, can then be transmitted more easily through these open sores. Furthermore, an immune system suppressed by HIV can make infection with

Syphilis A sexually transmitted disease that is caused by corkscrew-shaped bacterium called spirochetes. Syphilis is highly treatable and curable with the antibiotic penicillin.

Neurosyphilis A variation of syphilis that infects the nervous system.

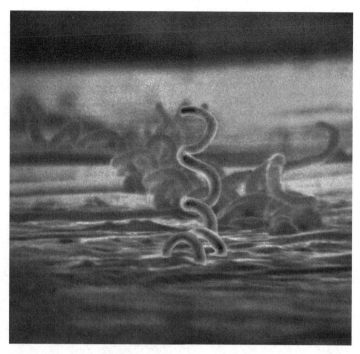

Figure 3-7 Micrograph of *Treponema pallidum.*

Source: Courtesy of David Cox, Department of Health and Human Services Centers for Disease Control and Prevention.

syphilis a far more dangerous and serious condition than usual.

Poliomyelitis

Poliomyelitis, commonly known simply as polio, is caused by a virus. Polio is highly preventable with a vaccine. Polio reached epidemic proportions in the United States during the early 20th century prior to development of an effective vaccine (Cono & Alexander, 2002). The polio virus primarily attacks children and is transmitted primarily by fecal matter in drinking water. Although polio is now rare (though still present) in the United States and United Kingdom, it is still an active threat in many developing countries. The polio virus attacks efferent nerve tracks of the PNS. ▶ For an interview with a woman who experienced polio as a child see the video *Poliomyelitis.* Polio is usually categorized by the sections of the PNS that it affects. Polio affecting the spinal nerves and the muscles innervated by the spinal

nerves is referred to as **spinal polio**. Polio affecting the cranial nerves and the muscles innervated by the cranial nerves is referred to as **bulbar polio**. If both spinal and cranial nerves are affected, it is termed **bulbospinal polio** and affects all muscles of the body to some degree.

Characteristic symptoms of polio are nonsymmetrical paralysis with diminished or absent reflexes (Cono & Alexander, 2002). The paralysis and weak reflexes reflect the inability of the PNS to deliver volitional and nonvolitional commands of movement from the CNS to the muscles. The machine known as

Poliomyelitis A virus that attacks the PNS and causes paralysis and absent reflexes. Also known as polio.

Spinal polio
Poliomyelitis that affects the spinal nerves and the muscles innervated by the spinal nerves.

Bulbar polio
Poliomyelitis that affects the cranial nerves and the muscles innervated by the cranial nerves.

Bulbospinal polio
Poliomyelitis that affects both spinal and cranial nerves and the muscles they innervate.

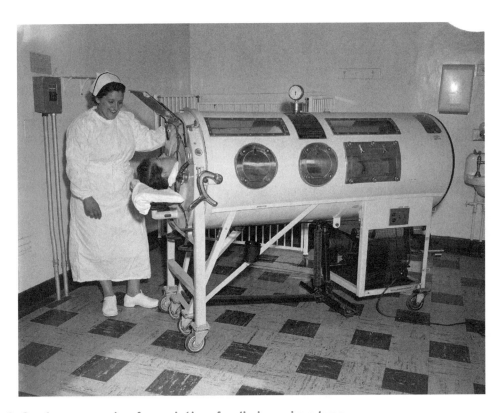

Figure 3-8   A nurse caring for a victim of polio in an iron lung.
Source: Courtesy of Department of Health and Human Services Centers for Disease Control and Prevention.

Post polio syndrome   Symptoms of muscle weakness, muscle pain, and fatigue within those limbs that were affected by a previous polio infection.

the Iron Lung (Figure 3-8) was once a common sight in hospitals and was responsible for enabling patients with severe polio to breathe despite the paralysis of their respiratory muscles. Polio is fatal in 2–10% of cases. Major recovery of muscle function usually occurs within 6 months of infection, but symptoms can persist indefinitely and even reemerge in later life as post polio syndrome (Cono & Alexander, 2002).

Post polio syndrome arises in about 25–50% of individuals who recover from a previous infection with polio. It is characterized by muscle weakness, muscle pain, and fatigue of the limbs that were affected by the initial polio infection. Post polio syndrome can affect facial muscles involved in speech as well as muscles of the neck and larynx, resulting in difficulties with voice production and swallowing (Silbergleit, Waring, Sullivan, & Maynard, 1991; Soderholm, Lehtinen, Valtonen, & Ylinen, 2010). ▶ See the video *Post Polio Syndrome* for an interview with an individual living with this disorder.

Seizures

Certain infectious diseases and congenital disorders (such as epilepsy, of which there are many forms) produce seizures. However, seizures also often occur as a result of stroke, traumatic brain injury, tumor, or surgical trauma to the brain, and as such it is important for speech-language pathologists to understand and recognize them.

Seizure A sudden, often periodic, abnormal level of electrical discharge occurring within the brain.

Aura The period of time immediately preceding the full onset of a seizure in which a person might experience some warning signs that a seizure is imminent.

Ictus The main stage of the seizure during which the primary symptoms are experienced.

Post ictus The stage of seizure that follows the ictus and that can last for minutes or hours and during which people might display lethargy and confusion and experience memory loss, weakness, and depression.

Post-ictal confusion The short-lived cognitive deficits following the ictus stage of a seizure.

Interictal period The time between the end of one seizure and the beginning of the next seizure.

Status epilepticus A state of constant seizure. When an individual experiences one seizure that leads right into another seizure with no interictal period.

The brain uses electricity to communicate with itself and the rest of the nervous system. Neurons generate and send electrical signals to each other during normal operation. Electrical impulses constantly fly among the billions of neuronal connections in the brain. However, if too much electricity occurs in the brain, a seizure will result. A seizure is a sudden, often periodic, abnormal level of electrical discharge in the brain. Seizures are most succinctly described as storms of electricity in the brain.

Seizures can be mild in nature and produce only a slowly accumulating level of brain damage in the affected areas over time. Or they can be far more severe with the potential of a single seizure producing immediate and permanent brain damage and even death.

There are many different categorizations of the stages of seizure. By most accounts, the three primary stages include the aura, ictus, and post ictus. These stages are most evident in severe seizures. The **aura** is the period of time immediately preceding the full onset of a seizure in which a person might experience some warning signs that a seizure is imminent. Signs of

oncoming seizure are varied and include headache, déjà vu, panic, nausea, radical mood shifts, tingling in the limbs, or visual abnormalities. The **ictus** is the main stage of the seizure when the person experiences the primary symptoms. In a tonic clonic seizure (discussed later), this is the period when the individual loses consciousness and begins convulsing until the motor activity ceases and the affected individual begins to regain consciousness. After regaining consciousness, the individual enters the post-ictus stage. The **post ictus** is the period that comes after the ictus. It can last for minutes or hours. During the post ictus, individuals are often lethargic and confused, and they might experience memory loss, weakness, and depression. This stage is often characterized by **post-ictal confusion**, which is a short-term cognitive deficit. The time between seizures (after the post ictus and prior to the next aura) is known as the **interictal period**. **Status epilepticus** is when a person experiences seizures, one after another that lead directly into each other with no interictal period. Status epilepticus is a severe and life-threatening condition that very negatively affects quality of life.

This text contains two descriptions of cases involving status epilepticus. In both cases, radical surgery was performed to reduce seizure activity. The first is the clinical note of patient H.M., who had his hippocampi removed to reduce seizures but was left with profound memory deficits. The second is of a woman with Rasmussen's encephalitis who had her right cerebral hemisphere removed to stop the hundreds of seizures she was having each day. ▶ Go to the video *Rasmussen's Disease, Seizures, and Hemispherectomy* to hear this woman describe her problem, her seizures, and the surgery that saved her life and allowed her to grow up and become (of all things) a speech-language pathologist.

The kind of seizure experienced depends on which part of the brain is affected. Specialists typically categorize seizures as partial or generalized.

Partial seizure A seizure in which pathologic levels of electricity in the brain remain confined to a particular region of the brain.

Simple partial seizure A partial seizure during which the seizure activity within the brain is limited to a small area within one cerebral hemisphere and the individual experiencing the seizure remains conscious.

Complex partial seizure A seizure that occurs over a large section of a single cerebral hemisphere and that creates an altered state of consciousness.

Generalized seizures A seizure that affects the entire brain and is associated with a total loss of consciousness.

Tonic clonic seizure A seizure in which an individual passes through a stage of muscle contraction and loss of consciousness (tonic phase) followed by a phase of abnormal motor activity (clonic phase).

Tonic phase The initial phase of a tonic clonic seizure characterized by a sudden stiffening of the body and limbs due to muscle contractions and a loss of consciousness.

Partial Seizures

Individuals with epilepsy most commonly experience partial seizures. During a **partial seizure**, the pathologic levels of electrical activity are confined to a particular region of the brain. Partial seizures can be considered pathologic overstimulation of a certain part of the brain created by an excess of electrical activity in the affected area. Partial seizures can create just about any imaginable motor, sensory, or emotional symptom because these seizures can occur in practically any part of the brain, though some areas are far more prone to seizure than others.

The symptoms an individual experiences during a partial seizure depend on which area of the brain is seizing. For example, a partial seizure in the occipital-parietal visual processing areas of the brain can produce visual hallucinations or somatosensory and visual abnormalities. Similarly, a seizure isolated to the temporal lobes might produce auditory hallucinations, such as the sound of music, if they occur in the area of the temporal lobes dedicated to processing music. Sacks (1970) describes a case of partial seizures of the temporal lobe in which an elderly woman wakes in the middle of the night to find herself experiencing the auditory hallucination of a deafening string of Irish songs from her youth playing over and over. However, some patients hear environmental sounds such as doors slamming or glass breaking.

There are two primary forms of partial seizure, simple partial seizures and complex partial seizures. In a **simple partial seizure**, the seizure activity in the brain is limited to a small area in one cerebral hemisphere and the individual experiencing the seizure remains conscious. If a seizure occurs over a larger section of a single cerebral hemisphere and creates an altered state of consciousness, the seizure is categorized as a **complex partial seizure**. Complex partial seizures often create changes in level of awareness or result in a dreamlike state. Individuals might produce some speech or mumbling and perhaps execute some seemingly purposeful movement. Nonetheless, during a complex partial seizure speech makes little sense and movement is highly disorganized. Complex partial seizures might also lead to a generalized seizure.

Generalized Seizures

Whereas partial seizures affect a localized portion of the brain, **generalized seizures** affect the entire brain and are associated with total loss of consciousness or awareness. There are two forms of generalized seizure: the tonic clonic seizure (once known as the grand mal) and the petit mal seizure, also known as absence attacks.

The **tonic clonic seizure** is so named because it manifests two distinct phases during the ictus. These two phases are the tonic phase and the clonic phase. The **tonic phase** at the beginning of the ictus signals the onset of the seizure, and the affected individual loses consciousness and the body stiffens as a result

Clonic phase   The second phase of a tonic clonic seizure characterized by a shaking, jerking, extraneous body movement.

Petit mal seizure   A generalized seizure in which an individual loses awareness for a few seconds and might seem simply to stare off into space before coming to.

of muscle contractions. The limbs might be rigidly stiffened toward the body or extend away. If the individual is standing, he or she will fall. The mere risk of fall associated with tonic clonic seizures can be a serious threat. Often, the onset of the tonic clonic seizure is announced by an automatic loud moan or even a ragged scream as the vocal folds are adducted and air is simultaneously forced between the adducted vocal folds by the contracting thoracic muscles. The tonic phase is short, lasting only a few seconds, and leads into the clonic phase.

During the **clonic phase**, the individual begins to convulse and displays often violent twitching of the extremities and shaking of the entire body. The clonic phase usually lasts 2 to 3 minutes during which motor activity slowly decreases and leads to the post ictus. Tonic clonic seizures are almost always followed by a period of post-ictal sleep. Post-ictal confusion and amnesia are present when the individual regains consciousness and slowly wear off.

Whereas the chances of not recognizing the presence of a tonic clonic seizure are remote, petit mal seizures often go undiagnosed for years. The **petit mal seizure**, or absence attack, is a generalized seizure in which an individual loses awareness for a few seconds and seems simply to stare into space before coming to. There is no gross motor activity, shaking, or convulsing as seen in the tonic clonic seizure. In fact, parents and school teachers often mistakenly assume children who experience petit mal seizures are simply daydreamers and attribute their poor academic performance to not paying appropriate attention. In reality, the child is seizing and experiencing only bits and pieces of what is occurring in the classroom. During the time that these seizures go undiagnosed, they are also not being managed medically and are totally uncontrolled. Over time, these uncontrolled seizures can cause significant damage to the child's brain and lead to cognitive, language, and motor deficits.

Author's Note

How to Help a Person Experiencing a Seizure

If you are with someone who has lost consciousness as a result of a seizure, you should know a few simple items that will help you keep the person safe. First, be sure you never put anything in the mouth of an individual experiencing a seizure. Do not try to restrict the person's movements. Also, be sure to clear away any dangerous or sharp objects around the individual experiencing a seizure. Turn the person onto his or her side to keep saliva from falling into the airway, and place something soft under the individual's head, such as a pillow or a shirt. Finally, stay with the person until the seizure ends.

If you are a nonmedical professional, such as a speech-language pathologist, working in a medical setting and you are with a person who begins seizing, usually the most appropriate action is to get medical help immediately. Most often this takes the form of calling loudly for a nurse or doctor while staying with the patient. Protocols vary among institutions.

Main Points

- An etiology is the underlying medical cause of a symptom or deficit. An idiopathic etiology is one of unknown origin.
- Neurogenic communication disorders usually result from damage to the CNS and/or the PNS. Such damage can cause communicative, cognitive, language, and/or behavioral deficits. Etiologies of neurogenic communication disorders are often stroke, traumatic brain injury (TBI), surgical trauma, degenerative disorders, and infectious diseases.
- A stroke occurs when blood flow to a part of the brain is interrupted by a clot or hemorrhage within the brain. A stroke is also known as a cerebrovascular accident (CVA). There are two main categories of stroke: ischemic and hemorrhagic.
- Ischemic strokes occur when a blood vessel supplying bloodflow to the brain is occluded or blocked. This blockage deprives the brain tissue of blood supply necessary to survive. There are three main forms of ischemic stroke: thrombotic, embolic, and transient ischemic attacks.
- A thrombotic stroke is when an occlusion forms within a blood vessel and restricts blood flow to the brain. An occlusion that forms in a cumulative fashion and restricts blood flow to brain tissue is known as a thrombus. A thrombus is usually a result of atherosclerosis.
- An embolic stroke is when a mass traveling through the vascular system (an embolus) lodges in a blood vessel usually inside the brain and restricts blood flow to brain tissue. A thrombus can become an embolus if any piece of it breaks off the wall of an artery and travels to lodge elsewhere and create a blockage of blood flow to the brain.
- Transient ischemic attacks (TIAs), also known as mini strokes, are when a small ischemia within the brain occurs and is resolved by the body within 24 hours. TIAs do not cause permanent damage; however, recurring TIAs can cause language and cognitive deficits. TIAs can also be a warning sign of a larger oncoming stroke.
- Hemorrhagic strokes occur when a blood vessel within the brain ruptures.
- Three mechanisms of damage to the brain are possible with hemorrhagic strokes. First, the blood supply to a portion of the brain is interrupted as a result of the broken or burst blood vessel. Second, the blood from the hemorrhaged vessel spills outside the circulatory system into the brain and damages the tissue it comes into contact with. Third, intracranial pressure increases because of the continued release of blood into the brain or between the skull and the cranium.
- There are two main forms of hemorrhagic strokes: subarachnoid and intracerebral.
- Subarachnoid hemorrhagic strokes occur when there is a bleed between the surface of the brain and the skull in an area known as the subarachnoid space.
- Intracerebral hemorrhagic strokes occur when a blood vessel bursts within the brain itself.
- An aneurysm is the abnormal stretching or ballooning of an arterial wall. Aneurysms can be the result of hypertension, disease, hereditary factors, or atherosclerosis. When an aneurysm ruptures, it becomes a hemorrhagic stroke. Aneurysms often occur within the circle of Willis.
- A traumatic brain injury (TBI) is when serious and life-threatening damage to the brain occurs as a result of an external and forceful event. A TBI is usually the result of a forceful event such as a fall, motor vehicle accident, violent assault, sports-related accident, or being struck on the head by an object. The language and cognitive deficits resulting from a TBI are complex and

vary depending on which areas of the brain are damaged and to what extent.

- A brain tumor is an abnormal growth of cells in the brain. A brain tumor is also known as a neoplasm. A primary tumor of the brain is a tumor that originates in the brain. A secondary tumor of the brain is a cancerous tumor that spreads from another part of the body to the brain. A secondary tumor is also called a metastatic brain tumor. The deficits produced by a brain tumor depend on the area of the brain the tumor affects and to what degree. A malignant brain tumor is brain cancer.

- Surgical trauma is damage to the delicate tissues of the brain that might occur with the surgical removal of a tumor or the repair of a hemorrhage in the brain to save a person's life. Those who have surgical trauma can experience acquired language and cognitive deficits.

- Infections can also cause damage to the CNS and PNS. Infections can be viral, fungal, bacterial, or parasitic. The deficits caused by infections depend on the site of the infection, the nature of the infection, and the extent of damage done by the infection. A multitude of infections of the nervous system can affect speech, language, and/or cognition. Some of these infections include encephalitis, HIV/AIDS, Creutzfeldt-Jakob disease, syphilis, and poliomyelitis.

- Encephalitis is a general term for an acute inflammatory infection of the brain or spinal cord. A viral or bacterial infection of the brain or spinal cord causes encephalitis. The symptoms of encephalitis vary depending on the type and location of the infection.

- Human immunodeficiency virus (HIV) leads to acquired immune deficiency syndrome (AIDS). HIV/AIDS can cause neurologic changes and deficits, which are known as neuroAIDS, HIV/AIDS dementia, or HIV-associated neurocognitive disorder. Some deficits include inability to learn new information, slow information processing, disfluent speech, impaired recall, and reduced attention ability. Mild to severe deficits in the use of functional language might also occur.

- A small infectious protein called a prion causes Creutzfeldt-Jakob disease. Prion diseases, including Creutzfeldt-Jakob disease, attack the CNS. The symptoms include dementia with rapid onset and involuntary movement disturbances called myoclonus. Certain Alzheimer-like neuropathologic changes, such as amyloid plaques, are present in the brain tissue of those affected by Creutzfeldt-Jakob disease.

- Syphilis is a sexually transmitted disease caused by a corkscrew-shaped bacterium called a spirochete. Neurosyphilis is a variation of syphilis that affects the nervous system. Some signs and symptoms of neurosyphilis include meningitis, visual difficulties or abnormalities, facial weakness, cognitive deficits, and motor problems.

- Poliomyelitis is caused by a virus that attacks the motor nerve tracks of the PNS. Symptoms of polio include nonsymmetrical paralysis with diminished or absent reflexes.

- Seizures are sudden, often periodic, and abnormal levels of electrical discharge in the brain.

- The three primary stages of a seizure are the aura, ictus, and post ictus. The aura is the period immediately before the seizure during which a person might experience warning signs of an upcoming seizure. The ictus is the main stage of the seizure that can include loss of consciousness and convulsions. The post ictus is the period right after the ictus during which a person can experience confusion, memory loss, weakness, and/or depression. The time between seizures is called the interictal period. Status epilepticus is when a person experiences seizures without an interictal period. There are main two categories of seizures: partial seizures and generalized seizures.

- Partial seizures occur when the abnormal levels of electrical activity remain within a particular region of the brain.
- The two primary forms of partial seizures include simple partial seizures and complex partial seizures. During a simple partial seizure, the affected individual remains conscious and the seizure is restricted to a limited region of the brain. During a complex partial seizure, the individual seizing experiences altered states of consciousness and larger or multiple regions of seizure activity occur in one single cerebral hemisphere.

- Generalized seizures occur when the abnormal levels of electrical activity affect the entire brain. A total loss of consciousness or awareness occurs with generalized seizures.
- There are two forms of generalized seizures: tonic clonic seizures and petit mal seizures. During tonic clonic seizures, the individual loses consciousness and the body stiffens and convulses. During petit mal seizures, an individual loses awareness for a few seconds and might assume the posture of a daydreamer or an absent stare. Petit mal seizures are usually a disorder of childhood.

Review Questions

1. Why are some etiologies called idiopathic?
2. Compare and contrast how ischemic and hemorrhagic strokes damage the brain.
3. What are the three main forms of ischemic strokes and how do they differ?
4. Why is saving the ischemic penumbra a priority for medical professionals?
5. What are the two main forms of hemorrhagic stroke and how do they differ?
6. What is an aneurysm and why is having one dangerous?
7. What is a traumatic brain injury? What are some common causes of traumatic brain injury?
8. How do primary tumors and secondary tumors differ?
9. How might a benign tumor cause damage to the brain?
10. What is encephalitis? Give one example of encephalitis and what its effect on speech, language, or cognition might be.
11. How might HIV/AIDS affect speech, language, or cognition?
12. List symptoms of Creutzfeldt-Jakob disease.
13. What is syphilis, what organism causes this disease, and what are some ways it can affect speech, language, or cognition?
14. What is a seizure?
15. Name and describe the three primary stages of seizure.
16. What is the term that describes a state of constant seizure?
17. How are simple partial seizures and complex partial seizures different?
18. How are generalized seizures different from partial seizures?
19. How are tonic clonic seizures different from petit mal seizures?
20. Describe how you would assist/help a person experiencing a tonic clonic seizure.

References

1. American Cancer Society. (2009). Cancer facts and figures, 2009. Retrieved from http://www.cancer.org/Research/CancerFactsFigures/cancer-facts-figures-2009

2. American Heart Association. (2010). Heart Disease and Stroke Statistics. 2010 update. Dallas, TX: American Heart Association.

3. American Heart Association. (2007). Let's Talk About Ischemic Strokes and their Causes. Dallas, TX: American Heart Association.

4. Anderson, L., Vilensky, J., & Duvoisin, R. (2009). Review: Neuropathology of acute phase encephalitis lethargica: A review of cases. *Neuropathology and Applied Neurobiology, 35*(5), 462–472.

5. Baumann, N., & Pham-Dinh, D. (2001). Biology of oligodendrocyte and myelin in the mammalian central nervous system. *Physiological Reviews, 81*(2), 871–927.

6. Bonita, R. (1992). Epidemiology of stroke. *Lancet, 339*(8789), 342.

7. Cono, J., & Alexander, L. (2002). Poliomyelitis. In S. W. Roush, L. McIntyre, & L. M. Baldy (Eds.). *Manual for the surveillance of vaccine-preventable diseases* (3rd ed., Chap. 10). Atlanta, GA: Centers for Disease Control and Prevention. Retrieved from http://www.cdc.gov/vaccines/pubs/surv-manual/3rd-edition-chpt10_polio.pdf

8. Faul, M., Xu, L., Wald, M., & Coronado, V. (2010). *Traumatic brain injury in the United States: Emergency department visits, hospitalizations, and deaths*. Atlanta, GA: Centers for Disease Control and Prevention, National Center for Injury Prevention and Control. Retrieved from http://www.cdc.gov/traumaticbraininjury/pdf/blue_book.pdf

9. Gozke, E., Erdal, N., & Unal, M. (2008). Creutzfeldt-Jakob disease: A case report. *Cases Journal, 1*(1), 146.

10. Grant, I., Sacktor, H., & McArthur, J. (2005). HIV neurocognitive disorders. in H. E. Gendelman, I. Grant, I. Everall, S. A. Lipton, & S. Swindells. (Eds.), *The neurology of AIDS* (2nd ed., pp. 357–373). London, England: Oxford University Press.

11. Guyomard, V., Fulcher, R., Redmayne, O., Metcalf, A., Potter, J., & Myint, P. (2009). Effect of dysphasia and dysphagia on inpatient mortality and hospital length of stay: A database study. *Journal of the American Geriatrics Society, 57*(11), 2102–2106.

12. Ho, E., & Lukehart, S. (2011). Syphilis: Using modern approaches to understanding an old disease. *Journal of Clinical Investigation, 121*(12), 4584–4592.

13. Jacob, M., Krolak-Salmon, P., Tilikete, C., Issartel, B., Bernard, M., & Vighetto, A. (2005). Beware of neurosyphilis. *Journal Neurology, 252*, 609–610.

14. Joint United Nations Programme on HIV/AIDS (UNAIDS) & World Health Organization. (2007). *AIDS epidemic update, December 2007*. Retrieved from http://data.unaids.org/pub/epislides/2007/2007_epiupdate_en.pdf

15. McCabe, P., Sheard, C., & Code, C. (2008). Communication impairment in the AIDS dementia complex (ADC): A case report. *Journal of Communication Disorders, 41*(3), 203–222.

16. Mortimer, P. (2009). Was encephalitis lethargica a post-influenzal or some other phenomenon? Time to reexamine the problem. *Epidemiology and Infection, 137*(4), 449–455.

17. Praveen, K., Sinha, S., Chandrasekhar, H., Vijayan, J., & Taly, A. (2006). Sporadic onset Creutzfeldt-Jakob disease: Interesting MRI observations. *Neurology India, 54*(4), 418–420.

18. Rosamond, W., Flegal, K., Furie, K., Go, A., Greenlund, K., Haase, N., . . . American Heart Association Statistics Committee and Stroke Statistics Subcommittee. (2008). Heart disease and stroke statistics: 2008 update. *Circulation, 117*, e25–e146. Retrieved from http://circ.ahajournals.org/content/117/4/e25.full

19. Sacks, O. (1970). *The man who mistook his wife for a hat*. New York, NY: Summit Books.

20. Sacks. O. (1990). *Awakenings*. London, England: Harper Perennial.

21. Saigusa, L., Nagayama, H., Nakamura, T., Aino, I., Komachi, T., & Yamaguchi, S. (2008). A case of Creutzfeldt-Jakob disease with bilateral vocal fold abductor paralysis. *Journal of Voice, 23*(5), 635–638.

22. Sallustio, F., Diomedi, M., Centonze, D., & Stanzione, P. (2007). Saving the ischemic penumbra: Potential role for statins and phosphodiesterase inhibitors. *Current Vascular Pharmocology, 5*, 259–265.

23. Silbergleit, A., Waring, W., Sullivan, M., & Maynard, F. (1991). Evaluation, treatment, and follow-up results of post polio patients with dysphagia. *Otolaryngology—Head and Neck Surgery, 104*(3), 333–338.

24. Singer, E., Valdes-Sueiras, M., Commins, D., & Levine, A. (2010). Neurologic presentation of AIDS. *Neurologic Clinics, 28*(1), 253–275.

25. Soderholm, S., Lehtinen, A., Valtonen, K., & Ylinen, A. (2010). Dysphagia and dsyphonia among persons with post-polio syndrome: A challenge in neurorehabilitation. *Acta Neurologica Scandinavica, 122*(5), 343–349.

Chapter 4

The Aphasias

▶ *Where this icon appears, visit http://go.jblearning.com/ManascoCWS to view the corresponding video.*

In the United States, approximately every 40 seconds someone has a stroke (Rosamond, et al. 2008). Because a large proportion of strokes affect the left hemisphere and likely occur somewhere along the left middle cerebral artery, which supplies blood to the language areas of the brain, many of these stroke victims present with aphasia. This translates into a steady flow of individuals with aphasia into the caseload of speech-language pathologists who work in clinical settings.

Language is a system of symbols that is used to communicate meaning. Aphasia is a deficit in language abilities resulting from damage to the brain. Aphasia is an acquired disorder most often caused by stroke within the language-dominant (usually left) hemisphere, though any etiology that damages the left hemisphere can produce aphasia. Aphasia is not the result of motor, intellectual, or psychological impairment. It is strictly a deficit in language production, language comprehension, or both. Individuals with aphasia can display language deficits in any or all modalities of language (i.e., production and comprehension of spoken or written language).

Language deficits are generally divided into the categories of expressive language deficits and receptive language deficits. An expressive language deficit is a difficulty in formulation and production of language to communicate an intended meaning. Expressive language deficits usually arise from lesions in the anterior portion of the left cerebral hemisphere at or near Broca's area. However, lesions almost anywhere in the anterior portion of the left hemisphere are likely to produce some expressive deficits. A receptive language deficit is a deficit in the ability to derive meaning from language. Receptive language deficits include problems with verbal and/or written language and usually arise from lesions in the posterior portion of the left hemisphere at or near Wernicke's area.

The source of damage to the brain that most often produces aphasia is stroke. Small strokes often produce small and localized lesions in the brain. These small lesions can produce aphasia with few or no discernable concomitant

> **Aphasia** An acquired deficit in language abilities resulting from damage to the brain.
>
> **Expressive language deficit** Difficulty in formulation and production of language to communicate an intended meaning.
>
> **Receptive language deficit** A deficit in the ability to derive meaning from language.

cognitive or physical deficits. A similar isolated deficit profile of limited deficits can be produced by tumor or focal surgical trauma. However, aphasia is also associated with more generalized damage to the brain such as that often produced by traumatic brain injury or degenerative disease. In these scenarios, more and larger areas of the brain are damaged or degenerate. Etiologies that produce general damage or degeneration of the brain produce more cognitive and physical deficits along with aphasia.

Signs and Symptoms of Aphasia

Anomia

The most pervasive deficit in the aphasias is anomia. **Anomia** is a deficit in word finding ability. Some level of anomia is seen in all of the aphasias. A person with anomia knows the meaning he wants to communicate but cannot find the appropriate word or words to do so. Individuals with aphasia who display anomia often can describe an object in detail and maybe even use hand gestures to demonstrate how the object is used but cannot find the appropriate word to name the object. Anomia is a deficit of expressive language.

Verbal Comprehension Deficits

Whereas the term *receptive language deficit* can refer to a deficit in any modality of language interpretation (verbal language, written language, etc.), the term **verbal comprehension deficit** refers specifically to an inability to comprehend the verbal language others produce. In aphasia, verbal comprehension deficits are assumed to be acquired deficits resulting from neurologic damage. It is common for most individuals with

Anomia   A deficit in word retrieval for expression.

Verbal comprehension deficit   An inability to comprehend the verbal language produced by others.

aphasia to display some level of difficulty understanding verbal language. Most language used during social interactions is formulaic and predictable. Therefore, individuals with mild verbal comprehension deficits usually have no difficulty interacting socially and understanding or correctly guessing the meaning of most language presented to them. It might be only when presented with a lengthy or detail-heavy utterance that the verbal comprehension deficits of a person with aphasia begin to show. Individuals with more severe levels of aphasia display far more dramatic verbal comprehension deficits and might lack the ability to understand even a single word. This is illustrated anecdotally by individuals who have recovered from a stroke that produced moderate or severe receptive language deficits when they state that directly after the stroke the speech of others and even their own speech suddenly sounded like a foreign language.

Paraphasias

Even if individuals with aphasia can get around their anomia and find the words they want to say, they

Paraphasia An error in expressive language that is not related to motor deficits but that is linked to higher-level language deficits associated with aphasia.

Phonemic paraphasia An error in speech in which the word produced is discernible, mostly correct, and yet there are phoneme-level mistakes.

Neologism An error in speech that occurs when an individual produces a word that is entirely different from the intended word and is mostly unintelligible.

Semantic paraphasia An error in speech in which one word is substituted for another word that is similar in meaning.

might have difficulties producing these words error free. **Paraphasias** are errors in expressive language unrelated to motor deficits but linked to higher language–level deficits associated with aphasia. Goodglass, Kaplan, and Barresi (2001b) define paraphasias as syllables, words, or phrases produced unintentionally by an individual with aphasia. A **phonemic paraphasia**, also known as a literal paraphasia, is when the word produced is discernable, mostly correct, and yet there are phoneme-level mistakes. Phonemic paraphasias are phoneme "substitutions, omissions, or transpositions" (Goodglass et al., 2001b, p. 9). An example of a phonemic paraphasia is when an individual with aphasia intends to produce the word *staple* but transposes the initial /s/ phoneme to the final position and produces "taples."

A **neologism**, or neologistic paraphasia, occurs when an individual produces a word that is entirely different from the intended word and is mostly unintelligible. Goodglass and associates (2001b) define a neologism as when 50% or more of the intended word or utterance is indiscernible. An example of a neologism is when an individual with aphasia intends to produce the word *pencil* but instead produces "dowfler." A **semantic paraphasia** occurs when one word is substituted for another word that is similar in meaning (Goodglass et al., 2001b). Examples of semantic paraphasias are *glass* for *cup* or *airplane* for

helicopter. A substitution of a word that is unrelated in meaning to the intended word is categorized as an **unrelated verbal paraphasia** (Goodglass et al., 2001b). For example, substituting the word *lunch* for the word *bicycle* is an unrelated verbal paraphasia. ▶ For examples of many different types of paraphasias see the video interview *Recovering from Mixed Fluent Aphasia*.

Perseveration

To **perseverate** is to do something repeatedly, redundantly, and, more often than not, inappropriately. Although the word *perseverate* is commonly used in child language literature to refer to repetitive and obsessive behaviors of children with autism, it is also used in adult language disorders. In adult language disorders, such as the aphasias, a **perseveration** is a word that is said repeatedly and inappropriately. A **perseverative paraphasia** occurs when a word produced earlier is repeatedly and inadvertently produced by an individual instead of the intended word (Goodglass et al., 2001b, p. 9). An example of this is when an individual with aphasia correctly names a hammer as a "hammer" but then involuntarily continues to produce "hammer" when presented other items, despite knowing the correct names of the other items (see the Clinical Note on perseverative paraphasia). Perseverative paraphasias are very frustrating for people with aphasia. Often, speech-language pathologists can learn which words individual patients get stuck on and can avoid using those words in therapy.

Unrelated verbal paraphasia A verbal substitution of a word that is unrelated in meaning to the intended word.

Perseverate To do something repeatedly, redundantly, and, more often than not, inappropriately.

Perseveration A word that is said repeatedly and inappropriately.

Perseverative paraphasia A word that is produced repeatedly and inadvertently by an individual with aphasia instead of the intended word.

Agrammatism The lack of appropriate grammatical construction of language displayed by individuals with aphasia.

Function words The in-between words used to frame the major content words in a sentence.

Content words The words that carry the majority of meaning in a sentence.

Agrammatism

Agrammatism is a lack of grammar. This is often seen in individuals with aphasia who lack the ability to use language with appropriate grammatical construction. This most often arises because individuals with many kinds of aphasia systematically omit function words in their utterances. **Function words**, or functor words, are the in-between words used to frame the major content words in a sentence. **Content words** are the words that carry the majority of meaning. As a result of the omission of function words, the speech of individuals with aphasia might be grammatically incorrect while still conveying a great deal of meaning. The speech output of these individuals is often referred to as sounding telegraphic, which indicates that few words are used but the words that are used are generally used with some degree of efficiency. ▶ For examples of agrammatic speech of individuals with aphasia see the videos *Recovering from Mixed Fluent Aphasia* and *Recovering from Stroke and Nonfluent Aphasia*.

Repetition Deficits

Traditional models state that the ability to repeat words heard originates with the arcuate fasciculus, the white matter pathways stretching between Broca's area and Wernicke's area. These pathways enable a word to be heard and then transmitted from the posterior portion of the left hemisphere (Wernicke's area) that received the word for processing to the anterior portion (Broca's area) for verbal production of the word. In fact, babies begin mimicking verbalizations of their parents at the point in their brain development when their arcuate fasciculus has matured enough to begin to function.

Clinical Note

Perseverative Paraphasia

It does not take many years of clinical practice as a speech-language pathologist to witness countless examples of perseverative paraphasias. The most curious example that comes to mind from my own experience has to do with an older woman I saw years ago. She was about 75 years old and had experienced one left hemisphere stroke many years earlier that had left her mildly anomic. However, a more recent and severe left hemisphere stroke had transformed this mild anomia into a far more significant expressive language deficit consisting of severe anomia and a greatly reduced average length of utterance.

This woman's receptive language abilities were functional and, in light of her severe expressive language deficits, speech-language therapy focused primarily on reducing her anomia. We generally began each therapy session with her attempting, with my help, to name common objects. This patient generally had no perseverative difficulties.

However, that changed if her thoughts were directed to the object *hammer*. I quickly discovered in therapy that if she was presented with a hammer, a picture of a hammer, the word *hammer* written on a card, or even the gesture of how to use a hammer to drive a nail, the only word this woman would be able to produce verbally for the rest of the session was *hammer*, despite the fact that she knew very well that every other object presented to her was not a hammer. When she attempted to produce the target word to name any other objects, her brain would foil all attempts at success and to her amazement her mouth would produce the word *hammer*. The perseveration on the word *hammer* was devastatingly frustrating and usually lasted about 3 hours before she was able to produce any other words. Once I learned this, therapy progressed smoothly and this woman made great improvements, but we certainly avoided the use of the word *hammer*.

Lesions along the arcuate fasciculus create repetition deficits by impairing an individual's ability to move the auditory image of the word from the left temporal lobe where the word is received to the left frontal lobe where the word is selected for expression. However, just because a person cannot repeat a word does not mean that she cannot understand the meaning of the word she has been asked to repeat. See the discussion on conduction aphasia that follows to explore this type of deficit further.

Alexia and Agraphia

Reading and writing disturbances are common in aphasia. **Alexia** is an acquired impairment of reading,

Clinical Note

Alexia

Luria (1972) describes the experience of a man with receptive deficits in reading after being wounded in war. When looking for a restroom in the hospital following his injury he could not tell which restroom was the men's restroom. When speaking of the sign on the restroom door, he stated, "No matter how long I stared at it and examined the letters, I couldn't read a thing. Some peculiar foreign letters were printed there" (p. 62). Later this young man discovered that the letters were not written in a foreign language but that he had lost the ability to visually interpret writing in his native language.

More recently, the Canadian novelist Howard Engel experienced a stroke in the same part of his brain and stated that he had no idea he had experienced a stroke until he picked up his morning paper and was surprised to see it written in a foreign language, possibly "Serbo-Croatian or Korean" (Krulwich, 2010). Despite losing the ability read, his ability to write was preserved and eventually Engel produced the memoir *The Man Who Forgot How to Read*. An intact ability to write despite losing the ability to read occurs because writing abilities are preserved in motor memory which is stored in anterior, entirely different portions of the brain from the damaged language decoding and reading centers, which are located more posterior in the brain.

and there are many subtypes of alexia. Contrast the term *alexia* with the term *dyslexia*. Dyslexia is commonly used to refer to congenital or developmental reading deficits. (See the Clinical Note on alexia.) **Agraphia** is an acquired impairment in the ability to form letters or form words using letters. Lesions to the language-dominant hemisphere at the angular gyrus often results in alexia and agraphia. Often, but not always, individuals with deficits in auditory comprehension of language also display deficits in comprehension of written language. Similarly, individuals with anomia usually cannot find words for the production of verbal language or written language. However, there are exceptions and speech-language pathologists should always thoroughly test all language modalities.

Related Behaviors

Self-Repairs

A **self-repair** occurs when a speaker restates or revises a word or phrase in an attempt to produce it in an error-free fashion or refine it to reflect better the intended meaning (Levelt, 1983). Unimpaired speakers produce speech errors and repair them easily by restating words or revising phrases. Most unimpaired speakers are highly successful at correcting speech errors on their first attempt (Farmer, 1977; Levelt, 1983). Individuals with nonfluent aphasia make far more errors and therefore produce proportionately far more self-repairs and attempts at self-repairs to correct for these errors (Farmer, 1977; Liss, 1998). However, speakers with aphasia are far less successful at self-repairing errors in their speech than unimpaired speakers are (Farmer, 1977; Marshall & Tomkins, 1982). Farmer

Alexia An acquired impairment of reading.

Agraphia An acquired impairment in the ability to form letters or form words using letters.

Self-repair When a speaker restates or revises a word or phrase in an attempt to produce it in an error-free fashion or refine it to better reflect the intended meaning.

(1977) found that less than half of the self-repair attempts of her participants with nonfluent aphasia were successful.

These perseverative and unsuccessful attempts to self-repair semantic and phonetic errors can further compromise the ability of speakers with aphasia to communicate by decreasing their fluency of speech. Marshall and Tomkins (1982) and Whitney and Goldstein (1989) also observed that multiple attempts to self-repair an error within an utterance can slow the rate of speech as well as increase speaker frustration. (See the discussion of conduction aphasia later in this chapter for more information on possible negative impacts of unsuccessful perseverative self-repairs on the speech of those with aphasia.)

More recently, it has also been suggested that recurring attempts at self-repair by speakers with aphasia might actually contribute to maintenance of their long-term deficits. Fillingham, Hodgson, Sage, and Lambon Ralph (2003) studied the effects of errorless learning and errorless therapy on individuals with aphasia. These researchers suggest that the repetitive unsuccessful attempts of people with nonfluent aphasias to self-correct speech errors could function as a practicing and habituation of the production of speech errors. If true, then not only might the presence of a high number of attempts at self-repair decrease fluency, thereby contributing to the communicative difficulties of individuals with nonfluent aphasia (Marshall & Tomkins, 1982; Whitney & Goldstein, 1989), but they could also function to maintain the primary word finding and articulatory deficits of speakers with aphasia and/or apraxia of speech (AOS).

Speech Disfluencies

Certain kinds of speech disfluencies can inhibit the fluency of individuals with nonfluent aphasia (Brown & Cullinan, 1981, p. 358; Whitney & Goldstein, 1989). These behaviors consist of sound, word, part-word, or phrase repetitions, prolongations, and interjections (Brown & Cullinan, 1981). It should

be noted that the disfluency types associated with stuttering such as phoneme repetitions, syllable repetitions, or part-word repetitions are usually rare in aphasia. Individuals with aphasia most often produce the normal disfluencies such as interjections and self-repairs, but at pathologic levels of frequency.

Struggle in Nonfluent Aphasias

Most unimpaired individuals need not put forth any effort to express themselves verbally. Verbal expression is usually produced quite automatically and is, therefore, taken for granted almost universally by unimpaired speakers. However, when individuals acquire expressive language deficits, this automaticity of speech is lost to some degree. Most often, individuals respond to this loss by becoming frustrated and angry at suddenly having to expend incredible amounts of effort to produce and use language that formerly was effortless. For instance, as individuals with anomia attempt to overcome their word-finding difficulties and find the target word, they struggle visibly. Individuals with these deficits will display the struggle with their deficits and their frustration in different ways. Some clench their fists, grit their teeth, sigh, stare into space, or swear and curse whereas others simply acknowledge their difficulties verbally.

Preserved and Automatic Language

It is a long-established curiosity that even in severe cases of aphasia, it is common for some production of rote and overlearned language to be preserved. This can take the form of an intact ability to sing songs that the individual often heard or sang premorbidly. In fact, attempting to elicit a well-known song such as the "Happy Birthday" song is a fixture of aphasia evaluations. Preserved language skills might also take the form of intact abilities to recite rote language such as the days of the week, the months of the year, and counting to 10. Often, individuals with aphasia might be unable to begin the rote language task by themselves, but they can take over production of the task when provided with the first few words.

Language that is produced very automatically or that is associated closely with some stimulus might also be preserved. For instance, many individuals with aphasia who cannot produce any volitional expressive language might still be able to produce curse/swear words perfectly to express their pain and frustration when a nurse stabs them with a needle or a speech-language pathologist asks them to complete a task they are having difficulty with. Another example is when a speech-language pathologist asks the person with aphasia to say the word *Hey* the individual might not be able to do so but can promptly utter "Hey!" seconds later in direct response to someone entering the room.

The presence of preserved and automatic language often is used as a prognostic tool. The more preserved and automatic language an individual with aphasia has, the better their prognosis of recovery. Speech-language pathologists test for the presence of preserved or automatic language by simply asking the individual to produce the desired language (e.g., "Say the days of the week."). Automatic and preserved language is also useful clinically because when a person cannot produce any other verbal output, it can provide a useful starting point in therapy to begin rebuilding expressive language skills. See the following Author's Note for more on preserved language.

Associated Deficits

In the classroom, aphasia is usually spoken of as being a pure language disorder with no associated cognitive deficits. Theoretically and academically, aphasia is only a language disorder and students must first understand aphasia and how it affects communication before layering concomitant disorders and their potential effects on top of this definition. However, it is important to acknowledge that when a person's brain is damaged it is rare that only a single deficit

Author's Note

Preserved Language

It is important to note that the actual rote language preserved in individuals with aphasia varies by region and culture. Speech-language pathologists must consider cultural differences while testing for preserved language skills, especially if they are not native to the patients' region and culture.

For example, in a highly Protestant and religious community in the Deep South where most residents attended church, I found that I could elicit the recitation of the Bible verse John 3:16 from many, if not all, individuals with aphasia. These patients' progression through rehabilitation was often reflected by improvements in their ability to automatically produce this language as well as other preserved language.

To a religious individual who has lost all other language and expression the intrinsic value of being able to recite a bible verse should not be overlooked. Similarly, I have worked with patients with aphasia who were unable to produce any verbal language until we discovered their intact ability to sing church hymnals. Aside from indicating potential for improvement in lost language abilities, the ability to sing these hymnals gave these individuals hope for improvement and motivated them to get out of their house and reestablish a role for themselves in their communities. Also, it enabled these individuals to express themselves successfully and appropriately in song in their church setting. Given that the church setting was the only consistent social outlet in this particular rural setting, this seemingly minor skill proved very precious to these individuals.

such as aphasia arises. Most individuals with aphasia will also have deficits in cognition and motor skills that affect language production and/or swallowing.

Cognitive Deficits

Cognitive deficits do not always co-occur with aphasia. However, it is unlikely that most forms of brain damage create deficits restricted to any single ability such as language. Most etiologies that result in aphasia usually create some collateral damage to cognitive abilities as well. These cognitive deficits can be as severe as coma or as mild as an inability to balance the checkbook.

Cognitive deficits that often present concomitantly with aphasia are in the areas of arousal, attention, short-term memory, problem solving, inferencing, and executive functioning skills. Typically, the presence or absence of concomitant cognitive deficits is determined by the location and severity of damage to the brain.

Motor Deficits

It is also common for motor deficits to co-occur with some forms of aphasia. Motor deficits often arise with damage to the frontal lobes, which are responsible for initiating and gross planning of movement. Because the left frontal lobe also houses expressive language abilities, many aphasias that characteristically include expressive language deficits present with concomitant motor deficits. Examples of motor deficits that concern the speech-language pathologist are the dysarthrias, apraxia of speech, and the dysphagias (swallowing disorders).

Classification System

Different frameworks and models define aphasia and whether and how it can be classified into categories and subcategories. Most begin as dichotomous models reflecting the historical viewpoint that lesions to the anterior portion of the brain at or near Broca's area produce aphasia characterized by nonfluent speech while lesions to the posterior portion of the brain at or near Wernicke's area produce aphasia characterized by fluent speech.

In the field today, the most popular framework maintains this basic fluent/nonfluent aphasia tradition. This multidimensional view uses the major categories of fluent aphasia and nonfluent aphasia and

subdivides each into more specific aphasia subtypes. Major diagnostic tools such as the Boston Diagnostic Aphasia Exam (BDAE; Goodglass et al., 2001a) and the Western Aphasia Battery–Revised (WAB-R; Kertesz, 2006) use this framework to identify and categorize aphasia subtypes. Subtypes of nonfluent aphasia identified by the BDAE and the WAB-R include Broca's aphasia, transcortical motor aphasia, and global aphasia. Subtypes of fluent aphasia include classic Wernicke's aphasia, transcortical sensory aphasia, conduction aphasia, and anomic aphasia. These aphasias are primarily differentiated from one another based on the presence of expressive and receptive language deficits as well as deficits in repetition.

Although speech-language pathologists continue to use the fluent/nonfluent model, it is becoming more difficult to sustain based on new profiles of aphasia deficits that fall outside the fluent/nonfluent dichotomy. Researchers and speech-language pathologists now recognize a third major category of aphasia types that do not neatly fit into the traditional fluent/nonfluent system. Helm-Estabrooks (1992) created a "semi-fluent" category, while Hallowell and Chapey (2001) use "other forms of aphasia" (p. 8) in which to put nontraditional forms of aphasia. Another strike against the two-category system is that few patients actually display aphasia profiles that fit neatly into the subcategories. Goodglass, Kaplan, and Barresi (2001b) describe this system of classification as "rigid" (p. 58) when attempts are made to apply it clinically. The clinical reality is that patients' profiles of deficits usually fall between labels and are simply identified as displaying mixed aphasia or a nonspecific form of fluent or nonfluent aphasia. Also, the particular type of aphasia patients display usually evolves during their recovery and rehabilitation, so any initial labeling of a patient with aphasia is not static for long.

One purpose of having a system of classification,

Mixed aphasia A nonspecific form of fluent or nonfluent aphasia that combines attributes of more distinctive forms of aphasia.

even if it is an imperfect one, is to have a reference point for professionals to communicate information about patients. This enables standardization of knowledge and language among speech-language pathologists and streamlining of communication regarding patients' language deficits. For instance, if a patient is described as displaying a Broca's aphasia or a Broca's-like aphasia, with little further explanation most experienced speech-language pathologists can make an educated guess about the probable primary and secondary deficits that the patient displays.

Another reason to attempt to classify aphasia types and subtypes is for the purpose of lesion localization. **Lesion localization** is the practice of identifying the location in the brain of focal lesions based on the profile of deficits displayed by the patient. Goodglass, Kaplan, and Barresi (2001b) state that, historically, most major contributors to the science of aphasia have identified the same major configurations of aphasic symptoms as resulting from specific lesion locations. Accurate prediction of aphasic deficits from a specifically located lesion is not possible. However, prediction of lesion location by the aphasic deficits displayed by an individual is more reliable. The ability to estimate lesion location based on language deficits is valuable for confirming other professionals' estimates of where the damage occurred in the brain, augmenting brain imaging studies, and estimating the location of a lesion in the brain when no lesion is visible on imaging studies.

Cortical/Subcortical Aphasias

Aphasia is usually created by cortical lesions to or within the language-dominant hemisphere. Specifically, damage at or near Broca's area, Wernicke's area, and the arcuate fasciculus are known to create certain types of aphasia profiles. The **cortical aphasias** are aphasias that arise as a result of damage to the cortex. However, aphasia can also arise from and alongside damage to certain subcortical structures such as the thalamus and an area within the basal ganglia known as the striatocapsular region (Nadeau & Gonzalez Rothi, 2008). The term **subcortical aphasias** are used to describe aphasias that arise as a result of damage to subcortical structures.

> **Lesion localization**   The practice of identifying the location of pathology in the brain based on the profile of deficits the individual displays.
>
> **Cortical aphasia**   Aphasia that arises as a result of damage to the cortex.
>
> **Subcortical aphasia**   Aphasia that arises as a result of damage to subcortical structures.

The Cortical Aphasias
Nonfluent Aphasias

Individuals with nonfluent aphasia display very agramatic, halting, and effortful speech that consists mainly of content words. The expressive output of individuals with nonfluent aphasia can be as restricted as 10 words per minute to about 50 words per minute (Halpern & Goldfarb, 2013). These individuals usually speak in short phrases or single-word utterances. They are usually very well aware of their language deficits and are motivated to improve their expressive capabilities. Nonfluent aphasias arise from damage to the anterior of the language-dominant hemisphere near areas of motor control. As a result, most nonfluent aphasias exist alongside significant motor deficits contralateral to the site of lesion (e.g., a contralateral hemiparesis or a contralateral hemiparalysis). A breakdown of the cortical aphasias and profiles of their gross deficits are provided in Table 4-1.

Broca's Aphasia

Broca's aphasia is the result of damage to the inferior posterior frontal lobe of the left hemisphere (Broca's area) extending deep into the white matter. Broca's area is prerolandic (located just anterior to the fissure

Table 4-1   Gross Deficits of the Cortical Aphasias

Nonfluent Aphasias	Receptive Language Deficits	Expressive Language Deficits	Repetition Ability
Broca's	Grossly intact	Significant deficit	Significant deficit
Transcortical motor	Grossly intact	Significant deficit	Grossly intact
Global	Severe-profound deficit	Severe-profound deficit	Significant deficit
Fluent Aphasias	**Receptive Language Deficits**	**Expressive Language Deficits**	**Repetition Ability**
Wernicke's	Significant deficit	Grossly intact (though often devoid of meaning)	Significant deficit
Transcortical sensory	Significant deficit	Grossly intact (though often devoid of meaning)	Grossly intact
Conduction	Grossly intact	Grossly intact	Significant deficit
Anomic	Grossly intact	Mild-moderate naming deficits	Grossly intact

of Rolando), suprasylvian (just above the sylvian fissure), and receives vascular supply from the middle cerebral artery. A lesion entirely restricted to Broca's area is known to produce only mild aphasic symptoms. However, a larger lesion resulting in damage within and adjacent to Broca's area produces the more severe symptoms associated with this aphasia.

Broca's aphasia is the prototypical nonfluent aphasia and is characterized primarily by a halting, effortful, agrammatic, and often telegraphic verbal output. Those with Broca's aphasia have extreme difficulty producing grammatically correct expressive language. Their speech consists largely of content words with few or no function words. The speech of those with Broca's aphasia is also very disfluent. This is largely because of the pauses these individuals require to overcome or circumlocute their anomia. Repeated and unsuccessful attempts to self-repair speech errors also contribute to the disfluency of speech of these individuals. The prosody of those with Broca's aphasia is compromised by shortened length of utterances and the presence of self-repairs and disfluencies.

The written language of these individuals usually mirrors their verbal language output. Production

of written language is usually further hindered by a hemiplegia or hemiparesis contralateral to the lesion. An unfortunate manifestation of contralateral hemiplegia or hemiparesis among those with Broca's aphasia (and other nonfluent aphasias) is concomitant motor deficits in the dominant writing hand. This arises because most individuals write with their right hands, which are contralateral to their language-dominant hemisphere (their left hemisphere). Therefore, a left-hemisphere lesion might affect production of verbal language while also creating motor deficits of the writing hand.

Despite deficits in expressive language, individuals with Broca's aphasia display functionally intact receptive language abilities. These patients understand most of the everyday conversation around them. They usually can respond appropriately to simple questions using their limited speech output, intact gestural abilities, and body language. For example, a patient with Broca's aphasia can usually answer appropriately a question such as "Would you like the television on?" with a nod of the head or point at the door in response to the speech-language pathologist's request to do so. However, higher-level deficits in receptive language are often present and manifest in an inability to comprehend detail-heavy or syntactically complex language such as "Point to my ear, then your foot, but only after I point to my nose." These higher-level deficits in receptive language abilities often go unnoticed by family and even the patient until the speech-language pathologist diagnoses the presence of these deficits during the initial evaluation. Deficits in reading usually mirror receptive language deficits. However, possible visual deficits and hemispatial neglect must always be evaluated as primary or contributing factors in reading deficits.

Deficits in repetition are also present in Broca's aphasia. Despite mostly intact receptive language abilities, those with Broca's aphasia cannot repeat phrases or often even single words.

The general result of these deficits and intact abilities is that those with Broca's aphasia are very aware of their expressive deficits and use their intact receptive language and the limited forms of expression they have left very effectively. It is often said that, because of this profile, individuals with Broca's aphasia are very poor speakers but very good communicators. The following transcription is a short example of the speech of an individual with Broca's aphasia as the speech-language pathologist (SLP) targets his anomia in therapy:

> SLP: "Can you tell me what coin this is?" (The SLP presents a nickel.)
>
> Patient: "Yeah, I know. It's ... That's ... Yeah. It's ... It's a ... The money. I know what. I can't say."
>
> SLP: "I know you know what coin it is. Just try to find the word for me. That is what we're practicing."
>
> Patient: "Yeah, I know. It's five. The money. Five. It's ... A ..."
>
> SLP: "You're right, it is worth five cents and it is a bright and shiny new ..."
>
> Patient: "Bright and shiny ... A ... It's a five cents.... A ... nickel."

Transcortical Motor Aphasia

There are two primary locations of damage that produce transcortical motor aphasia: the supplementary motor cortex and the area just anterior to Broca's area (Freedman, Alexander, & Naeser, 1984). These lesions typically spare Broca's area. Articulation might be preserved in transcortical motor aphasia, but if the lesion reaches posteriorly into the area of the primary motor cortex that controls movement of the face, articulation deficits will be present (Freedman et al., 1984). Lesions producing transcortical motor aphasia result from occlusion of branches of the anterior cerebral artery or the most anterior branches of the middle cerebral artery in the left hemisphere.

In many ways, transcortical motor aphasia resembles Broca's aphasia. Those with transcortical motor aphasia display intact receptive language abilities paired with very disfluent speech patterns and likely anomia. The hallmark characteristic of transcortical motor aphasia that differentiates it from Broca's aphasia is preserved repetition abilities. It is generally accepted that preserved repetition in this aphasia is because the lesion is far enough anterior to spare the arcuate fasciculus and its connections with Broca's area.

As in Broca's aphasia, written language in transcortical motor aphasia often mirrors verbal language. Individuals with transcortical motor aphasia are very good communicators despite their expressive language deficits. Also as in Broca's aphasia, this is because of their use of gesture, facial expression, and what little expressive language remains.

Global Aphasia

Global aphasia is the result of damage to and loss of most of what is known as the zone of language. The **zone of language** comprises all of Broca's and Wernicke's

> **Zone of language** The anatomic area within the language-dominant hemisphere that houses Broca's and Wernicke's areas as well as the arcuate fasciculus.

areas, as well as the arcuate fasciculus. The etiology of such extensive damage to the left hemisphere is occlusion of a primary branch of the middle cerebral artery.

Global aphasia is a worst-case scenario for language. Those with global aphasia typically have little to no receptive language ability or expressive language ability. These individuals are often so impaired as to be unable to comprehend even the shortest spoken utterances. Expressively, these individuals might be unable to produce even a single word verbally, which renders them near mute.

Although those with global aphasia usually have lost most of their preserved and automatic language, they might retain the ability to produce one or two odd words or neologisms. These individuals can perseverate on these one or two words or neologisms and repeat them endlessly or produce them in response to every question. For example, a stroke patient I once saw presented with global aphasia and her only preserved word was the neologism "widgee"; she produced this neologism in response to every question she was asked.

It is important to note that global aphasia is listed as a nonfluent aphasia. However, as in the preceding scenario, these individuals might produce their one preserved word very fluently and might string together repetitions of this word or neologism fluently using intact prosodic abilities. However, this type of aphasia is easily differentiated from a fluent aphasia. Individuals with a fluent aphasia present with endless numbers of words and neologisms that they produce fluently.

So much of the brain is damaged from an occlusion of the left middle cerebral artery that those with global aphasia present with most, if not all, possible concomitant cognitive and motor deficits. These individuals might be so cognitively impaired that they can be difficult to arouse even to participate in therapy. Once aroused, they might be unable to follow events because of their attention and short-term memory deficits. Their language and cognition might be so impaired as to make them unable to understand that a symbol can represent an object or idea. Motor deficits in global aphasia are severe and usually consist of a hemiplegia on the side of the body contralateral to the lesion, severe dysarthria, buccofacial oral apraxia, apraxia of speech, and swallowing and mastication problems (dysphagia). Dysphagia is often so severe as to require the patient to be fed by a feeding tube.

Global aphasia, the most severe aphasia and resulting from the most severe damage to the brain, has the worst prognosis for recovery. Those with any other form of aphasia are more likely to recover a significant degree of lost abilities. Individuals with severe and persistent global aphasia usually never recover functional verbal language skills. These individuals often are candidates for interventions that use augmentative and alternative communication (AAC) strategies.

Fluent Aphasias

Individuals with fluent aphasias display fluent though often nonsensical speech. Fluent aphasias arise from damage to the midposterior of the language-dominant hemisphere. The locations of damage to the brain that produce the fluent aphasias are usually far from the more anterior areas of the brain that contribute to motor control. As a result, individuals who display fluent aphasia usually have no gross motor deficits. Table 4-1 provides a breakdown of the fluent aphasias and profiles of their gross deficits.

Wernicke's Aphasia

The prototypical fluent aphasia is Wernicke's aphasia. **Wernicke's aphasia** results from lesion to Wernicke's area within the posterior one-third of the superior gyrus of the temporal lobe of the left hemisphere. Lesions here often result from an occlusion in the

> **Wernicke's aphasia** A fluent aphasia with receptive deficits, repetition deficits, verbal output void of meaning, and a usual lack of awareness of the presence of these deficits.

inferior/posterior branches of the middle cerebral artery. The more the lesion reaches posteriorly toward the angular gyrus and into the visual association cortex of the occipital lobe, the more likely reading deficits are present resulting from impaired ability to process visual information effectively.

Those with Wernicke's aphasia present with significant receptive language deficits as well as impaired repetition. These individuals are often incapable of understanding even the most simple requests and statements and tend to have difficulty with conversational rules such as turn-taking. However, unlike those with Broca's or transcortical motor aphasia, those with Wernicke's aphasia are usually unable to recognize their deficits. This condition of having a deficit and not knowing it exists or denying that it exists is known as **anosognosia**. This condition is a neurologic problem, not a psychological one. Whereas individuals with Broca's or trancortical motor aphasia are very aware of their deficits, struggle against them, attempt to correct their errors, and become frustrated at their failures, those with Wernicke's aphasia usually remain completely unaware of even their most profound language deficits. When confronted with evidence of their deficits such as when they see and hear themselves recorded on video, these individuals are often very good at defending their errors and confabulating explanations for their mistakes.

Author's Note

Anosognosia

Anosognosia is a long word that is so similar to other words bandied about in health sciences that it requires a short explanation. The Greek root word *gnosis* means to know. The word *agnosia* is not to know. There are many cognitive and sensory deficits that the word *agnosia* is used to refer to. With a further expansion of the word we get *anosognosia*, which means not to know that you do not know. Anosognosia is always used to indicate a patient's pathologic inability to recognize his or her deficits.

Those with Wernicke's aphasia are very fluent speakers. However, their expressive language is usually tangential to any subject matter introduced during conversation. Their expressive language is often so heavily composed of neologisms and paraphasias as to be indecipherable.

Those with Wernicke's aphasia display losses of verbal pragmatic skills, and conversational turn taking becomes notoriously difficult for them. As a result, these individuals often display **logorrhea**, a near nonstop output of speech. Expressive language in Wernicke's aphasia is also largely devoid of any discernable meaning. The speech of these individuals is referred to as **empty speech**. Although those with Wernicke's aphasia are very fluent speakers, they are extremely poor communicators.

Following is a short transcription of an individual with Wernicke's aphasia working with the speech-language pathologist. The speech-language pathologist is trying to get the patient to answer her questions correctly. However, as is typical with Wernicke's aphasia and transcortical sensory aphasia (discussed later), the patient's answers are often neologistic, nonsensical, tangential, and very paraphasic. Despite the level of deficit, the patient is very anosognosic and maintains perfect confidence that he is responding correctly to the questions of the speech-language pathologist.

> SLP: "Where would you find this?" (The SLP presents a toothbrush to the patient.)
>
> Patient: "Which." (Spoken as a statement, not an inquiry.)
>
> SLP: "Where would you find this?"

Anosognosia The pathologic condition of having a deficit and not knowing the deficit exists or denying that the deficit exists despite evidence indicating otherwise.

Logorrhea A near nonstop, usually meaningless and tangential, output of speech.

Empty speech Speech often produced by those with fluent aphasia that is abundant yet lacking in meaning.

Patient: "Brushing a which." (Patient answers confidently and without hesitation.)

SLP: "Brushing where?"

Patient: "On film, of course. That's what you do."

SLP: "Where would you find it? In your bath . . . ?" (SLP gives first part of the word *bathroom* as a cue.)

Patient: "Absolutely. Here. In the blemma."

SLP: "Maybe in a bathroom?"

Patient: "Yes, bathroom."

SLP: "What do you use it for?"

Patient: "Brushing up the brusher."

SLP: "What do you brush with it?"

Patient: "A see. A see."

SLP: "What do you brush with this?"

Patient: "A shirt."

SLP: "You brush a shirt with this?"

Patient: "Sure you do. I've done lots."

SLP: "Teeth. You brush your teeth with it."

Patient: "Not necessarily."

A comparison of the transcript of the patient with Wernicke's aphasia with the previous example of Broca's aphasia reveals iconic differences. The patient with Broca's knows exactly what the SLP is asking him. There are meaningful exchanges between the patient with Broca's and his speech-language pathologist. The patient knows when he is being unsuccessful and he keeps trying until he produces the target word appropriately. However, in this example of Wernicke's aphasia it seems the patient is totally oblivious to what the SLP asks of him and, yet, has no idea that he is responding incorrectly and even bizarrely to the questions asked. This example of the speech of a patient with Wernicke's aphasia demonstrates that there is no meaningful exchange of information and absolutely no successful communication between the patient and the speech-language pathologist. Topping it off, at the end of this transcription the patient with Wernicke's aphasia defends his strange assertion that toothbrushes are used to brush shirts.

Transcortical Sensory Aphasia

Lesions that occur posterior to Wernicke's area at the temporo-occipital-parietal junction produce transcortical sensory aphasia. More anteriorly placed lesions in this area are within the watershed area between the middle and posterior cerebral arteries whereas slightly more posterior lesions are solidly in the realm of the posterior cerebral artery (Kertesz, Sheppard, & MacKenzie, 1982).

Transcortical sensory aphasia is characterized by poor auditory comprehension, relatively intact repetition, and fluent speech with semantic paraphasias present. Intact repetition abilities primarily distinguish transcortical sensory aphasia from Wernicke's aphasia. Because of the lesion location within the visual/occipital association area, visual deficits are often present (Kertesz et al., 1982). ▶ See the video *Recovering from Mixed Fluent Aphasia* for an interview with a woman working to overcome deficits associated with fluent aphasia.

Conduction Aphasia

Conduction aphasia is characterized by fluent speech and relatively intact auditory comprehension with significant deficits in repetition. Those with severe conduction aphasia often cannot repeat even single words. Although repetition is impaired, it is important to note that these individuals display relatively intact comprehension of language. Despite their inability to repeat language received auditorily, those with conduction aphasia can paraphrase the meaning of the language heard because of their intact auditory comprehension and expression. For instance, when asked to repeat the sentence "The people ate fish and danced" an individual with conduction aphasia may not be able to repeat the sentence. However, when asked what the sentence means, this same person may be able to state, "There were fish being eaten . . . and people dancing."

The major lesion site that creates conduction aphasia is on the supramarginal gyrus of the parietal lobe, posterior to the primary sensory cortex and just above Wernicke's area. The traditional explanation of conduction aphasia is that lesions at the supramarginal gyrus damage the arcuate fasciculus and thereby disconnect Wernicke's area from Broca's area while leaving both intact. The intactness of Wernicke's and Broca's areas accounts for the mostly intact receptive and expressive language of those with conduction aphasia. However, the disconnection between these two areas resulting from damage to the arcuate fasciculus accounts for the person's inability to repeat. It is thought that without the direct connection between Broca's area and Wernicke's area provided by the arcuate fasciculus, the brain cannot transfer language heard from the temporal lobe to the frontal lobe for direct repetition. There are alternate explanations of conduction aphasia but most explanations are characterized by the hypothesis of a disconnection between posterior and anterior areas of the brain as a central explanation.

Although the speech of those with conduction aphasia is fluent, it is often characterized by phonemic paraphasias as well as anomia. These patients are highly aware of the paraphasias present in their speech. Because of this awareness, the normally fluent paraphasic speech of those with conduction aphasia at times is rendered disfluent by self-repair attempts; they might halt verbal expression at every speech error and attempt to correct it. As patients struggle with repeated attempts at self-repair, they slowly zero-in on the correct production of the target word. This behavior is known as **conduit d'approche** and is not restricted to conduction aphasia, though that is where it is most often seen. The following transcription typifies conduit d'approche as a person with conduction aphasia struggles to say *banana*:

> SLP: "Okay. What is this?" (SLP holds up a picture of a banana.)
>
> Patient: " Budda, ana … budda, ana … buddafly … budda, ann … banadud … bana, nud, na … bana, na … banana."

Although this patient was ultimately successful at producing the target word (*banana*), individuals with aphasia are often unsuccessful at correcting their speech errors. Goodglass and Kaplan (1972) suggest that because of conduit d'approche those with conduction aphasia might be as disfluent as those with Broca's aphasia.

Conduit d'approche A zeroing-in behavior in which a person with aphasia correctly produces a target word after several repeated and unsuccessful attempts where each failed attempt is closer to the correct production of the target word than the last.

Anomic aphasia An aphasia characterized by fluent speech and intact receptive language but a disproportionately severe deficit in naming abilities.

Anomic Aphasia

Although anomia is present in most forms of aphasia, it has been noted to occur, at times, in disproportionate severity relative to other deficits present or even in isolation. When this occurs, the label *anomic aphasia* is often applied. **Anomic aphasia** is characterized by fluent speech, intact receptive language, and a significant deficit in naming. Anomia can be produced by damage anywhere within the language areas.

Subcortical Aphasias

Until recently, it was thought that subcortical structures, being far from the primary language areas of the cortex, could play no part in higher-level cortical processes such as language. In some cases, this is true. Nonetheless, speech-language pathologists and researchers have noted and documented the presence of aphasia as a result of damage to the thalamus and alongside damage to parts of the basal ganglia. The mechanisms behind the production of aphasia as a result of damage to most subcortical structures are still poorly understood. The most well documented subcortical aphasia profiles that have arisen are thalamic aphasia and striatocapsular aphasia.

Thalamic Aphasia

Ischemic stroke within the left or dominant side of the thalamus often produces thalamic aphasia. **Thalamic aphasia** is characterized by almost fluent speech, significant anomia in spontaneous speech but less so in confrontational naming tasks, impaired receptive language, perseverative semantic paraphasias, normal articulation, hypophonic voice, intact repetition, and intact grammar (Kuljic-Obradovic, 2003; Nadeau & Gonzalez Rothi, 2008). Note that, although speech output is usually well articulated and grammatically intact, speech output is reduced and only semifluent.

Striatocapsular Aphasia

Ischemic stroke within a part of the basal ganglia known as the striatum can produce **striatocapsular aphasia**. Striatocapsular aphasia is characterized by loss of fluency, rare phonemic paraphasias, and preserved repetition (Kuljic-Obradovic, 2003). Anomia is present but is usually mild compared to the naming deficits found in thalamic aphasia.

Although the mechanisms behind thalamic aphasia are still mostly theoretical, those behind the occurrence of striatocapsular aphasia are better understood. Nadeau and Crosson (1997) examined a number of cases of striatocapsular aphasia and concluded that, as was traditionally thought, the basal ganglia have nothing to do with language. Rather, they found that the aphasia observed alongside lesions to the striatum of the basal ganglia was a result of hidden concomitant reduced blood flow to the primary language areas. This disruption in blood to the language cortices was simply invisible on neuroimaging studies. In other words, infarcts that damage the striatum can at times also disrupt blood flow to the primary language cortices, enough to create aphasia but not enough for the outright and immediate cell death that shows up immediately on neuroimaging studies used in hospitals.

Atypical Aphasias

Progressive Nonfluent Aphasia and Semantic Dementia: Primary Progressive Aphasias

Frontotemporal dementia is a condition in which the frontal and temporal lobes of the brain atrophy while the parietal and occipital lobes remain intact. Frontotemporal dementia is largely hereditary and runs in families (Chow, Miller, Hayashi, & Geschwind, 1999). Degeneration of the brain in frontotemporal dementia is progressive and eventually terminal. Progressive nonfluent aphasia and semantic dementia are two variants in the subcategory of frontotemporal dementia known as the primary progressive aphasias (**Figure 4-1**).

The degeneration of the frontal and temporal lobes seen in the primary progressive aphasias create signature language disturbances that are initially present in the absence of any accompanying significant cognitive deficits. This is in contrast to other dementias such as Alzheimer's that begin with a degeneration of cognition and memory and affect language only in later stages. As atrophy of the frontal and/or temporal areas of the brain progresses in the primary progressive aphasias, language deficits worsen and other cognitive deficits begin to arise and become more severe. Over time individuals with these disorders lose the ability to carry out acts of daily living.

Thalamic aphasia Language deficits as a result of lesion at the thalamus that is characterized by almost fluent speech, significant anomia in spontaneous speech but less so in confrontational naming tasks, impaired receptive language, perseverative semantic paraphasias, normal articulation, hypophonic voice, intact repetition, and intact grammar.

Striatocapsular aphasia Language deficits associated with lesion at the striatum that occur as a result of a lack of blood flow to the cortical language areas.

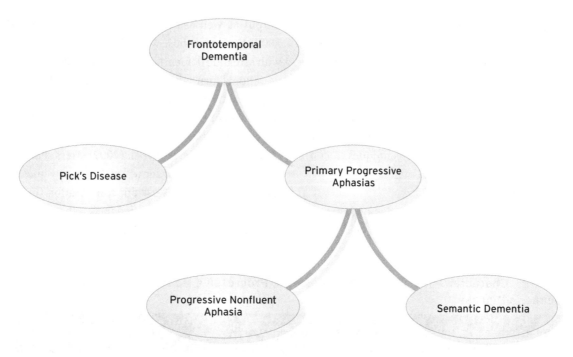

Figure 4-1 Frontotemporal dementias.

Progressive nonfluent aphasia and semantic dementia have an insidious onset that occurs slowly over time. These disorders are easily differentiated from the stroke-based aphasias because of the usual acute onset of stroke-based aphasias. Onset of progressive nonfluent aphasia and semantic dementia usually occurs prior to the age of 65 years (Chow et al., 1999).

There is often confusion regarding the terminology used in reference to these conditions, and many terms are used as synonyms. However, the most widely used terms are *progressive nonfluent aphasia* and *semantic dementia*. Nonetheless, students should note that many researchers and speech-language pathologists refer to progressive nonfluent aphasia as *nonfluent primary progressive aphasia* and semantic dementia as *fluent primary progressive aphasia* even though sometimes individuals present with forms of these disorders that are not entirely fluent or nonfluent, but somewhere in between. These forms can

be described as mixed progressive aphasia (Kertesz, Jesso, Harciarek, Blair, & McMonagle, 2009).

The neuroanatomic basis for progressive nonfluent aphasia is degeneration of the frontal lobes, with the left hemisphere usually more affected (Knibb, Woollams, Hodges, & Patterson, 2009; McMillan et al., 2010; Nestor et al., 2003). Assumed relevant atrophy is noted to occur in the perisylvian region of the left hemisphere, which includes areas above the sylvian fissure, including Broca's area.

The speech of those with progressive nonfluent aphasia is characterized by phonemic paraphasias, anomia, and grammatical errors (Knibb et al., 2009). These individuals often, but not always, display slow rates of speech, simplified syntax, and reduced phrase length (Knibb et al., 2009). Although receptive language is mostly intact, deficits in the ability to comprehend complex syntax also present in progressive nonfluent aphasia.

The neuroanatomic basis for semantic dementia is an initial greater degeneration of the temporal lobes than the frontal lobes, with greater atrophy in the left hemisphere than right hemisphere (Kertesz et al., 2009). Over time, atrophy in the frontal lobes becomes significant as well. Kertesz and associates (2009) warn that language and cognitive testing should be used in conjunction with neuroimaging techniques to confirm a diagnosis of semantic dementia.

The general language characteristics of semantic dementia are an excessive and disinhibited verbal output as well as semantic jargon (Kertesz et al., 2009). Similar to those with Wernicke's aphasia, those with semantic dementia also have difficulty with conversational turn-taking and characteristically will not stop speaking to listen to others. Turn-taking difficulties and logorrhea present early in semantic dementia but can be subtle or go unnoticed. Significant anomia is also present. Kertesz et al. (2009) stress that individuals with this disorder will so frequently question the meaning of words used in conversation (usually nouns) that this could be called the " 'What is _____?' disease" (p. 488). Table 4-2 compares and contrasts

Table 4-2 Characteristics of Semantic Dementia, Progressive Nonfluent Aphasia, and Alzheimer's Disease

Characteristics	Semantic Dementia	Progressive Nonfluent Aphasia	Alzheimer-Type Dementia
Age at onset	Commonly < 65 years	Commonly < 65 years	Usually > 65 years
Disease progression	Generally rapid	Slow	Variable
Spontaneous speech	Fluent and grammatically correct, but empty of content words	Labored, telegraphic with long word-finding pauses and frequent phonological and grammatical errors	Initially normal in most instances
Paraphasias	Semantic	Phonological	Semantic (early), phonological (late)
Comprehension: Single words	Impaired	Intact	Initially intact
Syntax	Intact	Impaired	Initially intact
Repetition	Normal for single words	Phonemic errors	Generally intact
Episodic memory	Preserved for recent events	Intact	Severely impaired early in course
Frontal executive functions	Intact in early stages	Intact	Might be impaired
Visuospatial and perceptual skills	Intact	Intact	Often impaired from early on, sometimes severely
Behavior	Appropriate initially, but frontal features invariably appear later	Appropriate until very late	Normal in early stages, but commonly disturbed in later stages
General neurologic findings	Usually none	Buccofacial apraxia and unilateral limb signs commonly seen	Usually normal until late stage
MRI findings	Focal polar and inferolateral temporal lobe atrophy, often worse on the left	Left perisylvian atrophy	Hippocampal ± medial temporal atrophy

Source: Reprinted with permission of Taylor & Francis Ltd. from Gerrard and Hodges, Semantic dementia: Implications for the neural basis of language and meaning, Aphasiology 13 (1999).

characteristics of semantic dementia, progressive nonfluent aphasia, and Alzheimer's dementia.

Crossed Aphasia

In most people, the language-dominant hemisphere (usually the left hemisphere) is contralateral to their dominant hand (usually the right hand). This relationship ensures that the language-dominant hemisphere is usually responsible for the motor control of the dominant hand for writing. Because Broca's area, which is highly involved in expressive language, is very close to the superior projections of the descending motor tracts (i.e., the upper motor neurons) coursing through the left frontal lobe, a lesion at Broca's area usually damages these descending motor tracts in the left cerebral hemisphere as well. This single lesion then produces aphasia because of damage at or near Broca's area and a contralateral hemiplegia or hemiparesis because of damage to these descending motor tracts. The contralateral hemiplegia or hemiparesis disables the right hand (usually the dominant hand for writing) with spasticity. This is the profile for most individuals with nonfluent aphasias.

However, in some individuals the language-dominant hemisphere does not control the dominant hand. In these cases, the dominant hand is ipsilateral to their language-dominant hemisphere. What this usually means is that the hemisphere nondominant for language (usually the right hemisphere) controls the dominant hand. In these cases, a lesion to Broca's area and the left upper motor neurons creates nonfluent aphasia and incapacitates the contralateral hand (usually the right). Nonetheless, in this scenario the left hand (the one ipsilateral to the damaged hemisphere) is used to write and it is preserved because the right hemisphere innervating it is undamaged. This condition of having a nonfluent aphasia that, despite the contralateral hemiplegia or hemiparesis, leaves the ipsilateral dominant writing hand preserved is known as **crossed aphasia**. See **Figure 4-2** for an illustration of what constitutes crossed aphasia.

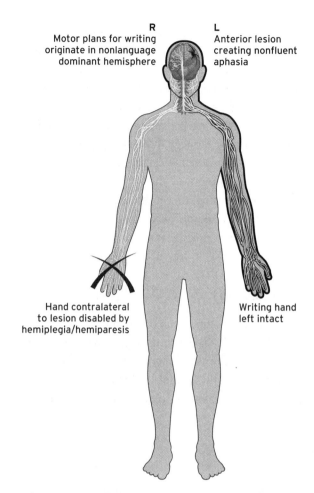

R Motor plans for writing originate in nonlanguage dominant hemisphere

L Anterior lesion creating nonfluent aphasia

Hand contralateral to lesion disabled by hemiplegia/hemiparesis

Writing hand left intact

Figure 4-2 **Crossed aphasia occurs when the damaged language-dominant hemisphere does not control a person's dominant writing hand.**

Because individuals with fluent aphasia usually have no concomitant hemiplegia/hemiparesis to disable the hand they use for writing because the lesions are too far posterior in the brain to produce motor deficits, the idea of crossed aphasia does not apply to those with fluent aphasia.

> **Crossed aphasia** The condition of having a nonfluent aphasia that, despite the contralateral hemiplegia or hemiparesis, leaves the dominant writing hand ipsilateral to the brain lesion motorically intact (i.e., the damaged language-dominant hemisphere does not control the dominant writing hand).

Crossed aphasia is important to recognize because it means that an individual has preserved motor abilities in their writing hand when a left hemisphere stroke renders them aphasic. An intact writing hand offers great potential for use in therapy as a means to reclaim language or establish a compensatory communication strategy. Whereas most individuals with typical nonfluent aphasia cannot even draw a picture to communicate their thoughts, individuals with crossed aphasia have the motor ability to use drawings to communicate and even use potentially preserved writing skills for communication.

Assessment of Aphasia

The primary components of an aphasia assessment usually include taking an in-depth case history, the assessment of functional communication and connected speech, the administration of a standardized test of aphasia, as well as some substantive evaluation of cognition.

Case History

As in all assessments by the speech-language pathologist, the first and perhaps most important step is gathering a case history through a thorough chart review and patient/family interview. The speech-language pathologist gathers basic demographic information including name, age, race, gender, as well as more detailed information regarding social and medical history. A good chart review is accomplished by the careful analysis and reading of the patient's medical chart as well as any additional medical records. It is important to read a patient's entire chart and not simply the last given report. In this way, the clinician can be sure that everything mentioned in the last entry is accurate and no dangerous misstatements or false assumptions have been made about the individual.

The second part of an informative and thorough case history is an interview with the patient with aphasia and family members or caregivers. Given that the patient might have an array of cognitive deficits, family members must be present during the initial interview to confirm or refute anything the individual with aphasia says.

Assessment of Functional Communication and Connected Speech

The interview portion of the case history gives the speech-language pathologist an opportunity to assess functional communication and connected speech of the individual with aphasia. The speech-language pathologist observes how the person with aphasia is using residual language abilities to communicate. This important baseline information can be compared later on with the results of a formal assessment of language ability. Whereas standardized tests of aphasia produce results indicating level of language ability and deficit, the assessment of functional communication and connected speech illustrates how these deficits affect the communicative abilities of the patient.

Administration of a Standardized Test of Aphasia

In addition to the case history and patient/family interview, the aphasia evaluation usually involves the administration of some form of standardized or formal assessment of aphasia. Standardized aphasia assessments usually assess multiple modalities of language including verbal reception of language, verbal expression, reading (visual reception of language), and writing (written expression of language). Different standardized tests of aphasia have different strengths and weaknesses that make them more or less appropriate in various practice settings. The patient's deficits also dictate the appropriateness of specific standardized tests. Choosing which standardized aphasia assessment to administer to which patient in a particular setting is a judgment call of the speech-language pathologist.

An experienced speech-language pathologist makes preliminary assumptions about the deficits of the person with aphasia throughout the chart review and patient/family interview well before administering any formal assessment. A formal aphasia assessment allows for the confirmation, refutation, and triangulation of preliminary conclusions so that the therapist can set appropriate goals and establish the best trajectory of therapy for the affected individual. A list of commonly used tests of aphasia follows (Shipley & McAfee, 2009):

- Aphasia Diagnostic Profiles (ADP; Helm-Estabrooks, 1992)
- Boston Diagnostic Aphasia Examination (3rd edition, BDAE-3; Goodglass et al., 2001a)
- Communication Activities of Daily Living (2nd edition, CADL-2; Holland, Frattali, & Fromm, 1999)
- Western Aphasia Battery–Revised (WAB-R; Kertesz, 2006)
- Quick Assessment for Aphasia (Tanner & Culbertson, 1999)
- Comprehensive Aphasia Test (CAT; Swiburn, Porter, & Howard, 2004)

Evaluation of Cognition

A necessary step in the evaluation of an individual with aphasia is the assessment of cognition. As previously mentioned, some level of cognitive deficit is almost universally present in those with aphasia. The ultimate goal of assessment is to set goals and a trajectory for therapy to improve deficits. Because cognition, language, and communication are intimately intertwined it is necessary to assess aspects of cognition as well as all primary modalities of language. If a speech-language pathologist operates on an incomplete knowledge of an individual's deficits, the likelihood of the patient benefiting from therapy is significantly reduced.

Aphasia Therapy

After stroke or other damage to the brain that produces aphasia, individuals experience a period of spontaneous recovery that lasts approximately 6 months post onset. During this time, individuals with aphasia improve to some degree even with no intervention. However, therapy for aphasia during this time of spontaneous recovery facilitates even greater levels of recovery and cues further improvements past the level achieved with spontaneous recovery alone.

There are three very broad categories of therapy interventions for aphasia: restorative therapy approaches, compensatory therapy approaches, and social therapy approaches. Restorative therapy is meant to help a patient regain a lost ability or skill by reducing the actual level of deficit. In contrast, compensatory therapy is used to help patients increase their level of function despite their deficits. Social approaches focus on reducing an individuals' barriers to communication. All three of these approaches are necessary and legitimate. During recovery and rehabilitation, patients usually benefit from restorative, compensatory, and social therapies and require them to maximize their recovery.

Restorative Therapy Approaches

Twenty to thirty years ago, it was believed that once a person's brain matured in adulthood it was essentially hardwired and unchangeable. Therefore, if part of the brain was damaged, little could be done to help that person recover from the damage. However, we now know that the brain is highly changeable and that when one part is damaged and ceases to function, other parts of the brain try to take on the role of the damaged part. In this way, the brain attempts to reorganize itself to optimize function. **Neuroplasticity** is the ability of a part of the

Neuroplasticity The ability of a part of the brain to change its previous function and to take on and learn a new and previously unknown role.

brain to change its function, take on, and learn new and previously unknown roles. One big reason for the brain to change its function is to compensate for brain damage. The idea of neuroplasticity is central to the concept of restorative therapy.

Most restorative therapies practiced today at least in part derive from the ideas and work of Hildred Schuell. Schuell was a speech-language pathologist who in the 1960s and 1970s pioneered the idea in the United States that with appropriate intervention individuals with aphasia can regain lost abilities (i.e., a person's brain can recover and relearn how to function following stroke). Although we take it for granted now that a person with aphasia can make significant and long-term improvements in their language abilities through concentrated therapy, this was a controversial topic when Schuell was practicing. A colleague of Schuell's, James J. Jenkins, is credited with stating, "All the hot-shot neurologists think Hildred's theories are crap—but she's the only aphasiologist in the world that can cure a patient" (Halwes, 2000). For a discussion of Hildred Schuell's contributions and principles of her philosophy regarding therapy, interested readers are directed to read *Schuell's Stimulation Approach to Rehabilitation*, by Coelho, Sinotte, and Duffy (2008).

Schuell's Stimulation Approach

What is now considered traditional aphasia therapy is based heavily on Schuell's stimulation approach. The stimulation approach focuses on using the auditory modality of language to stimulate the reacquisition of language in other modalities. This approach focuses on reestablishing disrupted language skills by presenting certain stimuli to the patient. As noted earlier, the idea that language abilities could be reestablished following brain damage by presenting stimuli to patients and eliciting responses was groundbreaking in its day. Principles of Schuell's stimulation approach include the following (Coelho et al., 2008):

1. Auditory stimulation of language should be intensive. Other modalities of language can also be stimulated, but auditory stimulation should be ever present.
2. The difficulty level of the stimulus presented to the patient must be controlled and be presented just at or below the patient's ability level.
3. Sensory stimulation must be repetitive and present, even if the patient does not seem to respond to it at first.
4. Every stimulus presented should elicit a response.
5. If a patient is unable to produce a response, it is because the speech-language pathologist needs to provide more stimulation (cues).
6. During therapy, a maximum number of responses need to be elicited from the patient. The more responses elicited, the more opportunities for the patient to experience success, progress, and be given useful feedback from the speech-language pathologist.
7. Feedback from the speech-language pathologist is necessary. The speech-language pathologist must highlight success with feedback and use feedback to promote further success and encourage the patient.
8. Therapy should be intensive and systematic.
9. Therapy sessions should begin with easy tasks and progress to more difficult tasks once success has been established.
10. Therapy materials should be varied enough to avoid boredom and frustration on the part of the patient.
11. As the patient progresses, new therapy tasks should build on previously mastered therapy tasks.

Following are examples of therapy tasks used in Schuell's stimulation approach:

- *Point-to tasks*. During these tasks, the speech-language pathologist asks the patient to point to something or to many things sequentially. The higher the verbal comprehension levels of the patient, the longer the point-to utterance he should be able to understand and hold in memory long enough to complete. Examples of point-to tasks are "Point to the door" as an easy task versus "Point to the door, ceiling, and your nose, after I touch my nose," which is a far more difficult task for persons with anything but a mild level of receptive deficits.

- *Following directions with objects.* Similar to point-to tasks, during following directions tasks the speech-language pathologist gives the patient a simple task, such as, "Pick up the flashlight," to more difficult tasks such as, "Pick up the flashlight and put it down beside the mirror, after I touch the pencil." Once again, the shorter utterance is far more easily accomplished by someone with receptive deficits than the longer, more complex utterance is.

- *Yes/no questions.* Questions that require a simple yes or no response from the patient are classic tasks of aphasia therapy. The difficulty level of the questions is easily manipulated from very simple to very complex. Also, same as the point-to and following directions tasks, the patient can complete these tasks successfully with no expressive language.

- *Paraphrasing/retelling.* In these tasks, the patient must retell a story or paraphrase a paragraph that she read quietly to herself or heard read aloud by the speech-language pathologist. This is a far more difficult therapy task than the previous three tasks. The retelling of a story, a paragraph, or even a sentence requires the patient to comprehend the material, remember it long enough to retell it, and find the words to communicate the meaning appropriately.

Melodic Intonation Therapy

Melodic intonation therapy (MIT) was begun as an attempt to use the intact melodic/prosodic processing skills of the right hemisphere in those with aphasia to help cue retrieval of words and expressive language. Albert, Sparks, and Helm (1973) did a preliminary study on the use of MIT and examined the reliance on melody in eliciting expression. In this study, therapy was effective for six out of eight participants. Since the publication of this study the formal process of MIT has been revised and refined. Even with written protocols for MIT, it is believed that almost all speech-language pathologists use the technique in their own fashion (Norton, Zipse, Marchina, & Schlaug, 2009).

Nonetheless, MIT universally involves modeling and eliciting, at first, functional words or short function phrases in a slow and sing-song manner that varies by only two notes. The speech-language pathologist gives visual cues using the hand to illustrate and emphasize the change in intonation of the target word or utterance or by tapping the left hand along with the syllables of the target utterance. The successful patient progresses through various levels of the MIT program as envisioned by Helm-Estabrooks and Albert (1991). The first level of MIT focuses on successful elicitation of verbal utterances. Level two of MIT focuses on elicitation of verbal utterances after a delay in cues from the speech-language pathologist. In the third and last level of MIT, the speech-language pathologist attempts to push the patient into producing more complex and spontaneous utterances while fading out the use of MIT cues and intonation patterns and slowly replacing them with normal prosody.

Constraint-Induced Aphasia Therapy

Similar to the idea once held that improvement of aphasia was not possible after the spontaneous recovery period, it was once believed that recovery from loss of movement in a limb affected by hemiplegia was not possible after a year post onset (Meinzer, Elbert, Djundja, Taub, & Rockstroh, 2007). However, studies of constraint-induced movement therapy (CIMT) dispute this. Studies initially in primates and then in humans document that, if an individual's method of compensation for a hemiplegic arm is constrained (by tying the intact arm behind the back, thereby forcing the patient to use the weakened limb), the individual's ability to use the hemiplegic hand and arm increases substantially. The underlying assumption of CIMT is reversal of **learned nonuse** (Lillie & Mateer, 2006), that individuals with hemiplegia can improve the movement of a weakened limb by using it instead of compensating for weakness by not using it enough to cue improvement.

The primary principles of constraint-induced movement therapy are the following:

- The use of constraints to restrict compensation for the target deficit
- Massed practice
- Shaping of the behavior

Given the success of CIMT, it was not long before researchers attempted to apply the same theoretical basis to aphasia therapy and created constraint-induced aphasia therapy (CIAT). CIAT applies the principles of CIMT to the rehabilitation of aphasia. Pulvermuller et al. (2001) give an example of CIAT in which they establish a card game with blind barriers set up between the individuals with aphasia. Participants with aphasia must request individual cards from each other and must verbally deny possessing cards not in their hand when asked by other participants (like Go Fish). A constraint in this game is use of the blind barrier that keeps participants with aphasia from compensating for their lack of verbal language production by using gestures or other nonverbal communication. This game was performed by participants intensively over time (massed practiced). As the individuals improved at the game, the speech-language pathologists increased the difficulty level of the tasks (shaping of behavior).

Although studies suggest that CIAT is successful (Meinzer et al., 2007; Pulvermuller et al., 2001), it is a relatively new approach to treating aphasia and research is still being conducted to determine its level of efficacy as compared with more traditional aphasia therapy approaches.

Errorless Learning Therapy

Most forms of learning are **errorful**, meaning people learn by trial and error. For example, in the forms of aphasia therapy discussed previously, patients with aphasia are allowed and expected to produce some number of errors on their way to relearning language production. This is because traditionally the difficulty level of therapy tasks is set just at or slightly above the ability level of the patient so that the patient must expend effort and strive for success.

The primary concept of errorless learning therapy is to prevent the individual with aphasia from producing any errors in therapy so as to avoid reinforcement of error production. Although the use of errorless learning is primarily supported in the realm of treating memory deficits, it has recently begun to be studied in the treatment of anomia (Fillingham, Sage, & Lambon Ralph, 2006; McKissock & Ward, 2007). For instance, say an individual with aphasia is shown a picture of a dog. He then tries to find and produce the appropriate word to name the object in the picture. However, by using trial and error he produces the word *cat* nine times before successfully finding and producing the word *dog*. In this simplified example, the patient has essentially practiced saying the word *cat* in response to a picture of a dog nine times more than he has practiced producing the word *dog* in response to the picture of the dog. In essence, he has practiced producing an error and, it is believed by some, the odds of him now saying the word *cat* in response to an image of a dog is greater than before.

Learned nonuse When an individual learns to compensate for a deficit by employing other intact abilities and, in doing so, ceases to exercise the physical or intellectual ability in which the deficit is present.

Errorful learning Learning in a way that produces some level of failure. Learning by trial and error.

It should be emphasized here that in any type of therapy, controlling and minimizing the number of errors patients produce is the role of the speech-language pathologist. What is different in errorless therapy is that the focus of therapy tasks is to elicit verbal production of language from the patient while avoiding any possibility of error production. An example of an errorless learning therapy task is when a patient is shown a picture of a dog 10 times and each time is told to say the word *dog*. Here, the patient has correctly produced the word *dog* 10 times in response to being shown a picture of a dog and has not practiced any errors.

To achieve errorless therapy for errorless learning, the difficulty level of therapy tasks is set very low so as to avoid any possibility of error production. Errorless learning therapy also uses large amounts of repetition and drill and difficulty level rises slowly over time only when the patient can succeed 100% at a higher level of difficulty.

Compensatory Therapy Approaches

The communicative needs of people with aphasia vary widely among individuals. Using restorative therapies alone is often inappropriate and the speech-language pathologist must concentrate on developing an augmentative or alternative form of communication (AAC), especially for individuals with severe to profound aphasia who might not regain functional speech.

Augmentative and Alternative Communication

The primary form of compensatory therapy used in aphasia is AAC. AAC strategies assist the person with aphasia to communicate by either replacing their language system entirely (alternative) or complementing their remaining language abilities (augmentative). AAC systems can be high tech or low tech.

Low-tech AAC strategies are often used at some point in rehabilitation. Common low-tech AAC strategies are having the patient use gestures, draw pictures, or point to pictures or symbols on a communication board or folder to communicate. High-tech AAC options include programmable voice-generating computer devices such as the Lingraphica. Lingraphica also recently released apps for the iPhone and iPad that allow a person with aphasia to use the iPhone or iPad in a similar manner to the Lingraphica system. A forerunner among these apps is Proloquo2Go.

Social Therapy Approaches

Individuals with aphasia often lose confidence in themselves as communicators. They can become isolated in their communities and may not engage others in conversation for fear of experiencing rejection when people discover and fail to understand their communication deficits. Social therapy approaches primarily address these types of problems. The goal of social therapy approaches is to reduce the limitations to communication in the lives of those with aphasia and to improve overall quality of life. This is accomplished by increasing the confidence level of the individual with aphasia as a speaker, increasing the opportunities the person has to communicate, and increasing the person's overall sense of being valued and accepted by others.

Communication Partner Training

In communication partner training, the spouses, caregivers, healthcare professionals, or other individuals in the everyday environment of those with aphasia are trained to facilitate the participation, language, or communication of the individual with aphasia. Communicative partner training is the most prevalent form of social therapy for aphasia (Simmons-Mackie, Raymer, Armstrong, Holland, & Cherney, 2010) and targets changing the behavior not of the individual with aphasia but of individuals in the environment of the person with aphasia. It is a form of manipulating the environment external to the person with aphasia. Some strategies often taught to communication partners are the following (Simmons-Mackie, 2008):

1. Speak slowly.
2. Pause between conversation topics.
3. Speak using shorter utterances and avoid long, complex sentences.
4. Repeat and rephrase often and when not understood.
5. Use gestures and facial expression to augment speech.
6. Paraphrase the utterances of the individual with aphasia back to him or her for confirmation to ensure you grasp the meaning of what the person is trying to say.
7. Use multiple modalities when communicating with an individual with aphasia, including

Author's Note

The Importance of Communicative Partner Training

It certainly is true that many nonaphasic speakers do not understand the communicative needs of those with aphasia, hence the importance of communication partner training. This might be surprising to students of speech-language pathology, but keep in mind that most people do not spend as great a portion of their lives thinking about aphasia as you do.

Recently, there walked into my clinic a delightful older married couple. About a year and a half before our meeting, the husband had experienced a stroke and became severely aphasic. After speaking on the phone with his wife, I had the impression that he had improved little, if at all, since his stroke. At our first therapy session, I, two student speech-language pathologists, and this couple sat face to face for an interview and a formal evaluation of the husband's aphasia deficits. In the interview, I became acutely aware that the wife answered every question asked, even those we directed to her husband. When I asked the wife to let him reply, she was able to restrain herself only a moment or two before interjecting her answers into her husband's burgeoning attempts to respond. Once his wife interjected her answers, the husband obediently sat back in his chair quietly off the hook.

I let the issue slide for a while. But after 15 minutes, I stole outside the therapy room, motioning the wife to follow me so that we could speak behind the two-way mirror that looked into the therapy room where her husband and the two students were. I made small talk with the wife and asked a few questions. This freed the husband to be interviewed without interruption by the students. Being deprived of the ability to answer questions put to her husband caused this very caring and very loving wife to be visibly nervous, bordering on agitated, but she did not want to be rude to me, so she answered my questions shortly while watching her husband through the glass out of the corner of her eye.

In less than 5 minutes, the anxiety had left the woman and in its place was a staring and pure dumbfounded amazement. Seemingly against all odds, in the very next room her husband was conversing quite well for a man with severe aphasia. In fact, he had come alive and was all talk with smiles and jokes whereas before he was morose and silent as a statue. What was the explanation? It was no miracle. The husband had certainly been aphasic after his stroke, but that was not why he was not speaking these days. The wife's look of joy and amazement quickly turned to a look of guilt and shame as she grasped the harsh reality of the situation. She had not heard her husband speak since his stroke simply because she never allowed him to speak. Unbeknown to his wife, the husband had recovered a great deal from his previously severe aphasia. Yet she, now so used to speaking for him, had continued speaking for him and, in doing so, kept him from speaking for himself. Therapy for this man primarily focused on pushing him to be an advocate for himself while also training his wife to be a more effective communication partner.

writing key words, to ensure comprehension and expression.

8. Always create equality in the relationship by allowing input from the person with aphasia.

9. Avoid speaking to people with aphasia in a pedagogic (teaching) fashion or tone of voice.

Often, the spouses or caregivers who communicate the most with the individual with aphasia do not realize how best to communicate or facilitate overall communication with their partner. In fact, communicative partner training often involves correcting inhibiting behaviors of individuals. The short anecdote in the preceding Author's Note provides a good example of the importance of creating equality in the relationship between speakers with aphasia and speakers without aphasia.

Group Therapy for Aphasia

A social therapy approach for aphasia is group therapy that includes multiple individuals with aphasia and perhaps even multiple speech-language pathologists. The social therapy approach to group therapy emphasizes a departure from the traditional speech-language pathologist–patient relationship. All participants in the group session, patients and speech-language pathologists alike, are equals and everyone participates equally. Persons with aphasia, though often lacking self-confidence in their communication abilities to speak or attempt to speak in front of a group of individuals without aphasia, are far less inhibited among others with similar problems. This dynamic creates a safe place for people with aphasia to speak in front of a group. This allows many therapeutic opportunities to occur that are not available with other therapy techniques. ▶ See the video *Living with Alzheimer's Disease* to hear a man and his wife talk about the value of the group therapy approach.

There is a strong psychoemotional component to group therapy. In most group sessions, individuals present with varying deficits at varying levels of severity. This dynamic allows those individuals with more recent strokes and often more severe aphasia to see and interact with other individuals who have already worked through the severe stage of recovery. Individuals still in the grip of severe aphasic deficits can use the model of someone else having been through what they are going through to establish hope that they can recover. Hope for recovery facilitates participation in therapy and improves the prognosis for recovery. Brookshire (2007) uses the term *psychosocial groups* to refer to these sessions and lists common group activities as follows:

- Roundtable discussions of emotions, attitudes, personal problems, or social issues
- Group problem-solving activities where members give advice to those seeking help with their personal and life issues
- Role playing to act out common situations and interactions
- Group activities such as language or memory games or field trips where everyone participates to build confidence and stimulate language abilities

A social approach to group therapy for those with aphasia allows many goals that must be left unaddressed in individual one-on-one therapy sessions to be targeted. Group therapy also allows persons with aphasia to practice refining their pragmatic language among peers and practice the functional use of the language and communication skills being retrained in individual therapy (carryover from individual therapy). In this way, speech-language pathologists often use group therapy sessions as a transition between direct restorative therapy sessions and the patient being sent back into the community. Group therapy sessions present opportunities for the speech-language pathologist to address the social therapy goals of increasing individuals' self-confidence as communicators, increasing their sense of self-value, and finally increasing opportunities for communication.

Main Points

- Aphasia is an acquired deficit in language as a result of brain damage. Aphasia is most often caused by a stroke to the left cerebral hemisphere. Aphasia is not the result of motor, intellectual, cognitive, or psychological impairment.
- Language deficits are grossly divided into expressive language deficits and receptive language deficits.
- Expressive language deficits are characterized by difficulty in formulating or producing language to communicate an intended meaning. Expressive language deficits are usually caused by lesions in the anterior left cerebral hemisphere often at or near Broca's area.
- Receptive language deficits are characterized by difficulty deriving meaning from verbal and/or written language. Receptive language deficits are usually caused by lesions in the posterior left hemisphere often at or near Wernicke's area.
- Signs and symptoms of aphasia include anomia, verbal comprehension deficits, paraphasias, perseveration, agrammatism, repetition deficits, alexia, and agraphia.
- Anomia is word-finding deficit.
- Verbal comprehension deficits are the inability to understand verbal language produced by others and are deficits of receptive language.
- Paraphasias are errors of expression that occur at the syllable, word, or phrase level and are produced unintentionally. A phonemic paraphasia is an error made at the phoneme level. A neologistic paraphasia is an error made when the word produced is entirely different from the word intended and is 50% or more indiscernible. A semantic paraphasia is when one word is substituted for another word that is similar in meaning. An unrelated verbal paraphasia is an error made when one word produced is substituted for another word that is not similar in meaning.
- A perseveration is a word that is said repeatedly and inappropriately. A perseverative paraphasia occurs when a word produced earlier is repeatedly and inadvertently produced by an individual with aphasia instead of the intended word.
- Agrammatism is the lack of appropriate grammatical construction of language. Agrammatical speech is caused by the omission of function words, which are the in-between words used to frame content words of a sentence. Content words are the words that carry most of the meaning. Agrammatical speech generally sounds telegraphic because few words are used, though the words are usually used with efficiency.
- Repetition deficits are caused by lesions along the arcuate fasciculus. The arcuate fasciculus consists of white matter pathways stretching between Broca's area and Wernicke's area.
- Alexia is an acquired impairment of reading. Agraphia is an acquired impairment in the ability to form letters or words for written language.
- Behaviors related to aphasia include self-repairs, speech disfluencies, struggle in nonfluent aphasias, and preserved or automatic language.
- Self-repairs occur when a speaker restates or revises a word or phrase to produce it error free or refine a word's meaning. Individuals with aphasia are unsuccessful at self-repair far more often than unimpaired individuals. Multiple unsuccessful attempts at self-repair often compromises the prosody and speech fluency of individuals with aphasia.
- Speech disfluencies produced by those with aphasia consist of sound, word, part-word, or phrase repetitions, prolongations, and interjections. These are normal disfluencies that escalate in frequency to pathological levels.
- Individuals with nonfluent aphasia often visibly show struggle when attempting to produce expression.

- Preserved language is the intact production of rote and overlearned language. This can include the ability to recite days of the week or months of the year or counting to 10.
- Automatic language is language that is associated with and produced somewhat reflexively in response to a stimulus.
- Some cognitive deficits that can co-occur with aphasia include problems with arousal, attention, short-term memory, problem solving, inferencing, and executive functioning skills.
- Some motor deficits that occur alongside aphasia and directly concern the speech-language pathologist include the dysarthrias, apraxia of speech, and also dysphagia.
- The cortical aphasias are those aphasias that arise as a result of damage to the cortex. The nonfluent cortical aphasias include Broca's aphasia, transcortical motor aphasia, and global aphasia.
- Broca's aphasia is the result of damage to the inferior posterior frontal lobe of the left hemisphere. Individuals with Broca's aphasia have mostly intact receptive language abilities with deficits in repetition and expression.
- Transcortical motor aphasia is a result of damage to the supplementary motor cortex or the area just anterior to Broca's area. Individuals with transcortical motor aphasia display mostly intact receptive language abilities and relatively intact repetition with deficits in expressive language.
- Global aphasia is a result of damage to a large area of the zone of language within the left cerebral hemisphere. Global aphasia is characterized by severe to profound deficits in expressive language, receptive language, and repetition.
- The fluent cortical aphasias include Wernicke's aphasia, transcortical sensory aphasia, conduction aphasia, and anomic aphasia.
- Wernicke's aphasia is a result of lesion to the cortex at or around Wernicke's area. Wernicke's aphasia is characterized by receptive language deficits, fluent but empty speech, and repetition deficits.
- Transcortical sensory aphasia is a result of damage just posterior to Wernicke's area. Transcortical sensory aphasia presents with deficits in receptive language, relatively intact repetition, and fluent and often empty speech resembling Wernicke's aphasia.
- Conduction aphasia is a result of damage to the supra marginal gyrus of the parietal lobe that is posterior to the sensory cortex above Wernicke's area. This damages the arcuate fasciculus, but leaves Broca's and Wernicke's areas intact. Conduction aphasia typically presents with relatively intact receptive and expressive language but with deficits in repetition.
- Anomic aphasia can result from damage anywhere within the language areas of the left hemisphere and is characterized by mild to moderate word-finding deficits in absence of other deficits.
- The subcortical aphasias are those aphasias that arise as a result of or alongside damage to the subcortex. The subcortical aphasias include thalamic and striatocapsular.
- Thalamic aphasia is a result of an ischemic stroke to the left side of the thalamus. Some signs include almost fluent speech, significant anomia in spontaneous speech, impaired receptive language, perseverative semantic paraphasias, normal articulation, hypophonic voice, intact repetition, and intact grammar.
- Striatocapsular aphasia is language deficits associated with lesion at the striatum of the basal ganglia but which occurs as a result of a lack of blood flow to the cortical language areas.
- Atypical aphasias include crossed aphasia and the primary progressive aphasias. The primary progressive aphasias are the result of a degenerative pathology rather than acute pathology and include progressive nonfluent aphasia and semantic dementia.

- Progressive nonfluent aphasia is a result of degeneration of the frontal lobes in the left hemisphere. Some signs include phonemic paraphasias, anomia, grammatical errors, slow speech rate, simplified syntax, reduced phrase length, and mostly intact receptive language.
- Semantic dementia is a result of degeneration that begins in the temporal lobes. Some signs include excessive and disinhibited verbal output, semantic jargon, pragmatic deficits, significant anomia, and questioning the meaning of words.
- Crossed aphasia is when damage to the language-dominant hemisphere is ipsilateral to the individuals writing hand and therefore does not impair motor functioning of the individuals writing hand.
- Assessment of aphasia usually includes the following: a case history, assessment of functional communication and speech, a standardized aphasia test (or the administration of formal diagnostic tasks), and a cognitive evaluation.
- Aphasia therapy facilitates spontaneous recovery. Spontaneous recovery can occur up to 6 months post onset.
- The three categories of aphasia therapy are restorative, compensatory, and social.
- Restorative approaches are based on the idea of neuroplasticity. Neuroplasticity is the ability of a part of the brain to change its function to take on a new role.
- Restorative approaches include Schuell's stimulation therapy, melodic intonation therapy, constraint-induced therapy, and errorless learning.
- Schuell's stimulation therapy reestablishes lost language abilities through the use of auditory stimuli to evoke a response.
- Melodic intonation therapy is the use of the intact melodic/prosodic processing of the right hemisphere to cue word retrieval and production in the left hemisphere.
- Constraint-induced therapy constrains a patient's ability to compensate for deficits and forces the person to use the weakened skills, thereby directly exercising and improving the areas of weakness.
- Errorless learning therapy is a technique that focuses on reducing the number of errors produced by patients in therapy by setting the difficulty of therapy tasks very low for the client to succeed.
- Compensatory approaches enable patients to increase their level of function despite their deficit.
- Compensatory approaches for aphasia usually take the form of augmentative and alternative communication (AAC).
- Compensatory approaches can include both low-tech techniques and high-tech AAC devices. Low-tech techniques include gestures, drawings, and pointing to pictures on a communication board. High-tech devices include programmable voice-generating computers such as Lingraphica as well as applications for the iPhone and iPad.
- Social approaches revolve around increasing an individual's self-confidence, opportunities to communicate, and overall sense of value and acceptance as a communicator.
- Social approaches include communication partner training and group therapy.
- Communication partner training changes the behavior of those in the environment who most interact with those with aphasia to facilitate the communication of the person with aphasia.
- Group therapy is a dynamic setting in which hope, psychosocial emotional support, pragmatics, self-confidence, and additional goals are addressed with multiple clients and clinicians present. Group therapy for those with aphasia allows for the targeting of many goals, such as pragmatics, left unaddressed in individual one-on-one therapy sessions.

Review Questions

1. Define aphasia.
2. How are phonemic, neologistic, semantic, and unrelated verbal paraphasias different from one another?
3. How might self-repairs produced by a person with aphasia reduce fluency?
4. What are three cognitive and three motor deficits that can co-occur with aphasia?
5. Why is it useful to use a classification system for the aphasias?
6. Detail the three cortical nonfluent aphasias, their lesion location(s), and signs/symptoms of each.
7. Explain the role of the arcuate fasciculus in conduction aphasia.
8. Detail the four cortical fluent aphasias, their lesion location(s), and signs/symptoms of each.
9. Detail two subcortical aphasias, their lesion location(s), and signs/symptoms of each.
10. How might a lesion at the striatum be associated with aphasia?
11. Why is it important to recognize crossed aphasia?
12. What should be included during an aphasia assessment? Why is each component important?
13. Why is neuroplasticity important to aphasia rehabilitation?
14. How does aphasia therapy facilitate spontaneous recovery?
15. What are the three categories of aphasia therapy? Give an example of each.
16. How does Schuell's stimulation therapy differ from melodic intonation therapy?
17. How does constraint-induced therapy differ from errorless learning?
18. How might learned nonuse inhibit rehabilitation?
19. Why is communication partner training important?
20. How does group therapy facilitate hope and recovery?

References

1. Albert, M., Sparks, R., & Helm, N. (1973). Melodic intonation therapy for aphasia. *Archives of Neurology, 29,* 130–131.
2. Brookshire, R. (2007). *Introduction to neurogenic communication disorders* (7th ed.). St. Louis, MO: Mosby-Elsevier.
3. Brown, G., & Cullinan, W. (1981). Word-retrieval difficulties and disfluent speech in adult anomic speakers. *Journal of Speech and Hearing Research, 24,* 358–365.
4. Chapey, R., & Hallowell, B. (2001). Introduction to language intervention strategies in adult aphasia. In R. Chapey (Ed.), *Language intervention strategies in aphasia and related neurogenic communication disorders* (4th ed., pp. 341–382). New York, NY: Lippincott Williams & Wilkins.
5. Chow, T., Miller, M., Hayashi, V., & Geschwind, D. (1999). Inheritance of frontotemporal dementia. *Archives of Neurology, 56,* 817–822.
6. Coelho, C., Sinotte, M., & Duffy, J. (2008). Schuell's stimulation approach to rehabilitation. In R. Chapey (Ed.), *Language intervention strategies in aphasia and related neurogenic communication disorders* (5th ed., pp. 403–449). New York, NY: Lippincott Williams & Wilkins.
7. Farmer, A. (1977). Self-correctional strategies in the conversational speech of aphasics and nonaphasic brain damaged adults. *Cortex, 13,* 327–334.
8. Fillingham, J., Hodgson, C., Sage, K., & Lambon Ralph, M. (2003). The application of errorless learning to aphasic disorders: A review of theory and practice. *Aphasiology, 13*(3), 337–363.

9. Fillingham, J., Sage, K., & Lambon Ralph, M. (2006). The treatment of anomia using errorless learning. *Neuropsychological Rehabilitation, 16*(2), 129–154.

10. Freedman, M., Alexander, M., & Naeser, M. (1984). Anatomic basis of transcortical motor aphasia. *Neurology, 34*, 409–417.

11. Goodglass, H., & Kaplan, E. (1972). *The assessment of aphasia and related disorders*. Philadelphia, PA: Lea and Febiger.

12. Goodglass, H., Kaplan, E., & Barresi, B. (2001a). *Boston Diagnostic Aphasia Examination* (3rd ed.). Baltimore, MD: Lippincott Williams & Wilkins.

13. Goodglass, H., Kaplan, E., & Barresi, B. (2001b). *The assessment of aphasia and related disorders* (3rd ed.). Baltimore, MD: Lippincott Williams & Wilkins.

14. Hallowell, B., Chapey, R. (2001). Introduction to language intervention strategies in adult aphasia. In R. Chapey (Ed.). *Language intervention strategies in aphasia and related neurogenic communication disorders* (4th ed.) (pp. 341–382). New York, NY: Lippincott Williams & Wilkins.

15. Halwes, T. (2000). Schuell's aphasia therapy. Retrieved from http://www.dharma-haven.org/five-havens/schuell.htm

16. Halpern, H., Goldfarb, R. (2013). Language and motor speech disorders in adults (3rd ed.). Burlington, MA: Jones & Bartlett Learning.

17. Helm-Estabrooks, N. (1992). *Aphasia diagnostic profiles*. Austin, TX: Pro-Ed.

18. Helm-Estabrooks, N., & Albert, M. (1991). *Manual of aphasia therapy*. Austin, TX: Pro-Ed.

19. Holland, A., Frattali, C., & Fromm, D. (1999). *Communication activities of daily living* (2nd ed.). Austin, TX: Pro-Ed.

20. Kertesz, A. (2006). *Western Aphasia Battery: Revised*. San Antonio, TX: Pearson Publishing.

21. Kertesz, A., Jesso, S., Harciarek, M., Blair, M., & McMonagle, P. (2009). What is semantic dementia?: A cohort study of diagnostic features and clinical boundaries. *Archives of Neurology, 67*(4), 483–489.

22. Kertesz, A., Sheppard, A., & MacKenzie, R. (1982). Localization in transcortical sensory aphasia. *Archives of Neurology, 39*(8), 475–478.

23. Knibb, J., Woollams, A., Hodges, J., & Patterson, K. (2009). Making sense of progressive non-fluent aphasia: An analysis of conversational speech. *Brain, 132*, 2734–2746.

24. Krulwich, R. (2010, June 21). The writer who couldn't read. *Krulwich wonders: An NPR science blog*. National Public Radio.

25. Kuljic-Obradovic, D. C. (2003). Subcortical aphasia: Three different language disorder syndromes? *European Journal of Neurology, 10*, 445–448.

26. Levelt, W. J. M. (1983). Monitoring and self-repair in speech. *Cognition, 14*, 41–104.

27. Lillie, R., Mateer, C. (2006). Constraint-based therapies as a proposed model for cognitive rehabilitation. *Journal of Head Trauma Rehabilitation, 2*(21), 119–130.

28. Liss, J. M. (1998). Error-revision in the spontaneous speech of apraxic speakers. *Brain and Language, 62*, 342–360.

29. Luria, A. R. (1972). *The man with a shattered world*. Cambridge, MA: Harvard University Press.

30. Marshall, R., & Tomkins, C. (1982). Verbal self-correction behaviors of fluent and non-fluent aphasic subjects. *Brain and Language, 15*, 292–306.

31. McKissock, S., & Ward, J. (2007). Do errors matter? Errorless and errorful learning in anomic picture naming. *Neuropsychological Rehabilitation, 17*(17), 355–373.

32. McMillan, A., Gunawardena, D., Avants, B., Morgan, B., Gee, J., & Grossman, M. (2010). Speech errors in progressive non-fluent aphasia. *Brain and Language, 113*(1), 13–20.

33. Meinzer, M., Elbert, T., Djundja, D., Taub, E., & Rockstroh, B. (2007). Extending the constraint-induced movement therapy (CIMT) approach to cognitive functions: Constraint-induced aphasia therapy (CIAT) of chronic aphasia. *NeuroRehabilitation, 22*, 311–318.

34. Nadeau, S., & Crosson, B. (1997). Subcortical aphasia. *Brain and Language, 58*, 355–402.

35. Nadeau, S. E., & Gonzalez Rothi, L. J. (2008). Rehabilitation of subcortical aphasia. In R. Chapey (Ed.), *Language intervention strategies in aphasia and related neurogenic communication disorders* (5th ed.). New York, NY: Lippincott Williams & Wilkins.

36. Nestor, P., Graham, N., Fryer, T., Williams, G., Patterson, K., & Hodges, J. (2003). Progressive non-fluent aphasia is associated with hypometabolism centered on the left anterior insula. *Brain, 126*(11), 2406–2418.

37. Norton, A., Zipse, L., Marchina, S., Schlaug, G. (2009). Melodic intonation therapy: Shared insights on how it is done and why it might help. *Ann N Y Acad Sci, 1169*, 431–436.

38. Pulvermuller, E., Neininger, B., Elbert, X., Mohr, B., Rockstroh, B., & Iaub, I. (2001). Constraint-induced therapy of chronic aphasia following stroke. *Stroke, 32*, 1621–1626.

39. Rosamond, W., Flegal, K., Furie, K., Go, A., Greenlund, K., Haase, N., . . . American Heart Association Statistics

Committee and Stroke Statistics Subcommittee. (2008). Heart disease and stroke statistics: 2008 update. *Circulation, 117*, e25–e146. Retrieved from http://circ.ahajournals.org/content/117/4/e25.full

40. Shipley, G., McAfee, J. (2009). Assessment in Speech-Language Pathology (4th ed.). Clifton Park, NY: Delmar, Cengage Learning.

41. Simmons-Mackie, N. (2008). Social approaches to aphasia intervention. In. R. Chapey (Ed.), *Language intervention strategies in aphasia and related neurogenic communication disorders* (2nd ed.). Philadelphia, PA: Lippincott Williams & Wilkins.

42. Simmons-Mackie, N., Raymer, A., Armstrong, E., Holland, A., & Cherney, L. (2010). Communication partner training in aphasia: A systematic review. *Archives of Physical Medicine and Rehabilitation, 91*, 1814–1837.

43. Swiburn, K., Porter, G., & Howard, D. (2004). *Comprehensive aphasia test*. New York, NY: Psychology Press.

44. Tanner, D., & Culbertson, W. (1999). *Quick assessment for aphasia*. Oceanside, CA: Academic Communication Associates.

45. Whitney, J., & Goldstein, H. (1989). Using self-monitoring to reduce disfluencies in speakers with mild aphasia. *Journal of Speech and Hearing Disorders, 54*, 576–586.

Chapter 5

Right Hemisphere Disorders

▶ *Where this icon appears, visit http://go.jblearning.com/ManascoCWS to view the corresponding video.*

Damage to the right cerebral hemisphere produces some of the most strange and bizarre deficits and behaviors seen in brain-damaged populations. For instance, these patients might be unable to acknowledge their deficits, even when profound. They might be unable to process sensory information coming from the left side of their body or the left side of their environment and in extreme cases are incapable of even grasping the concept that there is a left side of the environment. They can believe that their loved ones have been replaced by identical imposters. They might have vivid hallucinations, depression, delusions, or display any number of other behaviors or problems.

Until the last 30 years, the history of the study of the brain has largely been the history of the study of the left hemisphere. Paul Broca's and Carl Wernicke's discoveries of the localization of language abilities to the left hemisphere led to a century of exploration of left hemisphere abilities while the right hemisphere,

Author's Note

History of the Right Hemisphere

A large part of the historical hyperfocus on the left hemisphere and the loss of language following damage to it must surely be the result of how easily left hemisphere disorders are to conceive and, therefore, to acknowledge for study. It is simple to imagine the loss of language. Students new to speech-language pathology grasp the idea of aphasia almost immediately. It is as straightforward as this: I had an apple, and then I lost my apple; now I am appleless.

But how are we to imagine and make suitable as a subject for study the loss of something far more fundamental to the human experience such as the ability to recognize one's own body, the ability to recognize the existence of the left side of one's environment, or the belief that one's family and loved ones are genuine and have not been replaced by aliens? I have spent entire class periods with students peppering me with deep and penetrating questions regarding the nature of right hemisphere disorders. The existence of these disorders can lead to deep scientific and philosophical contemplation regarding human perception of the world and what is in it. It is no surprise that scientists conveniently ignored this entire half of the brain for a hundred years.

despite being half of the brain, was virtually ignored. Whereas the left hemisphere was deemed the "unique flower of human evolution" (Sacks, 1970, p. 2), the right hemisphere was referred to, often contemptuously, as the *subordinate*, *minor*, or *unconscious* hemisphere. As previously mentioned, neglect of the right hemisphere ended in the 1960s when a surgery known as corpus commissurotomy, which involves cutting the corpus callosum to relieve intractable seizures, allowed for the study of the capabilities of each cerebral hemisphere independent from the other (Myers, 2009).

Normal Right Hemisphere Function

Whereas the left hemisphere is dominant in language processing, the right hemisphere nonetheless plays very important roles in communication. The right hemisphere processes certain nonlinguistic and emotional elements of communication. These nonlinguistic elements of communication include prosody and facial expression, gesture, and body language. The ability to understand the meaning of the prosodic qualities of speech and the facial expressions of others is a very important social skill. This skill, together with body language, allows us to comprehend the ever important emotion behind verbal language and the true and intended meaning of spoken language. Without knowledge of the emotional content of an utterance, the true meaning of the communication is likely to be lost or misinterpreted. For instance, sometimes the emotion with which a speaker delivers words can be more relevant than the literal meaning of the words.

The right hemisphere also plays very important roles in math and visuospatial skills such as perception of depth, perception of distance, perception of shapes, localizing targets in space, and identifying figure–ground relationships (Joseph, 1988). This hemisphere is responsible for processing the melody of

music. The right hemisphere also puts together the many small details for the perception of a larger picture (i.e., the macrostructure, or gestalt).

Something for speech-language pathologists to remember is that the cerebral hemispheres do not normally operate in isolation but in tandem. Connectionist theories suggest that different areas of the brain normally all work together to accomplish a single purpose. This includes the two cerebral hemispheres. Although one hemisphere might play a dominant role in a task, the processes of one hemisphere support and augment processes in the opposite hemisphere. As the saying goes, it takes two to tango, and this is true in the normal functioning of the brain.

The Right Hemisphere's Role in Communication

Right hemisphere disorders are a group of deficits or changes that occur following insult to the right cerebral hemisphere. Note that a group disorders—not a single disorder—is being discussed here. Typically, right hemisphere disorders are not involved in linguistic (language-related) deficits. An individual who has experienced a right hemisphere stroke might still have intact and functional language abilities because those skills localized in the left cerebral hemisphere remain untouched. Nonetheless, just because an individual's language abilities are intact does not mean the person has no difficulties communicating. There is certainly a great deal more to communication than language. A study by Glosser, Wiener, and Kaplan (1988) indicates that speakers with aphasia can use their intact right hemisphere functions of processing nonlinguistic cues (i.e., prosody, body language, facial expression) to communicate with others (to some degree) despite their language deficits. So, these are powerful means used to communicate, and when the right hemisphere is damaged and the ability to process these signals is lost it can significantly impair an individual's social pragmatic communication abilities.

Also, the right hemisphere regulates many cognitive functions that subserve language, such as sustained and selective attention that make effective linguistic communication possible. A loss of these cognitive processes that normally creates a mental state where effective linguistic communication is possible negatively affects an individual's ability to use intact language skills.

Etiology of Right Hemisphere Disorders

The source of damage to the brain that is most often responsible for right hemisphere damage is stroke. In aphasia, the stroke occurs in the left hemisphere. In right hemisphere disorders, the stroke obviously occurs in the right hemisphere.

Different etiologies of right hemisphere damage create different deficits. The level of deficit or disorder

Author's Note

Right Hemisphere Disorder

I was working in a hospital when I received a referral from nursing to evaluate Mrs. T. after she experienced a left hemisphere stroke. Upon walking in and introducing myself, I was surprised to find Mrs. T. speaking quite well for someone who had experienced a left hemisphere stroke. What a lucky woman, I thought to myself as I began my evaluation of aphasia and cognition, assured that I would find no evidence of deficits.

Mrs. T. was very alert. She excelled on the language portions of my evaluation. I would even go as far as to say that she blew the language portions of my test out of the water. I was a busy speech-language pathologist and did not need to waste anymore time evaluating this woman, who so clearly had come through her stroke remarkably unscathed. I reasoned that I would finish the present task we were doing, do a quick picture description task so that I could get a better sense of her connected speech, and then I would call it quits, congratulate her on her luck, and hurry off to my next appointment.

I pulled out the Cookie Theft picture from my copy of the Boston Diagnostic Aphasia Examination (see **Figure 5-1**) and showed it to Mrs. T. with the simple request, "Tell me what you see here." In contrast to what I was expecting, which was a fluent and accurate description of the picture, the response I received gave me quite a shock.

A person with a nonfluent aphasia understands perfectly what is going on in the picture but can have difficulty finding the appropriate words to describe it. A person with a fluent aphasia might begin strong by describing what is going on in the picture but then might quickly jump to an unrelated topic, and then another, and then another. However, Mrs. T. was not aphasic in any way, as I had already surmised from her evaluation so far.

Mrs. T. looked at the picture and without a pause launched into her response:

> The woman washing dishes is the wife. The boy on the stool is her husband. The girl standing behind the boy on the stool is the husband's mistress with whom he is having an illicit love affair. Together they are pulling the microwave out of the cabinet to hit his wife over the head with to kill her. Next, they plan on pulling her body through the window and burying her in the backyard. They are doing this so they can run off and be happy together.

Upon finishing, Mrs. T. sat back against her pillow, apparently very pleased with herself for giving such a thorough answer. Meanwhile, I sat confused and shocked. This was not the answer a woman with a left hemisphere stroke would give, but one of a patient with right hemisphere stroke. I returned to the nursing station and, after making some phone calls and researching, found, indeed, that Mrs. T.'s chart was incorrect—somehow the misinformation had appeared during her transfer between the nursing home and the hospital. I was certainly surprised at Mrs. T.'s gross misinterpretation of the Cookie Theft picture, but more so, I was shocked that I had almost allowed this woman with profound deficits to pass unrecognized through my evaluation.

So, let me dissect her response. Of course, Mrs. T. gave a gross misinterpretation of the image. Was her answer thorough and complete? Yes, it was. Was her answer well stated? Very much so. She clearly was not aphasic in any sense of the word. But was her response appropriate? Not by a long shot! How did Mrs. T. make such grievous errors? One explanation is that because of the stroke she experienced in her right hemisphere Mrs. T. had a deficit in her ability to perceive individual details and then piece them together appropriately to generate an accurate comprehension of the picture. One disorder she might have been displaying here is simultagnosia (discussed later). Simultagnosia is an inability to perceive appropriately many visual details

together (simultaneously). I could also assume that she displayed a deficit in her ability to put together a correct perception of the whole (inferencing deficit leading to a loss of macrostructure, also discussed later). In other words, she was unable to perceive all the individual details of the picture and put them together correctly in her head to create a correct understanding of the meaning of the entire picture.

Mrs. T. was able to perceive some details correctly such as the gender of the people in the picture. However, some details she gathered were erroneous, for instance, she mistook the cookie jar for a microwave. Once she had gathered what details she could, she attempted to make sense of the picture. In doing so, she came to a grossly incorrect conclusion regarding what is happening in the picture. She was also perfectly oblivious to her substantial and tragic errors, indicating possible anosognosia (discussed later) probably with a healthy dose of impulsivity and lack of reflection on one's performance thrown in for good measure.

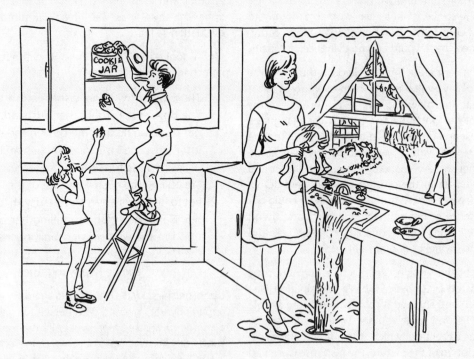

Figure 5-1 The Cookie Theft.

Source: From Boston *Diagnostic Aphasia Examination*—Third Edition (BDAE-3), by Goodglass, H. in collaboration with Kaplan, E. and Barresi, B., 2001, Austin, TX: PRO-ED. Copyright 2001 by PRO-ED, Inc. Reprinted with permission.

an individual with right hemisphere damage displays depends on the location and extent of the damage. A small focal right hemisphere stroke can produce a very specific deficit and leave most other cognitive and perceptual processes intact, whereas a very large stroke in the right hemisphere more than likely results in multiple profound deficits.

Any etiology that damages the right hemisphere, such as trauma, disease, seizure disorders, infection, and toxicity, can produce right hemisphere deficits. When both hemispheres are damaged it is common to have left hemisphere deficits such as aphasia present simultaneously with right hemisphere deficits. This is often the case in traumatic brain injury or multiple strokes.

Right Hemisphere Damage versus Aphasia

It is beneficial in a discussion of right hemisphere disorders to draw a distinct line between right hemisphere disorders and aphasia. The preceding Author's Note is a description of a patient who displays deficits associated with right hemisphere damage. This is merely one possible manifestation of right hemisphere damage. In reality, very rarely are the deficit profiles of any two individuals with right hemisphere damage (or aphasia) exactly alike. Most disorders present in a myriad of combinations in a myriad of ways, and furthermore the patient can react to deficits in any number of ways.

Deficits and Syndromes Following Right Hemisphere Damage

Now that a general picture of the possible manifestation of right hemisphere disorders has been illustrated, this section provides a more detailed

Table 5-1 Disorders and Deficits Associated with Right Hemisphere Damage

Communication Deficits
Facial recognition (prosopagnosia)
Comprehending facial expressions and expressing using facial expressions
Prosodic deficits
Inferencing deficits
Discourse deficits
Visuoperceptual Deficits
Simultagnosia
Cerebral achromatopsia
Attentional Deficits
Neglect
Sustained and selective attention deficits
Neuropsychiatric Disorders
Anosognosia
Depression
Capgras delusion
Visual hallucinations
Paranoid hallucinations

discussion of the relevant individual disorders that might present. However, fair warning is issued to the reader: How the right hemisphere functions is relatively poorly understood as are many of the problems that arise from damage to it. Many different disorders and deficits are associated with right hemisphere damage, and most are known by many different names. Often, these deficits are interpreted differently by different people depending on discipline and theoretical point of view. To be as clear as possible, I list in Table 5-1 the individual conditions (deficits or symptoms of a greater problem) that are discussed in this chapter. Although some of the conditions discussed fit nicely into multiple categories, I have tried to reach a functional presentation of the material for the early speech-pathology student.

Communication Deficits

Communication deficits resulting from right hemisphere damage often work together to create communication difficulties that manifest primarily in the realm of pragmatics. Others often perceive individuals with right hemisphere damage as odd and difficult to communicate with. The manifestation of pragmatic deficits in communication is more subtle than the wholesale language deficits of those with aphasia.

Facial Recognition (Prosopagnosia)

The ability of a human to recognize a familiar face is of great importance. Aside from the obvious social-pragmatic functions of recognizing faces, consider the use of this ability in basic survival. Imagine a Paleolithic man who has to get close enough to another person to hear that person's voice to know whether it is a friend or foe. This poor man probably would not last long. Or imagine a young child lost in a crowded mall, unable to recognize the face of his mother. In both of these situations, the ability to recognize familiar faces is a basic survival tool used to discriminate familiar individuals from unfamiliar and potentially threatening individuals.

The ability to process visual information about facial features and the spatial relationships between them and then to use that information to recognize a person is a skill that humankind has developed and specialized in for a millennia. It is also a skill that, like all skills, can be lost. **Visual agnosia** is a general term used to describe an inability to perceive visual stimuli appropriately as a result of damage to the central nervous system and not peripheral damage to the eyes or optic nerve.

Visual agnosia An inability to appropriately perceive visual stimuli resulting from damage to the central nervous system, not peripheral damage to the eyes or optic nerve.

When the specific ability to recognize faces is lost, in the absence of any other visual agnosia, it is known as prosopagnosia. Prosopagnosia is a deficit specifically in the ability to recognize faces. In severe cases, this can manifest as an individual's inability to recognize the faces of even close loved ones. It is important to emphasize that the individual's eyes are working fine, but the brain is having trouble because the visual association cortex within the occipital lobe that processes and interprets visual information from the eyes regarding faces has been damaged. Individuals with true prosopagnosia have no difficulty recognizing any other objects other than faces. Although individuals affected with prosopagnosia might not recognize a familiar person by sight of the face, they can still recognize a person by voice, smell, clothing, or other distinctive features of the individual.

Comprehending Facial Expressions and Expressing Using Facial Expressions

The conclusion that the right hemisphere allows people to properly evaluate facial expressions is based on the observation that those with right hemisphere lesions are less adept at interpreting facial expressions correctly (Benowitz et al., 1983; Blonder, Bowers, & Heilman, 1991; Bowers, Bauer, Coslett, & Heilman, 1985; DeKosky, Heilman, Bowers, & Valenstein, 1983; Harciarek & Heilman, 2009). Individuals with right hemisphere damage are less adept at correctly identifying the emotions being conveyed on the faces of speakers. Of course, this deficit in processing emotional expression of faces is intertwined with prosopagnosia.

The importance of facial expression in verbal communication should not be underestimated. Facial expression can be used, as prosody may, to reinforce or to completely alter the meaning of a verbal utterance. The inability to process the emotions expressed on the face restricts an individual to a less informed and more literal interpretation of verbal utterances.

Individuals with right hemisphere damage might also have deficits in their ability to use their face for the appropriate expression of emotion (Blonder, Burns, Bowers, Moore, & Heilman, 1993; Borod,

Koff, Lorch, & Nicholas, 1986). The right cerebral hemisphere controls the left side of the face. As it turns out, in general people display more emotional expression on the left side of their faces than on the right side of their faces (Sackheim, Gur, & Saucy, 1978). Therefore, damage to the right cerebral hemisphere can limit expressivity on the most expressive portion of the face. As a result, individuals with right hemisphere damage can present with a flat facial affect and reduced facial expression. It should come as no surprise that the social interactions of these individuals suffer if they cannot correctly interpret the emotions on the faces of others and cannot correctly use their face to express their own emotions.

Prosodic Deficits

Speech contains a linguistic component—the language used—as well as an additional layer of meaning on top of the actual words spoken: prosody. Prosody is the changes in pitch, stress, timbre, cadence, and tempo a person uses to infuse spoken words with emotional content (Tucker, Watson, & Heilman, 1977). In other words, humans hear the words that are said and how the words are said and consider this additional information when determining the overall meaning of the utterance.

Individuals with right hemisphere damage, specifically parietotemporal damage of the right hemisphere, have difficulty comprehending the emotional content of speech because they cannot process the prosodic component of speech (Heilman, Scholes, & Watson, 1975; Tucker et al., 1977). As a result of this deficit, they perform poorly at appropriately identifying the emotion behind a speaker's utterances, which leads to very literal interpretations of verbal language. A too literal interpretation of language can lead to misinterpretation or an entire lack of comprehension of figurative language such as sarcasm and idiom. These misinterpretations negatively affect the communication and create negative social experiences for the person with right hemisphere disfunction.

In addition to difficulties interpreting prosody, those with right hemisphere damage also have difficulty using prosody to express their own emotions (Tucker et al., 1977; Weintraub, Mesulam, & Kramer, 1981). As a result, listeners often perceive them as monotone and expressionless. Although these individuals can appear emotionless, they still possess the full range of emotions but cannot express them. Speech-language pathologists must realize that individuals with right hemisphere damage, despite not seeming to be upset, can be on the verge of an emotional crisis without giving any external sign because of their deficits in prosody.

Inferencing Deficits

Possibly underlying many manifestations of right hemisphere damage are inferencing deficits. Inferencing is the ability to take previous knowledge and experience and apply it to the interpretation of the meaning of details in a situation. This ability allows for the appropriate perception of macrostructure. Perception of macrostructure (or gestalt) is the accurate interpretation of the overall meaning of stimuli indicated by the details. The inability to read facial expressions is rooted partly in the inability to infer the meaning of the facial expressions. Also, the appropriate perception of humor, sarcasm, and other nonliteral expression is rooted in a person's ability to interpret the information in a nonliteral sense and infer the true meaning of the expression. For example, when given a complex picture or photograph to interpret, individuals with right hemisphere disorder often seem to perseverate on individual details of the picture without grasping the overall whole. An example of this is Mrs. T.'s gross misinterpretation described earlier. However, more often than not, individuals with right hemisphere disorders seem to get stuck on individual details of a picture and cannot form any overall interpretation of a picture, even an incorrect one. See the following Author's Note for another example.

Discourse Deficits

All the disorders discussed in this chapter contribute to the inability of the person with right hemisphere damage to participate effectively in discourse. Discourse is the exchange of communicative information between a speaker and a listener. Discourse involves a speaker, a listener, and the given situational context in which the exchange occurs. Myers (2009) states that for discourse to be effective participants must be aware of the following items and possess the following abilities:

- The general topic of the discourse
- The purpose for which the discourse is occurring
- The presence and limits of any knowledge shared between the participants in the discourse
- The cultural background of participants and the cultural appropriateness regarding the expression of certain ideas and emotions that might be perceived as taboo
- The ability to perceive breakdowns in the communicative exchange and make appropriate repairs
- The ability to make the appropriate inferences to comprehend the true meaning of the discourse

> **Discourse** The exchange of communicative information between a speaker and a listener or the back and forth among individuals participating in conversation.

Individuals with right hemisphere damage generally neglect the parameters of effective discourse. For instance, attentional deficits can limit a person's

---

Author's Note

Lack of Macrostructure/Gestalt and Discourse Deficits

Recently, during an evaluation of an older person, I cracked open a current edition of *National Geographic* (known for its visually complex photography, among other things) and found a humorous picture of a field mouse perched precariously and devastatingly high (for a mouse) above ground between two stems of green wheat against a beautiful blue sky. This mouse was acrobatically doing the splits, with its hind legs stretched between two tall stems of wheat, while using its front paws to munch placidly on a piece of grain. The outrageous physical position of the mouse contrasted with its apparently Zen-like calm as it ate makes this photo striking and humorous to any typical viewer. I placed the picture in front of this patient with right hemisphere damage and asked him to describe what he saw. His response was as follows:

> Well... what is that? It is an animal of some sort. Furry, brown, and with claws. The animal might be holding something. There is grass and sky. Probably a pretty day to go for a walk. I used to walk a lot with my daughter on good days. We've had a lot of good days this winter. Used to be 10 feet of snow around this time....

I prompted the patient by asking if there was anything funny or out of the ordinary about what was happening in the picture. He restated the details he had already observed and failed to perceive anything more about the photo. This patient displayed a very good example of a lack of perception of the macrostructure of the picture. He perceived a series of individual details that he was unable to piece together to realize that the central figure with brown fur and claws was a mouse or that the photo was taken in a field, much less the overarching theme of the humorous position of the mouse. Furthermore, he displayed discourse deficits in the form of inappropriate tangential utterances by speaking about his own experiences on pretty days, insensitive to the fact that he had steered well off course of the original topic of conversation, and that it was inappropriate to do so. This example gives a good indication of how multiple deficits can interact while a patient is producing a single response.

knowledge of the general topic of conversation. Lack of perception of the nonlinguistic affective features of communication (prosody, body language, facial expression) as well as lack of ability to make appropriate inferences reduce the person's ability to access the true purpose and true meaning of the discourse. The person with right hemisphere damage also might be limited in ability to infer the presence of any shared knowledge among communication partners, and as a result, those with right hemisphere damage are often perceived as pedantic or as stating the obvious. A reduced sensitivity to discourse can result in the person's inattention to breakdowns in conversation and lack of understanding of the need to make conversational repairs. Myers (2009) lists the most common discourse deficits of those with right hemisphere damage:

- Lack of sensitivity to shared knowledge
- Difficulties with turn-taking in conversation
- Difficulties with topic maintenance

Visuoperceptual Deficits

Simultagnosia

Often, those with lesions in the right parietal-occipital areas display a form of apperceptive visual agnosia known as simultagnosia. **Simultagnosia** is the inability to visually perceive many details at once, or simultaneously. As a result, individuals with simultagnosia might perseverate on individual details of a picture or object and cannot see how these details fit into the whole. Simultagnosia exists only in the visual processing domain. Although individuals with this disorder might be unable to recognize an object visually by the sum of its details, they might be able to make an accurate guess based on any distinctive features. For instance, a person with simultagnosia cannot perceive all the visual details of a coffee cup but recognizes the handle as the kind that might be on a coffee cup, and then may correctly infer that the object is a coffee cup. Also, if given the object to feel, the person can experience the object's features in a tactile sense, not a visual one, and might readily be able to perceive the object as a whole.

Of course, this disorder contributes to the macrostructure difficulties of a person with right hemisphere damage. In fact, simultagnosia is similar to prosopagnosia in that it is an inability to perceive simultaneously many individual details for perception and recognition of a whole visual image. It is likely that these two disorders share an underlying pathologic mechanism.

Cerebral Achromatopsia

Achromatopsia, also known as color agnosia, is color blindness. There are congenital as well as acquired forms of achromatopsia. The acquired form, cerebral achromatopsia, is rare and often results from trauma or damage to the cortex usually in the right cerebral hemisphere. Individuals with this disorder typically report that they see the world in shades of gray.

Attentional Deficits

Neglect

Neglect, also known as unilateral neglect, refers to a person's inability to attend to sensory stimuli from one side of the body or the environment. The side of the body or environment that is left unattended and unrecognized is contralateral to the damaged cerebral hemisphere. Because neglect is most often associated with right hemisphere lesions, the most commonly neglected side of the body or environment is the left side. However, right-side neglect has been noted following left hemisphere lesions, though it

---

Simultagnosia A neurologic disorder that produces the inability to visually perceive many details at once.

Achromatopsia Color blindness, also known as color agnosia.

Neglect A general term used to describe a deficit in the ability to attend to sensory stimuli from one side of the body or the environment.

Body neglect A deficit in the ability to attend to one side of the body. Also known as personal neglect.

Hemispatial neglect A deficit in the ability to attend to one side of the environment.

is far less common than left-side neglect (Beis et al., 2004). Buxbaum and associates (2004) found that of 166 patients with right hemisphere lesions, 49% (42 of 166) of these patients displayed some form of neglect.

As of yet, there is no popular consensus on the exact lesion locales necessary to produce unilateral neglect. This probably is because multiple unidentified subtypes of neglect result from lesions in different areas of the right hemisphere and subcortex. In the literature, multiple methods of categorizing and subcategorizing types of neglect and the many terms used to indicate the same deficit further muddy the water. However, it is generally accepted that lesions to the right hemisphere parietal-temporal-occipital area often result in neglect. Also, reports of damage to the basal ganglia resulting in neglect exist as well (Buxbaum et al., 2004; Vallar & Perani, 1986). As subtypes of neglect are more solidly defined, they will undoubtedly be linked more closely to lesions in certain neuroanatomic locations.

Generally speaking, there are two primary types of neglect: body and hemispatial. As mentioned, an individual might not be able to attend to one side of his or her own body. This subtype is called **body neglect**, or personal neglect (Bisiach, Perani, Vallar, & Berti, 1986; Guariglia & Antonucci, 1992). The subtype of neglect in which an individual cannot attend to one side of the environment is called **hemispatial neglect** but is also referred to as spatial neglect or extrapersonal neglect (Bisiach et al., 1986; Guariglia & Antonucci, 1992).

Individuals with body neglect cannot attend to tactile stimuli on one side of their own body. These individuals might not even recognize the existence of the neglected side of the body. In severe cases of body

neglect, an individual may exhibit somatophrenia. **Somatophrenia** is when individuals cannot perceive their own body parts as being parts of themselves. This can lead the individual to perceive the neglected side with confusion or even disgust. In profound cases of somatophrenia, the individual might initially come to believe that an extra arm and leg have been attached to their body. In body neglect, the neglected limbs often display a hemiparesis. However, even if motor function remains intact for the neglected limbs, this intact function can go completely unused as a result of the neglect. This condition of diminished use of a neglected limb despite the limb being motorically intact is referred to as **motor neglect**.

Somatophrenia A deficit in the ability to perceive parts of one's own body as belonging to oneself.

Motor neglect A condition of displaying diminished use of a neglected limb, despite the limb being motorically intact.

Clinical Note

Wheelchairs and Neglect

Patients with neglect often stay in rehabilitation facilities and nursing homes, and while in these facilities they are transported to and from therapy sessions in a wheelchair by staff. If a patient is unaware of the position of one side of the body or of the existence of that side of the body, it is the responsibility of a facility's staff to ensure that the patient's neglected body parts remain undamaged. It is always important to be sure a patient's neglected body parts are placed safely out of harm so that they are not injured. A wheelchair combined with an inattentive driver pose dangers to a patient with body neglect. The spokes of the wheelchair can break fingers or the wrist of a neglected limb if it is left dangling. Also, neglected feet and ankles can become lodged and broken beneath the wheels of a moving wheelchair. The healthcare professional pushing the wheelchair is responsible for ensuring the safety of all limbs of the individual sitting in the wheelchair.

Extinction A mild case of hemispatial neglect in which the affected individual can attend to stimuli within the neglected field of attention but only with prompting.

Those with hemispatial neglect cannot attend to one side of the environment. In short, they usually acknowledge the existence of only the nonneglected side of the world. Mild cases of hemispatial neglect can be referred to as extinction, in which a person might be able to attend to the neglected side but only with prompting. In severe cases, the individual with hemispatial neglect is totally unable to recognize or acknowledge the existence of the neglected side of the world, usually the left side. Visual and auditory information from the neglected side might go totally unattended to and unrecognized. Even olfactory information in the left nostril might be ignored. These individuals might eat food only from the nonneglected side of the plate. They might attend only to speakers standing on the nonneglected side. They often bump into objects, such as door frames, located within the neglected space. If they are in a wheelchair, they might run the wheelchair against the wall on the neglected side and might not be able to determine why the wheelchair is stuck. If given a book to read, they might read only the print that exists in their nonneglected field. These individuals also might be unable to turn their body toward the neglected space (i.e., they might not be able to look, direct their attention to, or rotate their body toward the neglected side of the world). This inability to turn toward the neglected space makes perfect sense in the context of hemispatial neglect. How can a person turn the body toward a side of the world that does not exist?

Individuals with hemispatial neglect or body neglect, but no motor neglect, can still walk, though with some difficulty, and usually run the neglected side of their body into objects and door frames on the neglected side of the environment. Individuals with motor neglect cannot walk at all because of the lack of volitional movement in their neglected limbs.

Clinical Note

Standing on the Right Side of the Bed

Here is one of the most important and practical clinical notes in this text. Before walking into the hospital room of a person who has unilateral damage to the brain, the speech-language pathologist must first be sure of which side of the bed it is best to stand on. Generally speaking, it is always best to stand on the side of the bed ipsilateral to the damaged hemisphere, at least until the clinician has determined the presence and extent of neglect. If a person has experienced damage to the left hemisphere, the prudent speech-language pathologist stands on the left side of the bed so as to avoid being in the potentially neglected right attentional field. If a person has experienced right hemisphere damage, the prudent speech-language pathologist stands on the right side of the bed to avoid being in the potentially neglected left attentional field.

Not taking into account the possible presence of neglect can negatively and profoundly affect cognitive and language testing and interviewing. How can you interview and test a patient effectively if that patient does not even know you are standing beside him or her?

The presence of body or hemispatial neglect worsens an individual's prognosis for rehabilitation following brain damage. Neglect is a very disabling condition that negatively affects the individual's basic skills of everyday living and basic attentional abilities, and it significantly increases caregiver burden (Buxbaum et al., 2004). The presence of neglect can be an even more important factor in determining overall possibility of recovery than the size of the lesion to the brain (Buxbaum et al., 2004).

Sustained and Selective Attention Deficits

Sustained attention can be thought of as the capacity to stay alert and to hold one's attention on a single stimulus over time (Saldert & Ahlsen, 2007).

A person attending to a film in a quiet theater is displaying sustained attention. This ability is often disordered in individuals with right hemisphere damage (Saldert & Ahlsen, 2007).

Selective attention is the ability to focus on one stimulus while ignoring another stimulus. A person attending to the words that characters in a film say while ignoring all the talk and noise coming from other people in the audience is displaying good selective attention abilities. This ignoring, or blocking out, of the competing stimuli while focusing on only the selected stimulus is an example of intact selective attention abilities and how they are used. Individuals with right hemisphere damage usually display deficits in selective attention (Stuss et al., 1999).

As mentioned earlier, sustained and selective attention are necessary for appropriate attention to, processing of, and understanding of language as well as important social cues and social interactions (i.e., discourse). Without intact sustained and selective attention, individuals with right hemisphere deficits miss relevant information or are distracted by irrelevant stimuli and further lose the thread of conversation. This leads individuals with right hemisphere damage to difficulties communicating or to acting inappropriately in social situations.

Although deficits in sustained and selective attention are often documented as occurring notably in individuals suffering from right hemisphere damage, any significant injury to the brain may cause attentional deficits. Following is a list of the primary levels of attention in hierarchical order:

- *Sustained attention.* The ability to hold attention on a single stimulus.
- *Selective attention.* The ability to hold attention on a stimulus while ignoring the presence of a competing stimulus.
- *Alternating attention.* The ability to move or alternate one's attention back and forth from one stimulus to another.

- *Divided attention.* The ability to attend to one stimulus while simultaneously attending to another stimulus. Divided attention is also known as multitasking.

Neuropsychiatric Disorders

Although fully describing the neuropsychiatric disorders discussed in this section (except for anosognosia) is outside the scope of this text, it is important for speech-language pathologists to be able to understand and recognize these disorders. Neuropsychiatric disorders often present alongside neurogenic communication deficits and disorders.

Anosognosia

Anosognosia is an individual's inability to recognize or realize she has a problem. Translated from Greek, *anosognosia* literally means *not to know* that you *do not know*. Individuals with right hemisphere damage often display anosognosia. Although they might behave bizarrely, misinterpret or ignore discourse, or even lose one side of their body, these people are usually calm and assured that, if there *is* a problem, it does not have anything to do with them. Patients with right hemisphere disorders might blame any problems in their performance on the speech-language pathologist or caregivers or confabulate explanations

Author's Note

Anosognosia

It is not uncommon for individuals to come to my clinic following a right hemisphere stroke. Typically, this person walks in and is pleasant and calm in demeanor despite displaying profound impairments. But when I ask him why he is at the clinic, I usually get some version of this reply: "I don't know why I'm here." This is also usually followed by the patient pointing a finger at his caregiver and issuing the accusation, "She brought me here."

for their failures while refusing to acknowledge the possibility that they have deficits. A person must be able to acknowledge she has a problem before therapy can really begin to address the problem. Therefore, the presence of anosognosia often severely limits an individual's recovery.

Depression

Following disease, surgery, stroke, or trauma, depression is common. However, in those with right hemisphere damage depression can go unnoticed or might be masked by other deficits. As mentioned earlier, these individuals can have difficulty expressing emotion indicative of their true emotional state. Speech-language pathologists must be careful to inquire earnestly into the emotional state of the person with right hemisphere damage. If depression is suspected, the speech-language pathologist must refer the patient to the appropriate professionals, such as counselors, psychologists, or psychiatrists.

The Capgras Delusion

The Capgras delusion is named after Joseph Capgras, who published the first formal description of this disorder in 1923 (Sinkman, 2008). Capgras first described a woman living in Paris whose case was, in great part, characterized by her belief that people she knew were disappearing and being substituted by duplicates. Hence, the Capgras delusion is primarily characterized by a belief that loved ones, significant others, or family members have been replaced by imposters.

This delusion occurs in psychological disorders but also presents as a result of neurologic pathology or injury. Although most often displayed by individuals with schizophrenia or Alzheimer's disease, the Capgras delusion does at times

Capgras delusion A neuropsychiatric deficit characterized by a belief that loved ones, significant others, or family members have been replaced by imposters.

present in those with epilepsy, traumatic brain injury, and stroke or acute lesion to the right cerebral hemisphere. The location of the lesion varies, but the damage is usually in the right hemisphere or both the right and left hemispheres and can be found in the frontal, parietal, or temporal lobes (Bourget & Whitehurst, 2004).

The pathologic mechanism underlying the Capgras delusion is unknown. However, many explanations have been proposed. Neurologic explanations for the Capgras delusion usually involve the hypothetical disconnection between one part of the brain and another. Hirstein and Ramachandran (1997) suggest that the delusion occurs when damage to the brain severs the link between the part of the temporal lobe responsible for processing facial recognition and the part of the limbic system (the amygdala) responsible for producing the normal emotional response in reaction to the face that is seen. As a result of this disconnect, for instance, a father could view his son and recognize the appearance of his son, but the father would not experience the usual emotional response to his son that he unconsciously expects upon seeing his son. This lack of expected emotional response leads this father to conclude that this person looks and sounds exactly like his son, but that he simply is not his son. Consistent with this theory is that, often, individuals with the Capgras delusion recognize the voice of their loved one as being the original person, but upon seeing the individual insist that the loved one is an imposter.

Individuals with the Capgras delusion admit that their loved one's imposter looks and sounds exactly like the original person, but that, despite this remarkable resemblance, the loved one is an imposter. Usually, the person confabulates an explanation of why a loved one has been replaced. These explanations are, by nature, illogical and nonsensical. For example, a woman with a right hemisphere stroke might believe that doctors replaced her husband in an attempt to steal her jewelry while she slept at night. Brighetti,

Bonifacci, Borlimi, and Ottaviani (2007) present a study in which a young woman views her father to have been replaced by an imposter. Her explanation for the presence of this imposter is that her mother and the imposter had killed her real father so that they could start a new life together.

Visual Hallucinations

A visual hallucination is when an individual perceives something visually that does not truly exist or that is not really there. Lesions or seizure activity in the right hemisphere can produce visual hallucinations. Often, the location of lesions or seizure activity is the posterior aspect of the right hemisphere among the visual processing areas. The nature of visual hallucinations varies widely and unpredictably among individuals.

Paranoid Hallucinations

In addition to visual hallucinations, those with right hemisphere brain damage can present with paranoid hallucinations. Unlike visual hallucinations, which are usually benign in nature, paranoid hallucinations can be visual and/or auditory and the individual experiencing them perceives them as threatening, ominous, or foreboding.

Assessment of Right Hemisphere Disorders

Appropriate assessment of an individual with right hemisphere damage includes taking an in-depth case history, informal tests for deficits associated with right hemisphere damage, and a formal test of right hemisphere damage.

Case History

Gathering information for a thorough case history is important and involves reviewing all available medical records on the patient in the medical chart and an interview with the patient and family.

Informal Testing of Right Hemisphere Disorders

Below is a list of disorders associated with right hemisphere damage and possible methods of assessing for these disorders.

- *Prosopagnosia.* Speech-language therapists can assess for prosopagnosia by presenting to the patient family members, photos of family members or friends, or photos of famous individuals whom the patient might know, and then asking the patient to name the individuals in the photos.
- *Facial affect.* The speech-language pathologist usually assesses comprehension of facial affect by simply making a face expressing a certain emotion and asking the patient to name the emotion conveyed by the facial expression. Although making faces sounds easy, it takes a little practice. The speech-language pathologist needs to master the ability to make emotional facial expressions at will (as opposed to automatically, which is how it is usually done). Photos of people with emotional expressions on their faces are also used as stimuli.

  The expression of emotion through facial affect can be assessed by asking the patient to produce a facial expression to match a certain emotion. However, this does not necessarily indicate that the patient will automatically use appropriate facial expressions to communicate their emotions while they are speaking. Oftentimes, informal observation of the patient while speaking will indicate the presence of deficits in the use of appropriate facial expression.
- *Prosodic deficits.* The appropriate comprehension of prosody can be informally tested by repeating a phrase or sentence, each time varying the meaning of the phrase or sentence not by

changing the words but by altering intonation, and then asking the patient to interpret the emotional meaning being conveyed (e.g., "Did I say this in a happy way? A sad way?").

The appropriate use of prosody is informally assessed by listening to the connected speech of the individual, checking for an abnormal level of monotone. Also, the therapist can ask the patient to vary the prosody of their utterances to convey different emotional meanings to assess a patient's stimulability.

- *Inferencing deficits.* The speech-language pathologist can informally assess inferencing abilities by presenting very simple inferencing tasks to the patient, such as, "It is snowing; the kids are wearing heavy coats. What season is it?" More complex inferencing tasks are also commonly used, such as the illustrations created in the 1950s by Norman Rockwell, which have found a curious home in the medical community for assessing inferencing abilities. Because the illustrations generally present people in very human and complex social situations they are quite useful in testing inferencing abilities. Although most unimpaired individuals automatically interpret the paintings correctly, those with inferencing deficits find perceiving and interpreting all the necessary information contained in the paintings to be difficult. **Figure 5-2** presents an illustration titled *Breaking Home Ties* by Norman Rockwell. At first glance, this illustration simply depicts a man and a boy

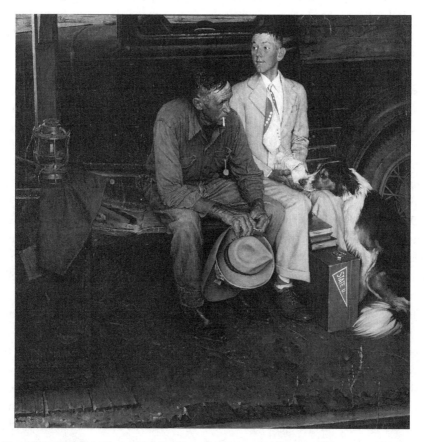

Figure 5-2 *Breaking Home Ties.* Illustration by Norman Rockwell.

Source: Printed by permission of the Norman Rockwell Family Agency. Copyright © 1954 The Norman Rockwell Family Entities. Image provided by the Norman Rockwell Museum Digital Collections.

sitting on a car. A person with inferencing deficits can usually gather that information but cannot grasp the deeper context of the story that the subtle details of the illustration depict. Intact inferencing enables a person to gather far more information from the illustration: the man and the boy are father and son; they are waiting on a bus; the dog belongs to the boy; the son is leaving for college and is quite eager to leave whereas the father and the dog are saddened by the situation; the father is a blue-collar worker who probably never had the opportunity to go to college and he has worked hard to give his son this opportunity.

- *Discourse deficits.* Observing and recording the patient as she communicates with others or engaging the patient directly in conversation for an extended period of time (usually the interview at the beginning of the assessment) is an appropriate method for assessing deficits in discourse or pragmatic use of language (Myers, 2009).

- *Neglect.* Therapists often use cancellation tasks, observation, line bisection, and line drawings to assess for neglect. In cancellation tasks, the patient is presented with a sheet of paper with various stimuli printed on the page and then is asked to mark certain stimuli, for example, asking the patient to circle all the Xs on a page covered in Xs and Os. The area where the patient does not circle the Xs might be an area of visual neglect. **Figure 5-3** shows an example of a cancellation task in which the patient was asked to strike through each mark on the page to create an X. The lack of marked through lines on the left portion of the page indicates some level of left neglect is present.

  Neglect can also be assessed by observing the patient for signs as he or she goes about activities of daily living, such as shaving, eating, putting on makeup, walking, and navigating a room.

  In line bisection, the speech-language pathologist draws a long line on a sheet of paper, centers the paper in front of the patient, and asks

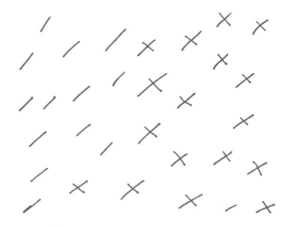

Figure 5-3 A cancellation task indicating presence of neglect.

the patient to put a mark in the center of the line. A mark too far to one side can indicate that the opposite side of the line is in neglected space.

Another common method of assessing neglect is for the speech-language pathologist to present the patient with a simple line drawing, such as a flower, clock, house, or tree, and then to ask the patient to copy it on another sheet of paper. Individuals with neglect typically leave out details on the neglected side of the drawing or try to draw all the details (such as numbers on a clock face) on the nonneglected side (**Figure 5-4**).

Myers (2009) suggests a baking pan task in which an individual is asked to distribute a number of blocks evenly within a baking pan. An uneven distribution of the blocks can indicate the presence of neglect.

- *Sustained and selective attention.* There are various informal tests of levels of attention. Commonly used are card-sorting tasks in which a number of cards are given to the patient and the patient is asked to sort them in various ways (depending on ability level). To assess sustained attention a patient can be asked to sort a stack of cards into the four categories of suit or the two categories of color with no competing stimuli to distract him. To accomplish this task the patient

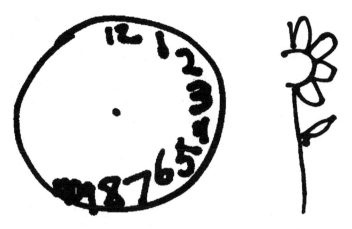

Figure 5-4   Line drawings copied by a patient that indicate presence of left neglect.

must be able to sustain attention on the task long enough to reach completion. Once competing stimuli are introduced, such as a radio or television playing in the background, the patient must block out the competing stimuli to keep his attention on the task at hand and it becomes a selective attention task.

- *Alternating and divided attention.* Card-sorting tasks can be modified to assess alternating and divided attention. For instance, to assess alternating attention the speech-language pathologist can instruct the patient to sort the cards by suit and, when given a cue, shift to sorting the cards by color or number, and then shift back, thereby testing the patient's ability to shift attention from one task to another. Divided attention can be assessed by asking the patient to sort the cards in a certain way and then, for instance, to simultaneously attend to a short story the speech-language pathologist tells during the card-sorting task.

Formal Testing of Right Hemisphere Disorders

The use of formal tests to assess for right hemisphere disorders is not as universal as issuing formal standardized tests for aphasia. This is probably because the aphasias are a single type of deficit whereas right

hemisphere disorders comprise a variety of deficits with different manifestations. Nonetheless, formal tests for right hemisphere disorders are useful in a thorough evaluation. Right hemisphere tests usually assess areas of language not evaluated by aphasia tests, such as the comprehension of humor, metaphor, sarcasm, facial expression, and prosody. Many tests meant to assess specifically for aphasia, dementia, or traumatic brain injury include sections or subsections that assess for right hemisphere disorders because patients with dementia and traumatic brain injury typically have damage in both hemispheres and present with a combination of left and right hemisphere syndromes. Following are tests useful for the assessment of right hemisphere disorders:

- The Right Hemisphere Language Battery (2nd edition) (Bryan, 1995)
- The Mini Inventory of Right Brain Injury (MIRBI; 2nd edition) (Pimental & Kingsbury, 2000)
- Communication Activities of Daily Living (2nd edition; CADL-2) (Holland, Frattali, & Fromm, 1999)
- Arizona Battery for Communication Disorders of Dementia (ABCD; Bayles & Tomoeda, 1993)
- Ross Information Processing Assessment (2nd edition; RIPA-2) (Ross-Swain, 1996)

Therapy for Right Hemisphere Disorders

Given the inherent strangeness of many disorders and deficits associated with right hemisphere damage, the family members of the affected individual often react with confusion or denial. It is not uncommon for family members to assume that their loved one has simply "lost their mind." As such, Halpern and Goldfarb (2013) point out that the first responsibility of the speech-language pathologist is to educate the family and caregivers regarding the nature of right hemisphere disorders. Then, it is appropriate to provide therapy to reduce or compensate for deficits and, finally, to encourage rehabilitation at home when formal therapy is discontinued. Although a period of spontaneous recovery follows damage to the right hemisphere, it is the role of the speech-language pathologist to maximize the patient's recovery and to facilitate a return to normal life, or as close as is possible, for the patient.

Treatment to Improve Facial Affect

Patients can be taught to express emotion through facial affect by consciously producing facial expressions that reflect their true emotional state. However, Myers (2009) suggests avoiding this kind of task on more severely impaired individuals whose lack of facial expression is related to a lower level of arousal and is not a true deficit in the use of facial expressions. Halpern and Goldfarb (2013) similarly caution that the clinician must rule out the possibility of a true emotional disorder before targeting the lack of emotional expression. They suggest referring the patient to a psychiatrist to rule out the presence of a true emotional disorder such as depression.

Treatment for Prosodic Deficits

For mildly impaired patients with prosodic expression deficits, Myers (2009) suggests educating these patients on the use of prosody and counseling them to identify their emotional state verbally to their families.

Myers (2009) also suggests a task in which patients are given a short story to read that ends with a quote by a character in the story. Given the emotional context set by the story, the patient must produce the final quote with the appropriate emotional prosody.

An example of a low-level treatment task for prosodic comprehension is teaching the patient to discriminate between changes in pitch or prosody. For example, the speech-language pathologist produces a single utterance multiple times, varying (or not varying) the prosody, and then asks the patient whether the productions were the same or different. If the patient can discern which productions were different, the speech-language pathologist cues the patient to produce the utterances and their differences verbally. This is usually followed by a discussion as to how the differences in pitch or prosody change the meaning. This task also allows for the simultaneous targeting of prosodic deficits in expression.

Treatment to Improve Discourse Deficits

As previously mentioned, a large part of the difficulty individuals with right hemisphere damage have with discourse is rooted in their decreased ability to make appropriate inferences. Therefore, successful treatment for inferencing deficits should improve comprehension of discourse. As mentioned, Norman Rockwell illustrations are commonly used to coach individuals to put together appropriate clues and details necessary to understand the overall meaning of a picture. A task given by Myers (2009) is to present short stories or pictures (from magazines, newspapers, websites) to the patient and have the patient generate appropriate titles for the stories or pictures. This task can be easily modified to an appropriate level of difficulty by lengthening or shortening the story and increasing or decreasing the complexity of the pictures presented.

Aside from inferencing deficits, therapy for discourse deficits targets increasing the patient's awareness of the listener's needs, increasing awareness of social conventions and expectations, and increasing theory of mind (the ability to see things from another's point of view; Myers, 2009). Tomkins (1995) and Myers (2009) elaborate on such treatments.

Treatment for Pragmatic Deficits

Brookshire (2007) describes a procedure in which the speech-language pathologist teaches the patient overt rules of social interactions and then asks the patient to view and analyze prerecorded interactions among individuals. Once the patient is adept at analyzing the social interactions of others, the individual is then taught to apply those skills of social analysis to herself and her own interactions to detect and repair problems she is having socially. Common targets are conversational turn-taking, maintaining eye contact, and maintaining topic. Role-playing tasks are often used to target these pragmatic deficits (Tomkins, 1995).

Treatment for Neglect

Traditionally used therapy strategies for neglect include visual scanning therapy (VST), in which a patient is given a task requiring a shift of attention toward or into neglected space. For example, the patient must shift attention and/or body position far enough left to find the edge of a book, and then read a complete line of text from left to right. Another example of VST is putting an object nearer and nearer and then into the patient's neglected space and directing the patient to shift his attention or body position toward the neglected space to find the object.

A general weakness of visual scanning therapy is that it requires the speech-language pathologist to

provide heavy verbal cues (e.g., "look left, look left") for the patient to succeed; generalization to activities of daily living can be poor because the patient has learned to rely on cues from the speech-language pathologist (Kerkhoff & Schenk, 2012).

Myers and Mackisack (1990) outline an alternative approach they call Edgeness that uses a flat container with raised edges (like a baking pan) and small cubes or blocks. The speech-language pathologist introduces the patient to the container and the edges of the container and then places the blocks in the container and asks the patient to find the blocks (see **Figure 5-5**). The more blocks placed into the neglected field as well as the more blocks used in total, the more difficult the task is. Foils can be added to increase difficulty. For instance, different colored blocks or blocks of different shapes can be placed in the container and the therapist can ask the patient to find a block of a certain color or shape. Edgeness has an advantage over VST because patients can monitor their own success—they know if they have found the block or not. Also, because there are discrete palpable borders within which the blocks are placed the patient can complete the task with little direct verbal cueing from the speech-language pathologist.

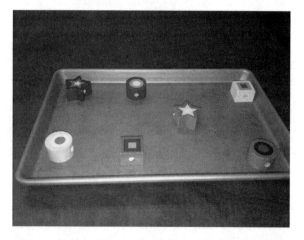

Figure 5-5 Edgeness task by Myers and Mackisack (1990).

Therapy Tasks for Sustained Attention Deficits

Treatment for sustained attention deficits typically involves drills that require patients to hold their attention on a task for successful completion. Examples are tasks in which an individual must hold his attention on a task to sort objects into any number of categories. Difficulty level is increased by increasing the number of categories into which the patient must sort. Trailmaking tasks are paper-and-pencil exercises that require an individual to connect randomly printed stimuli on a page in a sequential manner. For example, on a page printed randomly with the numbers 1 through 20, the individual must draw a line through the numbers in ascending order. An auditory drill for sustained attention is when the speech-language pathologist recites strings of names, letters, or numbers and instructs the patient to respond only to predesignated target stimuli (e.g., a certain name, number, or letter). Difficulty level of auditory drills is increased by increasing the number of target stimuli the patient is required to respond to and increasing the length between occurrences of the target stimuli.

Speech-language pathologists can also use simple games to improve sustained attention if the patient can comprehend the game and the rules. Games that can be used to target sustained attention are checkers, tic-tac-toe, and simple card games. The more rules the game has, the more difficult it is for the patient with cognitive deficits to play successfully.

Therapy Tasks for Selective Attention Deficits

Selective attention is often targeted using drills that add competing or distractor stimuli to sustained attention tasks. Examples of distractor stimuli are music from the radio or a television left on in the room. The Stroop task, which requires the patient to view a list of color words (*black*, *blue*, *red*, etc.), is also often used to target selective attention. Each word is printed in a color of ink that is inconsistent with the color each word names. Patients are then asked to tell the speech-language pathologist which colors the words are printed in, not which color the words name. To complete this task successfully, an individual must selectively ignore what the word says and verbally produce the word that names the color of the ink.

Therapy Tasks for Alternating Attention Deficits

Therapy to strengthen alternating attention abilities is usually composed of drills that require the patient to shift attention from one task to another quickly. For example, the patient must shift attention back and forth between two different sustained attention tasks such as sorting activities, or the patient must shift attention between two easy games such as Connect Four and tic-tac-toe.

Therapy Tasks for Divided Attention Deficits

Any activities that require multitasking strengthen divided attention abilities, for example, carrying on a conversation successfully while completing another task such as sorting or making change. Also, having the patient answer questions as he is completing a sustained attention task can help improve divided attention.

Environmental Manipulations to Facilitate Attention

Although restorative strategies are almost universally used to treat attention deficits, improvement using these strategies takes time. Speech-language pathologists must immediately implement strategies that allow the patient with attention deficits to capitalize on residual attention skills prior to beginning restorative therapy. This can take the form of manipulations of the environment. For example, the speech-language pathologist can reduce distractions in the environment by closing the blinds on the window, turning off the television or radio, or reducing clutter on the table or in the workspace. The speech-language pathologist can also instruct the family to speak clearly to the patient and to speak to the patient one person at a time when they are sure the patient is attending. The speech-language pathologist usually facilitates the patient's ability to pay attention by speaking in short and easy-to-follow sentences while also providing plenty of repetitions and frequent breaks (Mateer, Kerns, & Eso, 1996).

Treatment for Anosognosia

Treatment for anosognosia usually begins with counseling and coaxing the individual to recognize and take ownership of the deficits. This usually occurs naturally throughout the course of therapy as deficits are consistently targeted. However, in more overt cases of anosognosia a more direct approach can be successful. Although anosognosia must be approached carefully, a method of near last resort is to set up a video camera to record therapy during which the patient is presented with a simple task that someone without deficits could successfully complete. Prior to starting the task, the speech-language pathologist asks the patient to predict how she will perform on the task. Of course, because of the anosognosia, the patient will predict that she will be successful. Next, the patient attempts the task (and fails). At this point, the speech-language pathologist can review the video recording with the individual and it might lead the patient to the insight that she is not in touch with the reality of her deficits. However, it might also induce an extreme emotional reaction in the patient as she grasps the extent of her deficits, or the patient might attempt to confabulate a way of explaining the failure.

Cicerone and colleagues (2005) indicate that anosognosia need not always be addressed directly and that some deficits can be targeted even without targeting anosognosia. Furthermore, they argue that, at times, the presence of a lack of self-awareness can increase a patient's compliance with certain therapy tasks. These suggestions indicate that the presence of anosognosia does not necessarily dictate treatment targeting anosognosia but that each case must be dealt with on an individual basis.

Main Points

- Normal right hemisphere functions include the following:
  - Processing of nonlinguistic elements of communication such as prosody, facial expression, body language, and emotion
  - Math/visuospatial skills such as perception of depth, distance, and shapes
  - Localizing targets in space
  - Identifying figure–ground relationships
  - Processing melody of music
  - Perception of macrostructure or gestalt
- Right hemisphere disorders are a group of deficits or changes that occur following damage or pathology to a person's right cerebral hemisphere.
- Etiologies of right hemisphere disorders include anything that damages the right hemisphere, including stroke, disease, trauma, seizures, infections, and toxicity. The type and severity of resulting deficits or disorders depend on the location and extent of damage. Degenerative diseases can also produce right hemisphere disorders, though usually in the presence of left hemisphere syndromes as well. This is because degenerative diseases usually affect both hemispheres simultaneously.
- Communication deficits associated with right hemisphere damage include deficits in the following abilities:
  - Facial recognition
  - Comprehension of facial expression
  - Production of facial expression
  - Comprehension of meaning behind prosody
  - Production of normal prosody
  - Inferencing
  - Discourse
- Visuospatial deficits associated with right hemisphere damage include the following:
  - Simultagnosia, which is the inability to visually perceive multiple details at one time

- Cerebral achromatopsia, which is color blindness resulting from trauma or damage to the cortex that causes the individual to see in shades of gray
- Attention deficits associated with right hemisphere damage include the following:
  - Neglect, which is the inability to attend to or recognize the body/environment contralateral to the lesioned hemisphere
  - Body neglect, which is the inability to attend to sensory information concerning one side of the body
  - Hemispatial neglect, which is the inability to attend to sensory information from one side of the environment
  - Somatophrenia, which is an inability to recognize one's own body parts as being one's own
  - Motor neglect, which is the diminished use of a neglected limb despite it being motorically intact
  - Extinction, which is a mild form of hemispatial neglect in which a person is able to attend to objects within the field of neglect but only with prompting
  - Sustained and selective attention deficits, which can cause the affected individual to miss relevant information, become distracted by irrelevant stimuli, and further lose track of the topic of conversation
- Speech-language pathologists must understand and recognize neuropsychiatric disorders associated with right hemisphere damage because these can present alongside and interact with communication disorders. Neuropsychiatric disorders that result from right hemisphere damage include the following:
  - Anosognosia, which is the inability of the affected individual to recognize or realize that he or she has deficits. The affected

individual usually blames failures in therapy on the speech-language pathologist or caregivers and explains away failures by refusing to acknowledge the deficits.

- Depression is common in any population following disease, stroke, surgery, or trauma. However, emotional changes in individuals with a right hemisphere disorder can go unnoticed or can be masked by other deficits.
- The Capgras delusion is the affected individual's belief that loved ones, significant others, or family members have been replaced by imposters who look and sound like the original persons.
- Visual hallucinations are when an individual perceives something visually that does not truly exist or is not there. Visual hallucinations are caused by lesions or seizure activity in the posterior right hemisphere among the visual processing areas.
- Paranoid hallucinations are hallucinations that are perceived as threatening, ominous, or foreboding.
- Assessment of right hemisphere disorders usually includes the following techniques:
  - A case history, which includes gathering information from medical charts, medical records, and interviews with the patient and/or family members
  - Informal testing of cognitive deficits such as prosopagnosia, facial affect, prosody, inferencing, discourse, neglect, and attention deficits
  - Formal testing for right hemisphere disorders, which usually assesses language abilities not tested in formal aphasia tests such as humor, metaphor, sarcasm, facial expression, and prosody
- Treatment of right hemisphere disorders includes the following:
  - Tasks that target expression/comprehension of facial expressions, prosody, discourse, pragmatics, neglect, attention, and anosognosia
  - Environmental manipulations to reduce distractions, which might include closing the window blinds, turning off the television, instructing family members to speak clearly to the patient, speaking one person at a time, and speaking in short and easy-to-follow sentences while giving plenty of repetitions of important information and breaks for the patient to process what is being said

Review Questions

1. List and explain five functions of a normal right hemisphere.
2. Which surgical procedure led to a sudden resurgence of interest in the study of the right hemisphere during the 1960s?
3. List three common etiologies of right hemisphere disorders.
4. Where in the brain might a lesion produce prosopagnosia and how does prosopagnosia affect communication?
5. How do deficits in comprehension and production of facial expression affect communication?
6. How do deficits in comprehension and production of prosody affect communication?
7. How do deficits in inferencing and discourse affect communication and pragmatics?
8. How are body neglect and hemispatial neglect different?
9. How might neglect affect a patient's life and overall prognosis?

10. Name three neuropsychiatric disorders that can occur as a result of right hemisphere damage.

11. What are three usual components of assessment for right hemisphere disorders?

12. How can a speech-language pathologist informally assess comprehension and production of prosody?

13. How can a speech-language pathologist informally assess neglect?

14. How can a speech-language pathologist informally assess the four levels of attention?

15. Name two formal assessments for right hemisphere disorder.

16. How can a speech-language pathologist treat neglect in therapy?

17. How can a speech-language pathologist treat anosognosia in therapy?

18. How can a speech-language pathologist treat discourse deficits in therapy?

19. Name two environmental manipulations a speech-language pathologist can use to reduce distractions.

20. Name two instructions a speech-language pathologist can give family members to facilitate communication with their loved one with a right hemisphere disorder.

References

1. Bayles, K., & Tomoeda, C. (1993). *The Arizona Battery for Communication Disorders of Dementia*. Austin, TX: Pro-Ed.

2. Beis, J., Keller, C., Morin, S., Bartolomeo, M., Bernati, T., Chokron, S., . . . Azouvi, P. (2004). Right spatial neglect after left hemisphere stroke. *Neurology, 63,* 1600–1605.

3. Benowitz, L., Bear, D., Rosenthal., R., Mesulam, M., Zaidel, E., & Sperry, R. (1983). Hemispheric specialization in nonverbal communication. *Cortex, 19,* 5–11.

4. Bisiach, E., Perani, D., Vallar, G., & Berti, A. (1986). Unilateral neglect: Personal and extra-personal. *Neuropsychologia, 24*(6), 759–767.

5. Blonder, X., Bowers, D., & Heilman, K. (1991). The role of the right hemisphere in emotional communication, *Brain, 114,* 1115–1127.

6. Blonder, X., Burns, A., Bowers, D., Moore, R., & Heilman, K. (1993). Right hemisphere facial expressivity during natural conversation, *Brain Cognition, 21,* 44–56.

7. Borod, J., Koff, E., Lorch, M., & Nichols, M. (1986). The expression and perception of facial emotion in brain-damaged patients. *Neuropsychologia, 24,* 169–180.

8. Bourget, D., & Whitehurst, L. (2004). Capgras syndrome: A review of neurophysiological correlates and presenting clinical features in cases involving physical violence. *Canadian Journal of Psychiatry, 49*(11), 719–725.

9. Bowers, D., Bauer, R., Coslett, H., & Heilman, K. (1985). Processing of faces by patients with unilateral hemisphere lesions. *Brain and Cognition, 4,* 258–272.

10. Brighetti, G., Bonifacci, P., Borlimi, R., & Ottaviani, C. (2007). "Far from the heart far from the eye": Evidence from the Capgras delusion. *Cognitive Neuropsychiatry, 12*(3), 187–197.

11. Brookshire, R. (2007). *Introduction to neurogenic communication disorders* (7th ed.). St. Louis, MO: Mosby-Elsevier.

12. Bryan, K. (1995). *The Right Hemisphere Language Battery* (2nd ed.). London, England: Whurr.

13. Buxbaum, L., Ferraro, M., Veramonti, T., Farne, A., Whyte, J., Ladavas, E., . . . Coslett, H. B. (2004). Hemispatial neglect: Subtypes, neuroanatomy, and disability. *Neurology, 62,* 749–756.

14. Cicerone, K., Dahlberg, C., Malec, J., Langenbahn, D., Felicetti, T., Kneipp, S., . . . Catanese, J. (2005). Evidence-based cognitive rehabilitation: Updated review of the literature from 1998 through 2002. *Archives of Physical Medicine, 86*(8), 1681–1692.

15. DeKosky, S., Heilman, K., Bowers, D., & Valenstein, E. (1980). Recognition and discrimination of emotional faces and pictures. *Brain and Language, 9,* 206–214.

16. Glosser, G., Wiener, M., & Kaplan, E. (1988). Variations in aphasic language behaviors. *Journal of Speech and Hearing Disorders, 53,* 115–124.

17. Guariglia, C., & Antonucci, G. (1992). Personal and extrapersonal space: A case of neglect dissociation. *Neuropsychologia, 30*(11), 1001–1009.

18. Halpern, H., Goldfarb, R. (2013). Language and motor speech disorders in adults (3rd ed.). Burlington, MA: Jones & Bartlett Learning.

19. Harciarek, M., & Heilman, K. (2009). The contribution of anterior and posterior regions of the right hemisphere to the recognition of faces. *Journal of Clinical and Experimental Neuropsychology, 31*(3), 322–330.

20. Heilman, M., Scholes, R., & Watson, R. (1975). Auditory affective agnosia. *Journal of Neurology, Neurosurgery, and Psychiatry, 38,* 69–72.

21. Hirstein, W., & Ramachandran, V. (1997). Capgras syndrome: A novel probe for understanding the neural representation of the identity and familiarity of persons. *Proceedings: Biological Sciences, 264*(1380), 437–444.

22. Holland, A., Frattali, C., & Fromm, D. (1999). *Communication activities of daily living* (2nd ed.). Austin, TX: Pro-Ed.

23. Joseph, R. (1988). The right cerebral hemisphere: Emotion, music visual-spatial skills, body-image, dreams, and awareness. *Journal of Clinical Psychology, 44*(5), 630–673.

24. Kerkhoff, G., & Schenk, T. (2012). Rehabilitation of neglect: An update. *Neuropsychologia, 1*(24), 1072–1079.

25. Mateer, C., Kerns, K., & Eso, K. (1996). Management of attention and memory disorders following traumatic brain injury. *Journal of Learning Disabilities, 29*(6), 618–632.

26. Myers, P. (2009). *Right hemisphere damage: Disorders of communication and cognition.* Clifton Park, NY: Delmar Cengage.

27. Myers, P., & Mackisack, E. (1990). Right hemisphere syndrome. In L. LaPointe (Ed.), *Aphasia and related neurogenic disorders.* New York, NY: Thieme.

28. Pimental, P., & Kingsbury, N. (2000). *The Mini Inventory of Right Brain Injury* (2nd ed.). Austin, TX: Pro-Ed.

29. Ross-Swain, D. (1996). *Ross Information Processing Assessment* (2nd ed.). Austin, TX: Pro-Ed.

30. Sackheim, H., Gur, R., & Saucy, M. (1978). Emotions are expressed more intensely on the left side of the face. *Science, 202,* 434–436.

31. Sacks, O. (1970). *The man who mistook his wife for a hat.* New York, NY: Summit Books.

32. Saldert, C., & Ahlsen, E. (2007). Inference in right hemisphere damaged individuals' comprehension: The role of sustained attention. *Clinical Linguistics and Phonetics, 21*(8), 637–655.

33. Sinkman, A. (2008). The syndrome of Capgras. *Psychiatry, 71*(4), 371–378.

34. Stuss, D., Toth, J., Franchi, D., Alexander, M., Tipper, S., & Craik, F. (1999). Disassociation of attentional processes in patients with focal frontal and posterior lesions. *Neuropsychologia, 37,* 1005–1027.

35. Tomkins, C. (1995). *Right hemisphere communication disorders.* San Diego, CA: Singular.

36. Tucker, D., Watson, R., & Heilman, K. (1977). Discrimination and evocation of affectively intoned speech in patients with right parietal disease. *Neurology, 27*(10), 947–950.

37. Vallar, G., Perani, D. (1986). The anatomy of unilateral neglect after right-hemisphere stroke lesions: A clinical/CT scan correclation study in man. *Neuropsychologia, 24*(5), 609–622.

38. Weintraub, S., Mesulam, M., & Kramer, L. (1981). Disturbances in prosody: A right hemisphere contribution to language. *Archives of Neurology, 38*(1), 742–744.

Motor Speech Disorders: Apraxia of Speech and Evaluation of Motor Speech Disorders

▶ *Where this icon appears, visit http://go.jblearning.com/ManascoCWS to view the corresponding video.*

Disorders involving the effective manufacture, refinement, transmission, and execution of motor plans for speech are motor speech disorders. These disorders are strictly involved in the motoric component of speech. Remember that speech is simply the sounds made with the vocal and articulatory structures to verbally produce words whereas language is the actual words produced. The presence of a motor speech disorder does not necessarily imply the presence of cognitive or language disorders, though cognitive and language disorders do often present concomitantly with motor speech disorders. Categorized under the term *motor speech disorders* are apraxia of speech and the dysarthrias.

Apraxia of speech is a motor speech disorder so different from the dysarthrias that this whole chapter is dedicated to it. Since apraxia of speech was first recognized as a distinct disorder, researchers and speech-language pathologists have struggled to quantify, define, and treat this disorder and tease it apart from aphasia. Different opinions regarding apraxia of speech exist, probably more so than for any other disorder treated by speech-language pathologists. As such, apraxia of speech is often a contentious subject. Theories on the underlying nature of the disorder range from the idea that it is a motor speech disorder to the idea that it is purely linguistic in nature and a component of Broca's aphasia (Martin, 1974). Further muddying the waters, there are almost an absurd number of pseudonyms for this disorder, including dyspraxia, aphemia, peripheral motor aphasia, and apraxic dysarthria. However, the overwhelming majority of professionals have adopted the term *apraxia of speech*.

Terminology Notes

The root word of *apraxia* is *praxis*, which in Greek means to act or to move. By adding the prefix *a-*, which indicates *without*, it becomes the term *apraxia*, which means to not act or to not move, or without action or movement. Hence, the term apraxia of speech indicates a lack of movement or action for speech production. There are various kinds of apraxia, some that involve the inability to move limbs and eyes as well as oral structures. Even apraxia of speech is usually subdivided into two categories: *acquired apraxia of speech*, resulting from some form of brain damage; and the congenital form, *developmental apraxia of speech*, resulting from unknown etiology. For the sake of simplicity, the term *apraxia of speech* is used here to refer to the acquired/organic form of the disorder while discussion of developmental apraxia of speech is beyond the scope of this chapter.

Apraxia of speech   An acquired disorder of speech originating from an inability to create and sequence motor plans for speech.

Apraxia of Speech

Although there is more than one interpretation of the underlying nature of apraxia of speech, the most commonly held belief is that it is rooted in an inability to create and sequence (i.e., program) the neural impulses necessary to create appropriate motor movements for speech. In simpler terms, an individual's brain has lost the ability to produce plans that tell the muscles used to produce speech how to contract with the appropriate range, force, and timing to produce normal speech. So, apraxia is usually believed to be an inability to put together motor plans for speech. Contrast this with the dysarthrias, which are the result of a disruption or degeneration of an intact speech motor plan.

Apraxia of speech affects only the motor plans for movement intended to produce speech. Construction of appropriate motor plans for the articulators to produce nonspeech actions remains unaffected (hence, the term apraxia *of speech*). Even though an individual with apraxia of speech is unable to produce motor plans to coordinate muscles for speech production, the same individual shows no difficulty generating motor plans for the production of nonverbal actions with her articulators, unless there are concomitant problems creating nonspeech difficulties. The individual with apraxia of speech and no dysarthria displays no muscular weakness and usually can complete the nonverbal components of an oral-motor evaluation accurately and without difficulty, whereas deficits become obvious when the individual attempts speech.

Apraxia of speech usually occurs from damage to the inferior posterior left hemisphere, might co-occur with a dysarthria, and usually co-occurs with some level of aphasia. In fact, apraxia of speech is so often accompanied by aphasia that a professor of mine once told me that if a person displays apraxia of speech, I should assume and act as if the patient also has some level of aphasia, even if it is not immediately obvious (and this practical advice has served me well). However, so-called pure cases of apraxia of speech with no measurable language impairments have been documented (Sugishita et al., 1987), though they are rare.

Cases of pure apraxia with no associated aphasia lend support to the supposition that sound-level speech errors observed in apraxia of speech are the result of a motor programming deficit for speech and are not a

Motor speech programmer A network of neural structures that contribute to the function of creating appropriate motor plans for speech.

form of phonemic paraphasia (i.e., a linguistic deficit). Some view the high co-occurrence of apraxia of speech with Broca's aphasia as an indication that the speech errors commonly attributed to apraxia of speech are simply a linguistic component of Broca's aphasia and that apraxia of speech does not stand alone as a disorder distinct from Broca's aphasia. Martin (1974) began advocating for this alternative hypothesis that all the speech error patterns attributed in the early apraxia research to motor programming deficits (underlying the justification for establishing the term *apraxia of speech*) could be explained by the sound-level phonemic paraphasic errors ordinarily produced by those with aphasia. The debate about whether this is true continues, even though speech-language pathologists usually accept the premise that motor programming deficits are the underlying basis of apraxia of speech.

The perspective that apraxia of speech is a motoric disorder was solidified by the research of Darley at the Mayo Clinic (Darley, Aronson, & Brown, 1975). A definition given by Duffy (2005), an adherent to this model, defines apraxia of speech as follows:

> A neurologic speech disorder reflecting an impaired capacity to plan or program sensorimotor commands necessary for directing movements that result in phonetically and prosodically normal speech. It can occur in the absence of physiologic disturbances associated with the dysarthrias and in the absence of disturbance in any component of language (p. 5).

Motor Speech Programmer

Once language is formulated in the brain it becomes necessary for the central nervous system (CNS) to create sequences of neural impulses that command the muscles involved in speech production to produce the necessary movements at certain speeds, with certain forces, using certain ranges of motion to articulate speech. Darley, Aronson, and Brown (1975) conceive of apraxia of speech as being the

disruption of this function of the brain, which they term the **motor speech programmer**. The motor speech programmer is not a single structure in the CNS, but a network of structures that all contribute to the function of creating appropriate motor plans for speech. A thorough description of all components of the motor speech programmer is beyond the scope of this chapter. Nonetheless, certain left hemisphere structures such as Broca's area and the supplementary motor cortex play a large role in the motor speech programmer. The primary motor cortex, basal ganglia, and cerebellum are also involved in the appropriate production of motor plans for speech.

Speech Characteristics

The speech production of those with apraxia of speech is often very effortful and overtly characterized by a great deal of struggle and frustration. Apraxia of speech is characterized by articulation errors, limited prosody, slowed rate, and the visible groping about of the tongue, lips, and mandible. More often than not, resonance, coordination of respiration for speech, and phonation are left relatively intact. However, in severe cases these can be devastated alongside articulation and prosody.

Those with apraxia of speech are very aware of their speech errors. This awareness of errors often leads those with apraxia of speech to automatically slow their rate of speech considerably in an attempt to avoid production of speech errors. Also, when they produce speech errors, many individuals with apraxia of speech make several attempts at correcting them (self-repairs). The prosody of those with apraxia of speech is usually highly affected by the decreased rate of speech they adopt to avoid errors and fluency of speech is often disrupted by repeated attempts at self-repair. The oral groping behavior often displayed by those with apraxia of speech is a visible and audible trial-and-error behavior during which the individual moves the tongue, mandible, and lips to various, often inaccurate and seemingly outrageous, positions in an attempt to assume the appropriate acticulatory position for production of a certain phoneme or word.

As with all the neurogenic communication disorders, the impact that apraxia of speech has on the speech of an individual is largely determined by the severity of the disorder. Apraxia of speech can manifest at any level of severity from mild to profound. An individual with a mild case of apraxia of speech can experience barely noticeable articulation difficulties that she can easily disguise as normal and appropriate difficulties with articulation. In cases of moderate severity, the individual might continually struggle to articulate appropriately. In a severe case, an individual might be able to produce only a handful of words appropriately and will usually experience extreme difficulty producing appropriate speech. Profound cases of apraxia of speech usually render an individual completely mute with the inability to produce even a single phoneme.

The articulation errors of those with apraxia of speech are inconsistent and include various sound-level errors: phoneme substitutions, phoneme distortions, and voice-onset errors (Johns & Darley, 1970). Articulation errors of those with apraxia of speech often occur on the first phoneme of a word. In addition, the more motorically complex the target word, target phoneme, or target utterance, the more likely the individual with apraxia of speech will produce errors while attempting to articulate. If one assumes that apraxia of speech is a deficit in the ability to plan movements for speech, it is logical that the phonemes or phoneme combinations that require greater motor-planning abilities are more difficult to produce error free than those phonemes or phoneme combinations that require less motor planning abilities to execute successfully. For instance, single syllable words consisting primarily of stops and no consonant blends (e.g., dog, pop, dad), which require the coordination of fewer muscles and structures, may be produced error free and with greater ease than longer multi-syllabic words (e.g., tornado, automobile) or even more complex target words with consonant blends (e.g., Methodist, transplants). Johns and Darley (1970) report their participants with apraxia displayed the greatest difficulty on consonant clusters involving /s/ and /l/.

Articulation errors produced by those with apraxia of speech are varied and inconsistent (Johns & Darley, 1970). These speakers are said to have *islands of intact articulation*. This is in contrast to speakers with dysarthria, whose every utterance is consistently and predictably affected by their dysarthria. Whereas the errors of speakers with dysarthria are consistent and predictable, errors of speakers with apraxia vary wildly even among one individual's productions of the same phoneme. Someone with apraxia of speech might produce very different error patterns on repeated attempts of the same word (Johns & Darley, 1970).

Following are the attempts of a patient with a moderate-severity apraxia of speech to produce the word *vanishing*. Notice the trial-and-error behavior as the patient recognizes her errors and attempts to self-correct. Also, notice that the short and simple function words produced are error free whereas the more phonetically difficult word *vanishing* is produced only with great effort:

> SLP: Okay, here we go. Let's do *vanishing*. See if you can say *vanishing*.
>
> Patient: Okay, uh. Vanis. Vanis. Vani, schwing. Vanishwing.
>
> SLP: *Vanishing*.
>
> Patient: It's vanis, schwing. Vanishwing.
>
> SLP: Not *wing*. Not *vanishwing*. *Vanish- ing*.
>
> Patient: I know, its vanishwing. Vanis- wishing. Vaniwishing.
>
> SLP: *Vanish. Ing*.
>
> Patient: Yeah, uh. Vanish. Ing. Vanish. Ing. Vanishing. Vanishing.
>
> SLP: Nice.

See Table 6-1 for a listing of common articulatory difficulties experienced by those with apraxia of speech.

Table 6-1 Articulation Errors of Apraxia of Speech

Consonant and vowel distortions (consonant distortions are more prevalent)
Phoneme substitutions
Perseverative substitutions
Anticipatory substitutions
Phoneme additions
Phoneme prolongations
Voicing errors

Source: Adapted from Duffy, J. (2005). Motor speech disorders: Substrates, differential diagnosis, and management (2nd ed.). St. Louis, MO: Elsevier-Mosby.

Lesion Sites and Etiologies

Generally speaking, apraxia of speech results from damage to the left hemisphere (Duffy, 2005). Left hemisphere lesions at or around the inferior-posterior frontal lobe (Broca's area) often produce apraxia of speech. Sometimes lesion to the left parietal lobe in conjunction with lesion at the left frontal lobe produces apraxia of speech (Duffy, 2005). However, considerable debate exists over the exact location of a single focal lesion site in the left hemisphere that creates apraxia of speech.

Square, Roy, and Martin (1997) suggest that apraxia of speech can result from lesion to the parietal or frontal cortex or the subcortex underlying the frontal cortex. Dronkers (1996) used computerized axial tomography (CAT scans) and magnetic resonance imaging (MRI) to identify a left hemisphere lesion site in the precentral gyrus of the anterior insula, which she concludes is specialized for the motor planning of speech and produces apraxia of speech when damaged. However, Hillis, Work, Barker, Jacobs, Breese, and Maruer (2004) take exception to Dronkers' (1996) methods. Hillis and associates (2004) argue that their results indicate that, despite the correlation between apraxia of speech and lesion of the precentral gyrus of the anterior insula, dysfunction of Broca's area is more likely the primary

lesion site that produces apraxia of speech. Hillis and colleagues (2004) also state that it is likely that in addition to Broca's, multiple areas are involved in motor planning of speech and damage to any might produce apraxia of speech.

The etiologies of apraxia of speech include any process or event that damages the left inferior-posterior frontal lobe. The usual etiology of apraxia of speech is stroke involving occlusion of the left middle cerebral artery (Hillis et al., 2004), which affects the left insula and Broca's area, among other areas. However, apraxia of speech is also produced by generalized head trauma as well as focal trauma such as surgical trauma resulting from removal of an aneurysm or tumor in the vicinity of Broca's area.

Other Apraxias

There are different forms of apraxia besides apraxia of speech. These disorders are impairments of the ability to perform skilled purposeful movement. Like apraxia of speech, the following disorders cannot be accounted for by abnormal muscle tone, lack of strength, cognitive deficits, sensory difficulties, or a lack of coordination. The terminology and definitions used in different professions to refer to these disorders vary. Other apraxias worth noting are the following:

- *Buccofacial-oral apraxia (nonverbal apraxia, oral apraxia):* An inability to program and carry out any volitional movements of the tongue, cheeks, lips, pharynx, or larynx *on command.* Although individuals with this disorder might be unable to move their articulators in a volitional fashion on command, they usually can accomplish the same actions automatically in a natural context. So, if an individual is asked to "pucker your lips like you are giving a kiss," he might be unable to accomplish the task but shortly thereafter might pucker his lips appropriately when leaning in to kiss his wife. Volitional speech can also be affected whereas more formulaic utterances might be left unimpaired (as in apraxia of speech).

- *Ideomotor apraxia:* The lack of ability to program motor movements for pantomiming gestures and for the use of tools despite possessing the knowledge of how the tools are used and their function. For instance, an individual with this disorder can explain the purpose of a hairbrush and how to brush one's hair, but if she is given a hairbrush, she is unable to accomplish the task on command. However, this same individual may wake up each morning and automatically brush her hair in the natural context of standing in front of the bathroom mirror (Unsworth, 2007).

- *Ideational apraxia:* An inability to conceptualize a task, formulate motor plans required for the task, or hold in memory the idea of the task long enough to accomplish it successfully. Individuals with this disorder can perform individual components of a task but lack the ability to perform a series of actions sequentially to accomplish an entire act. An individual with ideational apraxia, if handed a hairbrush, may be able to raise the brush to his head but then be unable to accomplish the remaining actions necessary to brush his hair successfully. The primary difference between ideational and ideomotor apraxia is that individuals with ideational apraxia cannot perform the task volitionally or automatically whereas those with ideomotor apraxia perform well automatically and spontaneously but not on command.

Concomitant Disorders

Lesion to the left cerebral hemisphere, not lesion to the brain stem or subcortical structures, produces apraxia of speech. Due to the location of lesions in the inferior-posterior frontal lobe of the left cerebral hemisphere, lesions that produce apraxia of speech are also likely to create a number of accompanying deficits and disorders:

- *Hemiplegia/hemiparesis:* Individuals with apraxia of speech usually also have hemiplegia or hemiparesis contralateral to the cerebral hemisphere where the lesion is located. Notably, because most lesions producing apraxia of speech occur in the left hemisphere and because the left hemisphere controls the right hand, which is often the dominant writing hand, the hemiplegia/hemiparesis affects the individual's ability to write. The unfortunate net effect here is that, even if language abilities are preserved, apraxia of speech can inhibit verbal expression, while the accompanying hemiplegia/hemiparesis can inhibit written expression.

- *Hyperreflexia:* A likely result of damage to the motor areas of the brain that produces apraxia of speech is also concomitant damage to the upper motor neurons, which transmit extrapyramidal impulses of reflex regulation to the brain stem and spinal cord. Without these impulses to inhibit overactive release of reflexes, many inappropriate reflexes are released and others are made hyperactive.

- *Dysarthria:* A lesion at or near motor areas of the left frontal lobe that produces apraxia of speech is also likely to damage descending motor tracts (upper motor neurons) located in the same vicinity, thereby producing a dysarthria. In fact, data gathered by Duffy (2005) at the Mayo Clinic indicates that 29% of patients with apraxia of speech sampled also displayed a dysarthria, usually spastic dysarthria or unilateral upper motor neuron (UUMN) dysarthria.

- *Buccofacial apraxia/ideomotor apraxia:* Other apraxias such as these can occur alongside apraxia of speech or in isolation.

- *Nonfluent aphasia:* As previously mentioned, apraxia of speech is often the result of lesion at or near Broca's area and the presence of language deficits following lesion to Broca's area is almost a given. These language deficits usually take the form of a nonfluent aphasia. Distinguishing apraxic from aphasic errors in these individuals can be difficult.

Differentiation from Dysarthria

At times, differentiating apraxia of speech errors from dysarthric errors can prove challenging. However, there are notable distinctions between the two, as follows:

- Articulation errors produced by those with apraxia of speech are more likely to occur on longer and phonetically complex words. In contrast, dysarthric errors are consistent, predictable, and occur with the same frequency on shorter, phonetically simple words as on longer, phonetically complex words.
- Articulation errors produced by those with apraxia of speech are varied and inconsistent. These individuals can produce portions of utterances entirely free from errors, called islands of intact articulation. Articulation errors as a result of the dysarthrias are usually consistent and predictable.
- Individuals with apraxia of speech have greater difficulty producing less automatic and more volitional utterances whereas they can produce

automatic, nonvolitional utterances error free. For example, when a patient with apraxia of speech is given a card with the word *apple* written on it and is asked to say the word, he might be unable to produce it without error. However, while food shopping with his wife later this same patient can state that he likes *apples* with no errors or effort. (This phenomenon is usually followed by a quick look of exasperation on the patient's face.) In contrast, the dysarthrias usually negatively affect articulation equally across both natural and less natural, more volitional situations.

- Buccofacial-oral apraxia more often accompanies apraxia of speech than the dysarthrias.
- Impaired oral and velopharyngeal muscle strength, abnormal muscle tone, and limited range of movement suggest dysarthria. Whereas normal muscle strength, muscle tone, and appropriate range of movement of mobile articulators suggest apraxia of speech.

Table 6-2 shows percentage data on categories of errors produced by speakers with dysarthria and apraxia of speech. Both speakers with dysarthria and apraxia of speech often insert the schwa sound at times. However, dysarthric speech is overwhelmingly characterized by phoneme distortions, whereas apraxic speech is characterized more by phoneme substitutions and phoneme repetitions.

Table 6-2 **Percentages of Speech Errors Seen in Dysarthrias and Apraxia of Speech**

Speech Errors in Dysarthrias	Occurrence (%)	Speech Errors in Apraxia of Speech	Occurrence (%)
Distortions	65	Substitutions	32
Intrusive schwa	18	Repetitions	18
Substitutions	9	Intrusive schwa	18
Additions	5	Other	12
Other	2	Distortions	10
Repetitions	0.5	Additions	9
Omissions	0.5	Omissions	1

Source: Adapted from Johns, D. F., Darley, F. L. (1970) Phonemic variability in apraxia of speech. Journal of Speech and Hearing Research 13, 556–583.

Motor Speech Evaluation

A motor speech evaluation is undertaken to determine the presence of a motor speech disorder, if any, and to establish the severity of *any* motor speech disorder present not just apraxia of speech. The evaluation procedures discussed here may also be applied to diagnose the dysarthrias as well. However, an experienced speech-language pathologist often can immediately differentiate between errors resulting from apraxia of speech and those resulting from the dysarthrias, though achieving confirmation by further assessment procedures is always warranted.

The accurate evaluation and diagnosis of motor speech disorders serve multiple purposes:

- To identify the presence and establish the severity of any articulatory, resonatory, phonatory, or respiratory problems within the speech of the affected individual
- To validate a medical-neurologic diagnosis or to identify possible medical etiologies because the presence of a motor speech disorder often implies the presence of a problem in the nervous system
- To set goals for therapy and to determine the appropriate approaches used to achieve goals
- To develop a tentative prognosis for recovery of speech

Components of the Motor Speech Evaluation

The typical components of a motor speech evaluation are the following:

- A case history taken from medical records, and from patient and caregiver interviews
- An oral motor evaluation with maximum performance tasks
- Speech tasks that assess error patterns in speech
- Identification of confirmatory signs to support hypothesized motor speech diagnoses
- Instrumental measures

- Possibly, administration of a formal test of apraxia of speech, dysarthria, and/or intelligibility

Taking a Case History

It is useful to begin searching for diagnostic clues in the medical history and then in the speech of the affected individual. Gaining knowledge of the patient about to be evaluated begins with a thorough review of available medical records. This search for background information continues with the interview of the patient and caregivers. During a patient interview, speech-language pathologists typically ask questions that explore the nature of the illness or pathology producing speech problems as well as the perceived impact that speech deficits have on communication abilities and the patient's state of mind. In addition, an interview is useful for observing the speech capabilities, or lack thereof, of the patient in a natural context.

Oral Motor Evaluation with Maximum Performance Tasks

The **oral motor evaluation**, or oral mechanism evaluation, is the examination of the patient's individual oral structures and articulators and the observation of their nonspeech function. Put simply, this is the part of the evaluation when the speech-language pathologist asks the patient to move the tongue, lips, and mandible in certain ways so that the basic function of these structures and general appearance of the oral cavity can be evaluated. Speech-language pathologists employ a variety of nonspeech tasks to assess the integrity of the motor functions of the mobile articulators. Nonspeech tasks are used to isolate and test the functioning of any structure outside of the context of speech production for strength, mobility, range of motion, and symmetry of oral structures. Examples of nonspeech tasks include protruding and retracting the lips to assess the associated muscles as well

> **Oral motor evaluation** An evaluation of the oral structures and functions used in speech.

Table 6-3 Nonspeech Oral Motor Tasks Employed During Oral Motor Assessment

Oral Structure	Nonspeech Task
Lips	Labial protrusion, retraction, and lateralization against no resistance
	Labial protrusion, retraction, and lateralization against active resistance
	Puff checks and check for leaking of air at lips
Tongue	Lingual protrusion, retraction, and lateralization against no resistance
	Lingual protrusion, retraction, and lateralization against active resistance
Mandible	Elevation and depression of mandible against no resistance
	Elevation and depression of mandible against active resistance
	Lateralization of mandible with no resistance
	Lateralization of mandible with active resistance

as protruding, retracting, and lateralizing the tongue to assess the motor abilities of the lingual muscles.

The exact protocols for conducting oral motor evaluations differ greatly among speech-language pathologists according to personal preference. **Table 6-3** lists some common tasks employed during oral motor assessments. **Figure 6-1** is an example of an oral motor evaluation checklist.

Maximum performance tasks are often administered during oral motor evaluations. These tasks are used to test a patient's maximum limit of ability and to compare the patient's greatest effort on a task with a known average performance rate of unimpaired individuals. If a patient's maximum effort and performance fall short of those of unimpaired individuals, it can indicate a deficit.

A well-known example of a maximum performance task is diadochokinetic rates, also known as alternating motion rates (AMRs) and sequential motion rates (SMRs). Alternating motion rates are simple repetitive motor tasks that are used to test the speed and regularity of movement with which a single syllable can be uttered. The syllables usually employed in this diagnostic task are /pʌ/, /tʌ/, and /kʌ/ (i.e., "puh," "tuh," and "kuh"). A speech-language pathologist elicits the rapid repetition of each of these syllables individually. An unimpaired speaker usually can produce five repetitions of AMRs per second.

Sequential motion rates are the rapid repetition of more than one syllable at a time in sequence. Sequential motion rates test the individual's ability to move the articulators rapidly and precisely from one position to the next. The phoneme sequences used in sequential motion rates usually include /pʌtʌ/, /tʌkʌ/, /pʌkʌ/, and /pʌtʌkʌ/ (i.e., "puhtuh," "tuhkuh," "puhkuh," and "puhtuhkuh").

Some speech-language pathologists argue against the utility of AMRs and SMRs, stating that this practice only generates information about the nonspeech functioning of the involved structures, whereas therapy must always have a goal of improving actual speech function. Nonetheless, AMRs and SMRs are commonly employed alongside speech tasks in speech evaluations.

A maximum performance task that does employ speech production is the speech stress test. During a speech stress test, the patient is given a book to read aloud or is cued by the speech-language pathologist to speak continuously for up to 5 minutes to see if the person becomes fatigued and how this fatigue affects speech. The speech abilities of an unimpaired speaker do not degrade over 5 minutes of use. If speech production abilities do degrade over 5 minutes or less time as a result of muscle fatigue, that is indicative of pathology.

> **Maximum performance tasks** Tasks used to test an individual's maximum limit of ability and to compare the individual's greatest effort on a task with the known average performance rate of unimpaired individuals.

Speech Tasks

After the structures and functions of the articulators and speech systems have been examined in isolation using nonspeech tasks, it is useful then to observe how the patient performs when asked to coordinate these structures and functions to produce speech. Attempted speech is first

Speech-Language Pathology Clinic
Oral-motor Evaluation

Patient: _____ Age: _____

Date: _____ Examiner: _____

Room number: _____ c/o: _____

Circle appropriate options and note relevant abnormalities

Facial Symmetry at Rest: *Observe facial symmetry*

Symmetrical: Y/N   Asymmetrical: Eyes (right/left)   Cheeks (right/left)   Lips (right/left)

Notes: _____

Evaluation of Labial Movement: *Ask client to pucker*

Normal strength: Y/N   Reduced strength: (right/left)   Pucker deviates: (right/left)

Normal range-of-motion: Y/N   Reduced range-of-motion: (right/left)

Ask client to pucker against mild resistance of tongue depressor

Normal strength: Y/N

Ask client to smile

Symmetrical: Y/N   Smile deviates: (right/left)

Ask client to close lips and inflate cheeks to test labial seal

Strong labial seal (no air leaking between lips)   Weak labial seal (some air leakage): (right/left)

Notes: _____

Evaluation of Mandible: *Ask client to open their mouth*

Opens symmetrically: Y/N   Mandible deviates: (right/left)

Reduced range-of-motion: _____

Ask client to move mandible from side to side

Normal range-of-motion: Y/N   Reduced range-of-motion: (right/left)

Ask client to lower mandible against moderate resistance of your gloved hand

Normal strength: Y/N   Reduced strength: _____

Ask client to raise mandible against a mild resistance of your gloved hand holding chin down

Normal strength: Y/N   Reduced strength: _____

Notes: _____

Figure 6-1 A sample checklist for an oral motor evaluation.

Evaluation of Dentition

Teeth: Present/Absent/Dentures present/Owns dentures but does not wear/Owns dentures but are lost

Dental hygiene: _____

Occlusion: Normal occlusion/Malocclusion (Class I, Class II, Class III) _____

Notes: _____

Evaluation of Tongue: *Observe tongue at rest*

Color: Normal/Abnormal: _____

Appearance: _____

Extra/abnormal movements: _____

Ask client to protrude tongue

Extra/abnormal movements: _____

Symmetrical extension of tongue: Y/N   Tongue deviates: (right/left)

Ask client to protrude tongue and move tongue as far left and as far right as possible

Normal range-of-motion: Y/N   Reduced range-of-motion: (right/left)

Ask client to push left and then right against tongue depressor with extended tongue

Normal strength: Y/N   Reduced strength: _____

Ask client to push tongue against inside of left and right cheeks against resistance of your gloved hand

Normal strength: Y/N   Reduced strength: _____

Notes: _____

Evaluation of Hard Palate

Color: Normal/Abnormal: _____

Palatal arch: Normal/High/Low

Symmetrical: Y/N   Asymmetrical: _____

Noted abnormalities: Fistula/Cleft/Other _____

Notes: _____

Evaluation of Velum/Pharynx: *Observe velum*

Symmetrical: Y/N   Velum deviates: (right/left)

Color: Normal/Abnormal: _____

Appearance: _____

Extra/abnormal movements: _____

Figure 6-1 (Continued)

Observe tonsils

Appearance: Tonsils removed / Tonsils normal / Tonsils enlarged

Laryngeal Evaluation: *Ask client to cough as hard as they can*

Normal strong cough/Weak cough   Dry cough/Wet cough   Hypoadduction/
Hyperadduction

Ask client to sustain an /a/ for as long as possible

Greater than 20 seconds: _____   Less than 20 seconds: _____

Speech and Speech-like Tasks

Sequential and alternating motion rates

/pʌ/: _____   /tʌ /: _____   /kʌ/: _____

/pʌtʌ /: _____   /tʌkʌ/: _____   pʌkʌ: _____

/pʌtʌkʌ/: _____

Spontaneous Speech Sample: *Observe speech during interview*

Resonance (Normal/Abnormal): _____

Pitch/Loudness of voice (Normal/Abnormal): _____

Summary of Findings:

Figure 6-1 (Continued)

observed during the initial interview portion of the evaluation. For verbal repetitions, the speech-language pathologist asks the patient to repeat words, phrases, or sentences. For oral reading tasks (e.g., stress test), the speech-language pathologist asks the patient to read aloud and this production can be used to further gauge how the speech of the individual is affected.

It is important for the speech-language pathologist to be sure to assess the patient's ability to produce connected speech and spontaneous speech. This can be accomplished by asking open-ended questions (not yes/no questions) in the patient interview, by asking the patient to describe a picture presented to him or her, or by asking the patient to tell or retell a story.

Identification of Confirmatory Signs

Confirmatory signs are any observable physiologic characteristics displayed by the individual that support the speech-language pathologist's diagnosis. They can range from the presence of abnormal muscle tone (flaccid or spastic), to patterns of paresis/paralysis, to the presence of abnormal reflexes or involuntary movements.

Instrumental Measures

If possible, instrumental measures to accompany and support the observations of the speech-language pathologist are also warranted. Common instruments used to assess phonatory measures are Kay Elemetrics

Visi Pitch and Computerized Speech Lab (CSL). Speech-language pathologists can use Visi Pitch and CSL to assess the appropriateness of frequency (pitch) and intensity (loudness) of voice, range of frequency and intensity, as well as the regularity of vocal fold frequency and intensity during vocal fold vibration. Spectrographic analysis of speech, which can also be conducted using Visi Pitch or CSL or other products, generates useful data about the articulation, coarticulation, and voice onset times in speech.

Formal Tests/Assessments

Tests have been published to assist the speech-language pathologist in correctly identifying apraxia of speech, the dysarthrias, and their consequent impact on intelligibility. These tests often provide a standardized and methodical approach to diagnosis and assessment of severity. A test of apraxia of speech is the Apraxia Battery for Adults (Dabul, 2000).

Tests of dysarthria are as follows:

- Frenchay Dysarthria Assessment (FDA; Enderby, 1983)
- Dysarthria Examination Battery (DEB; Drummond, 1993)
- Quick Assessment for Dysarthria (Tanner & Culbertson, 1999)

Tests of intelligibility are as follows:

- Assessments of Intelligibility in Dysarthic Speakers (AIDS; Yorkston & Beukelman, 1981)
- Word Intelligibility Test (Kent, Weismer, Kent, & Rosenbek, 1989)

Therapy for Apraxia of Speech

Some general considerations when undertaking therapy for apraxia of speech are the presence of any concomitant deficits or other medical or emotional conditions that can complicate therapy. As mentioned previously, those with apraxia of speech very rarely do not have notable aphasia deficits as well as some level of dysarthria. It is often necessary for the speech-language pathologist to observe the patient and to determine the severity of all disorders affecting communication, the likelihood of decreasing the severity of these disorders, and the functional impact each disorder has on the patient's communication abilities. In other words, the speech-language pathologist might not have time to target all these problems at once and might have to choose to target the deficit that is most negatively affecting communication or the deficit most likely to resolve.

Prosthetics are of no use in remediating the disorder of apraxia of speech. Also, no pharmaceuticals can resolve this disorder, although many medicines are usually administered to combat the underlying medical etiologies, usually stroke, that create apraxia of speech. Three therapy treatment approaches are commonly applied for the treatment of communication deficits following apraxia of speech: articulatory-kinematic therapy, intersystemic reorganization, and alternative/augmentative communication strategies (AAC).

Articulatory-Kinematic Approaches

Perhaps the most commonly applied therapy for apraxia of speech is the articulatory-kinematic approach. This approach assumes that apraxia of speech is a disorder of the ability to create or retrieve motor plans for speech. Following this assumption, the articulatory-kinematic approach relies on motor learning theory and on the principle of neuroplasticity to attempt to reestablish motor planning abilities for speech. The principle of neuroplasticity assumes that the brain is changeable (plastic) and that it can rearrange itself to regain lost function after damage.

The articulatory-kinematic approach assumes, because the brain is plastic, that the lost motor abilities for speech can be retrieved or rebuilt by cueing the brain through therapy. Wambaugh amd Mauszycki (2010) state that to accomplish this goal this therapy approach relies heavily on three main components of motor learning: motor practice, modeling–repetition, and articulatory cueing. Motor practice is the intensive and repetitive production of movements (drill) to increase articulatory ability. Usually this centers on the repetitive production of target phonemes in isolation or within words or phrases, usually with verbal feedback from the speech-language pathologist. Modeling–repetition is when the speech-language pathologist produces the target phoneme, word, or phrase and instructs the patient to pay special attention to how the target word is articulated, and then to attempt to imitate the speech-language pathologist. Articulatory cueing is described by Mauszycki and Wambaugh (2011) as phonetic placement cues or phonetic derivations. Phonetic cues are descriptions given by the speech-language pathologist to the patient to increase the patient's awareness and understanding of articulatory requirements needed to produce the target. Phonetic derivations are when the speech-language pathologist teaches a patient to alter the distinctive features of one phoneme to produce another phoneme (also called shaping).

The articulatory-kinematic approach of Sound Production Treatment (SPT) by Wambaugh and colleagues employs the previously mentioned techniques and has been demonstrated by Wambaugh and Nessler (2004) to be effective in improving the speech of individuals with apraxia of speech. Sound Production Treatment is a therapy for apraxia of speech with research supporting its use (Wambaugh, 2004; Wambaugh & Nessler, 2004). A distinctive characteristic of SPT is the use of minimal contrast pairs in which the target phoneme is placed within an utterance and paired with an utterance that is minimally different (e.g., "The pear fell. The bear fell.") (Wambaugh, Doyle, Kalinyak, & West, 1996). The repeated practice of minimal contrast pairs in SPT gives the patient continuing and multiple opportunities to modify his or her speech patterns for the approximation of target phonemes or words. Which phonemes are targets for therapy are decided by the particular needs of the patient.

Another articulatory-kinematic therapy approach that seeks to reestablish motor plans for speech is

Clinical Note

Phonetic Derivation

An example of phonetic derivation is when the patient with apraxia of speech can produce the /z/ phoneme, and then the speech-language pathologist instructs the patient to change an aspect of /z/, say, to remove the voicing. Upon removal of the voicing, the phoneme produced is the /s/ phoneme. (When you whisper the /z/ phoneme, it turns into /s/.) Usually, even in severe cases of apraxia of speech the patient has one intact word or phoneme from which other words or phonemes can be derived and then practiced.

In the absence of the patient's ability to produce any phonemes, the speech-language pathologist must shape phonemes from nonspeech movements of the articulators. Care should be taken to focus on training movements for speech acts as quickly as possible rather than perseverating on perfecting the production of nonspeech movements.

known as PROMPT (Prompts for Restructuring Oral Muscular Phonetic Targets) (Hayden, 1984). The basis of the PROMPT method is to provide tactile kinesthetic cues, in addition to visual and auditory cues, to elicit production of the target phoneme or word. PROMPT therapy uses a system of touch and motion cues to help illustrate to the patient the features of the target sound. These cues involve the speech-language pathologist touching the head, face, or neck of the patient at various points to facilitate successful articulation. For instance, voicing on a phoneme is indicated by the speech-language pathologist placing four fingers to the side of the patient's neck at the larynx while articulation for a bilabial phoneme is cued by a tap of the lips. These tactile kinesthetic cues used in the PROMPT system as listed in Hayden (1984) can be used to illustrate such characteristics as the following:

- Place of articulation
- Muscles employed for phoneme production
- Level of tension required in muscles

- Voicing
- Nasality
- Movement of articulators
- Timing/speech of movement
- Degree of opening of mandible

A distinctive feature of the PROMPT system is that the speech-language pathologist's cues for each phoneme can be strung together to produce a continuous stream of cues to move a patient through an entire sequence of target phonemes. This technique was first developed in an attempt to treat developmental apraxia of speech in children (Hayden, 1984) but was later applied to acquired apraxia of speech (Bose, Square, Schlosser, & Van Lieshout, 2001; Square, Chumpelik, Morningstar, & Adams, 1986).

Melodic Intonation Therapy

It has long been observed that individuals with aphasia often have an intact ability to sing despite their loss of language. To capitalize on this intact melodic processing and to use it to facilitate speech, melodic intonation therapy was developed to teach the reacquisition of language by pairing exaggerated prosody and melodic components with production of phonemes and words. Studies examining the response of those with aphasia support this method's use in certain types of aphasia (Marshall & Holtzapple, 1976; Sparks, Helm, & Albert, 1974).

Although melodic intonation therapy was developed originally as a means of treating aphasia (Sparks et al., 1974), it has been applied successfully to the treatment of apraxia of speech. Dunham and Newhoff (1979) report the case of a man 7 months post stroke who was able to produce only a few phonemes. By learning a melody to pair with his phonemes, he was eventually able to imitate novel words and produce eight utterances using a written stimulus.

Intersystemic Reorganization

Intersystemic reorganization, a term coined by A. R. Luria, is the facilitation of speech by pairing the actions of an intact system (one not traditionally associated with speech) with the actions of the impaired speech system in an effort to facilitate operation of the speech system. Usually, this technique is used by routinely pairing a specific physical act (e.g., a gesture) that was not previously paired with speech with the simultaneous production of the target word (Rosenbek, Collins, & Wertz, 1976). The purpose of pairing these two actions is, once associated in the brain, the initiation of one action primes and increases the likelihood of initiation of the other. This is known as associative or Hebbian learning, and the popular mantra used to convey this principle is *neurons that fire together wire together*. When the use of gestures is used to retrain and facilitate speech the method can be referred to as gestural reorganization.

Research into intersystemic reorganization has classically focused on pairing sign language (specifically American Indian Sign Language [Amerind]) with verbal production of words (Skelly, Schensky, Smith, & Fust, 1974). However, intersystemic reorganization therapy can use any physical action paired with a verbal utterance, such as more meaningful gestures that an observer might understand even without an accompanying utterance (Goldstein & Cameron, 1952) or less meaningful gestures such as simple finger tapping (Simmons, 1978).

Augmentative and Alternative Strategies

Augmentative and alternative communication (AAC) strategies are commonly used to treat many communication disorders, including severe-profound apraxia of speech. Augmentative and alternative communication strategies can be low tech, such as picture exchange systems, letterboards, or pen and paper, or high tech, including speech output devices such as a Dynavox device or certain speech output apps now available on smartphones.

Usually, AAC is employed only in the long term for those individuals with severe or profound levels of apraxia of speech. However, these strategies can also be used as a stop-gap to establish functional communication until the individual with apraxia of speech has regained enough speech skills for functional verbal communication. Compensatory strategies such as AAC or alternative language modalities can also be used as long-term procedures to reestablish the functional communication of those individuals who are unlikely to regain lost speech skills.

Main Points

- Motor speech disorders involve inability in the effective manufacture, refinement, transmission, and execution of motor plans for speech. Motor speech disorders include apraxia of speech and the dysarthrias.
- Apraxia of speech is divided into two categories:
  - Acquired apraxia of speech, which is the result of damage to the brain
  - Developmental apraxia of speech, which is the result of an unknown congenital etiology
- Apraxia of speech is the inability to create and sequence (i.e., program) the neural impulses necessary to create appropriate motor movements for speech.
- Apraxia of speech is the result of disruption of the motor speech programmer, which is a network of structures that contribute to construction of motor plans for speech. Left hemisphere structures such as Broca's area, the supplementary motor cortex, primary motor cortex, basal ganglia, and cerebellum are involved in the appropriate production of motor plans for speech.
- Apraxia of speech is characterized by articulation errors, limited prosody, slowed rate, and the visible groping about of the tongue, lips, and mandible.
- The prosody of those with apraxia of speech is usually highly affected by the decreased rate of speech commonly adopted to avoid errors and attempts at self-repairing speech errors.
- The articulation errors of those with apraxia of speech are inconsistent and composed mostly of various sound-level errors: phoneme substitutions, phoneme distortions, and voice-onset errors.
- Phonemes or phoneme combinations that require greater motor planning abilities for successful execution are more difficult for those with apraxia of speech to produce than are phonemes or phoneme combinations that require less motor planning abilities.
- Individuals with apraxia of speech characteristically have islands of intact articulation.
- Left hemisphere lesions at or around the inferior-posterior frontal lobe (Broca's area) often produce apraxia of speech.
- The most common etiologies of lesions producing apraxia of speech is a stroke occluding portions of the left middle cerebral artery, generalized head trauma, or focal head trauma.
- Apraxia of speech often co-occurs with the dysarthrias and some level of aphasia.
- Other forms of apraxia include the following:
  - *Buccofacial-oral apraxia:* An inability to program and carry out any volitional movements of the tongue, cheeks, lips, pharynx, or larynx *on command.* However, individuals might be able to move the articulators in a less volitional, more natural and reflexive context.
  - *Ideomotor apraxia:* The lack of ability to program motor movements for the use of tools and the pantomiming of gestures despite possessing the knowledge of how the object is used and its function.

- *Ideational apraxia:* An inability to conceptualize a task, formulate motor plans required for the task, or hold in memory the idea of the task long enough to accomplish the task successfully.
- Concomitant disorders that can co-occur with apraxia of speech include hemiplegia/hemiparesis, hyperreflexia, dysarthria, buccofacial-oral apraxia, ideomotor apraxia, and nonfluent aphasia.
- Apraxia of speech differs from dysarthria in several ways: Apraxic articulation errors occur on longer and more phonetically complex words and errors are varied and inconsistent; dysarthric articulation errors occur on both short, phonetically simple words as well as long, complex words with consistent and predictable outcomes. Individuals with apraxia of speech often find less automatic utterances more difficult to execute than more automatic utterances whereas individuals with dysarthria will consistently produce errors across automatic and more volitional utterances. Buccofacial-oral apraxia is more likely to co-occur with apraxia of speech than with dysarthria. Normal muscle strength, muscle tone, and range of motion are present in apraxia of speech, whereas impaired oral/velopharyngeal muscle strength, abnormal muscle tone, and limited range of motion are often characteristic of dysarthria.
- A motor speech evaluation is used to accomplish the following:
  - Determine the presence and severity of a motor speech disorder
  - Determine the presence and severity of articulatory, resonatory, phonatory, or respiratory problems with speech production
  - Confirm or contradict medical-neurologic diagnosis
  - Determine prognosis for recovery of speech
  - Set goals and determine therapy approaches to be used
- The typical components of a motor speech evaluation include the following:
  - Case history
  - Oral motor evaluation
  - Speech tasks
  - Identification of confirmatory signs
  - Instrumental measures
  - Administration of a formal test
- Therapy for apraxia includes the following methods:
  - Articulatory-kinematic approaches, including strategies such as PROMPT, Sound Production Treatment, and Melodic Intonation Therapy
  - Intersystemic reorganization, the facilitation of speech by pairing the actions of an intact system (one not traditionally associated with speech) with the actions of the impaired speech system
  - Augmentative and alternative communication strategies, methods used to establish functional communication until the individual can verbally communicate again and for long-term use with those who have severe or profound levels of apraxia of speech

Review Questions

1. What is a motor speech disorder?
2. Define apraxia of speech.
3. Why does damage to the motor speech programmer create apraxia of speech?
4. What is a possible lesion site that produces apraxia of speech?
5. What is a common etiology of apraxia of speech?

6. How does apraxia of speech affect an individual's speech?

7. Describe the articulation errors that can occur in apraxia of speech.

8. Name and describe the three other discussed forms of apraxia.

9. What are three disorders that can occur alongside apraxia of speech?

10. How might one differentiate between dysarthria and apraxia of speech?

11. Why should a speech-language pathologist complete a motor speech evaluation on all patients?

12. What are the components of a motor speech evaluation?

13. What does an oral motor evaluation consist of?

14. Why are maximum performance tasks and speech tasks important during a motor speech evaluation?

15. What are two formal tests that can be used to determine the presence of apraxia of speech?

16. Why are prosthetics not useful in treating apraxia of speech?

17. How does articulatory-kinematic therapy work to remediate apraxia of speech?

18. What is a distinguishing characteristic of PROMPT therapy?

19. How does intersystemic reorganization therapy work to remediate apraxia of speech?

20. What are two reasons an individual with apraxia of speech might use augmentative and alternative communication strategies?

References

1. Bose, A., Square, P. A., Schlosser, R., & Van Lieshout, P. (2001). Effects of PROMPT therapy on speech motor function in a person with aphasia and apraxia of speech. *Aphasiology, 15*(8), 767–785.

2. Dabul, B. (2000). *Apraxia Battery for Adults* (2nd ed.). Austin, TX: Pro-Ed.

3. Darley, F., Aronson, A., & Brown, J. (1975). *Motor speech disorders*. Philadelphia, PA: W. B. Saunders.

4. Dronkers, N. (1996). A new brain region for coordinating speech articulation. *Nature, 384*, 6605.

5. Drummond, S. (1993). *Dysarthria Examination Battery (DEB)*. Tucson, AZ: Psychological Corporation.

6. Duffy, J. (2005). *Motor speech disorders: Substrates, differential diagnosis, and management* (2nd ed.). St. Louis, MO. Elsevier-Mosby.

7. Dunham, M., & Newhoff, M. (1979). Melodic intonation therapy: Rewriting the song. In *Clinical Aphasiology: Proceedings of the Conference 1979* (pp. 286–294). Minneapolis, MN: BRK.

8. Enderby, P. (1983). *Frenchay Dysarthria Assessment (FDA)*. San Diego, CA: Singular.

9. Goldstein, H., & Cameron, H. (1952). New method of communication for the aphasic patient. *Journal of the Arizona Medical Association, 9*, 17–21.

10. Hayden, D. (1984). The PROMPT system of therapy. *Seminars in Speech and Language, 5*(2), 139–156.

11. Hillis, A. E., Work, M., Barker, P. B., Jacobs, M. A., Breese, E. L., & Maruer, K. (2004). Re-examining the brain regions crucial for orchestrating speech articulation. *Brain, 127*, 1479–1487.

12. Johns, D. F., & Darley, F. L. (1970). Phonemic variability in apraxia of speech. *Journal of Speech and Hearing Research, 13*, 556–583.

13. Kent, R., Weismer, G., Kent, J., & Rosenbek, J. (1989). Toward intelligibility testing in dysarthria. *Journal of Speech and Hearing Disorders, 45*, 482–499.

14. Marshall, N., & Holtzapple, P. (1976). Melodic intonation therapy: Variations on a theme. In R. H. Brookshire (Ed.), *Clinical Aphasiology: Proceedings of the Conference 1976* (pp. 115–141). Minneapolis, MN: BRK.

15. Martin, A. D. (1974). Some objections to the term apraxia of speech. *Journal of Speech and Hearing Disorders, 39*, 556–583.

16. Mauszycki, S. C., & Wambaugh, J. (2011). Acquired apraxia of speech: A treatment overview. *ASHA Leader*. Retrieved from http://www.asha.org/Publications/leader/2011/110426/Acquired-Apraxia-of-Speech-A-Treatment-Overview/

17. Rosenbek, J. C., Collins, M., & Wertz, R. T. (1976). Intersystemic reorganization for apraxia of speech. In R. H. Brookshire (Ed.), *Clinical Aphasiology: Proceedings*

of the Conference 1976 (pp. 255–260). Minneapolis, MN: BRK.

18. Simmons, N. N. (1978). Finger counting as an intersystemic reorganizer in apraxia of speech. *Clinical Aphasiology, 1978*, 174–179.

19. Skelly, M., Schensky, L., Smith, R., & Fust, R. (1974). American Indian Sign (Amerind) as the facilitation of verbalization for the oral verbal apraxia. *Journal of Speech and Hearing Disorders, 39*, 445–456.

20. Sparks, R., Helm, N., & Albert, M. (1974). Aphasia rehabilitation resulting from melodic intonation therapy. *Cortex, 10*, 303–316.

21. Square, P. A., Chumpelik, D. A., Morningstar, D., & Adams, S. (1986). Efficacy of the PROMPT system of therapy for the treatment of acquired apraxia of speech: A follow-up investigation. *Clinical Aphasiology Conference*, 221–226.

22. Square, P. A., Roy, E. A., & Martin, R. E. (1997). Apraxia of speech: Another form of praxis disruption. In L. J. G. Rothi & K. M. Heilman (Eds.), *The neuropsychology of action* (pp. 173–206). East Sussex, England: Psychology Press.

23. Sugishita, M., Konno, K., Bake, S., Yunoki, K., Togashi, O., & Kawamura, M. (1987). Electropalatographic analysis of apraxia of speech in a left hander and a right hander. *Brain, 110*(5), 1393–1417.

24. Tanner, D., & Culbertson, W. (1999). *Quick Assessment for Dysarthria*. Oceanside, CA: Academic Communication Associates.

25. Unsworth, C. A. (2007). Cognitive and perceptual dysfunction. In S. B. O'Sullivan & T. J. Schmitt (Eds.), *Physical rehabilitation* (5th ed., pp. 1149–1188). Philadelphia, PA: F. A. Davis.

26. Wambaugh, J. L. (2004). Stimulus generalization effects of sound production treatment for apraxia of speech. *Journal of Medical Speech Language Pathology, 12*(2), 77–97.

27. Wambaugh, J. L., Doyle, P. J., Kalinyak, M. M., & West, J. E. (1996). A minimal contrast treatment for apraxia of speech. *Clinical Aphasiology Conference, 24*(97), 97–108.

28. Wambaugh, J. L., & Mauszycki, S. C. (2010). Sound production treatment: Application with severe apraxia of speech. *Aphasiology, 24*, 814–825.

29. Wambaugh, J. L., & Nessler, C. (2004). Modification of sound production treatment for aphasia: Generalization effects. *Aphasiology, 18*, 407–427.

30. West, C., Hesketh, A., Vail, A., & Bowen, A. (2009). Intervention for apraxia of speech following stroke. *Cochrane Database of Systemic Review, 4*, 1–12.

31. Yorkston, K., & Beukelman, D. (1981). *Assessments of Intelligibility of Dysarthria Speakers (AIDS)*. Tigard, OR: C. C. Publications.

Chapter 7

Motor Speech Disorders: The Dysarthrias

 Where this icon appears, visit http://go.jblearning.com/ManascoCWS to view the corresponding video.

Continuing the discussion of motor speech disorders, this chapter focuses on the dysarthrias. Whereas apraxia of speech is an inability to create the appropriate motor plans for execution of muscle movements for speech, the dysarthrias are the result of disturbances in the motor system that occur between the creation of an intact motor speech plan and the execution of those motor plans by the relevant musculature.

The Dysarthrias

The landmark research of Darley, Aronson, and Brown (1969a, 1969b, 1975) performed at the Mayo Clinic underlies and shapes our present-day understanding of the dysarthrias. The system of dysarthria classification created by Darley, Aronson, and Brown is now simply known as the Mayo Clinic model of dysarthria classification. The formal definition of

dysarthria presented by Darley, Aronson, and Brown (1975) is as follows:

> Dysarthria comprises a group of speech disorders resulting from disturbances in muscular control. Because there has been damage to the central or peripheral nervous system, some degree of weakness, slowness, incoordination, or altered muscle tone characterizes the activity of the speech mechanism. (p. 2)

Following in the tradition of these researchers, Duffy (2005) expands this earlier definition to recognize that a dysarthria can be produced by problems other than the "weakness, slowness, incoordination, or altered muscle tone" (Darley et al., 1975, p. 2). Duffy (2005) states the dysarthrias are

> a collective name for a group of neurologic speech disorders resulting from abnormalities in the strength, speed, range, steadiness, tone, or accuracy of movements required for the control of the respiratory, phonatory, or resonatory, articulatory, and prosodic aspects of speech production (p. 5).

> **Dysarthria** A group of disorders of speech caused by damage to the central or peripheral nervous system that creates weakness, slowness, incoordination, or abnormal muscle tone in musculature used to produce speech.

Therefore, the dysarthrias are a group of disorders produced by damage to the central nervous system (CNS) or peripheral nervous system (PNS) that results in disordered movement that affects speech production. Although it is important for speech-language pathologists to look for and note possible nonspeech or physiologic characteristics associated with the presence of a dysarthria, it is important to realize that the dysarthrias are disorders of speech production. Therefore, a person cannot "look" dysarthric, though he might have visible signs of the presence of dysarthria. A person can only sound dysarthric because dysarthria is a problem at the level of speech production.

Importance of Lesion Localization

In the past, the term *dysarthria* was used in medical and scientific fields to refer to essentially any disturbance in speech. Hence, being diagnosed with dysarthria had little diagnostic usefulness because the term was so general. The work of Darley, Aronson, and Brown (1969a, 1969b, 1975) popularized the idea that dysarthria was not a single disorder but a group of disorders and, furthermore, that each type has its own profile of speech and physiologic characteristics that results from the specific site of damage in the CNS or PNS. Therefore, it logically follows that if a speech-language pathologist is able to discern the differences between the dysarthrias, then the speech-language pathologist can use that information to localize where within the nervous system the lesion causing the dysarthria is located. The differentiation and identification of the dysarthrias by Darley, Aronson, and Brown (1969a, 1969b, 1975) suddenly gave speech-language pathologists an important tool: If a problem in the nervous system can be localized to a specific area using speech characteristics, a diagnosis of a specific dysarthria can confirm an accurate medical diagnosis or contradict an incorrect medical diagnosis.

Another valuable outcome of using the differential diagnosis of the dysarthrias for lesion localization is the early detection of diseases whose presenting symptom is a dysarthria. Many degenerative diseases initially present with disordered motor movements that can produce speech problems well before any other signs of disease arise. These changes in speech might be noticed earlier than other changes in motor abilities because speech is used so frequently. Therefore, the presenting signs of many diseases of motor degeneration occur in speech production but these signs often go unrecognized by healthcare professionals. As a result, individuals with these initial symptoms of disordered speech are referred to the speech-language pathologist, but no medical diagnosis is made. A knowledgeable speech-language pathologist can identify specific dysarthrias and, upon identification, localize the neurologic problem to a specific area in the nervous system. When communicated to a medical doctor or neurologist, this information can lead to early diagnosis and treatment of disease.

There are six primary forms of dysarthria: flaccid, spastic, unilateral upper motor neuron, ataxic, hyperkinetic, and hypokinetic. A mixed dysarthria occurs when a patient presents multiple dysarthrias simultaneously. The lesion sites and the neuromotor basis of the dysarthrias are listed in Table 7-1.

Terminology New and Old

Before moving into the main content of this chapter, it is important that students of speech-language pathology review and understand the meaning of these important terms:

Bilateral On both sides

Contralateral On the opposite side

Hyperkinetic An excess of movement, too much movement to be appropriate

---

Bilateral On both sides.

Contralateral On the opposite side.

Hyperkinetic An excess of movement; too much movement to be appropriate.

Hyperreflexia An excess of reflexes; overactive reflexes.

Table 7-1 The Dysarthrias, Their Neuromotor Basis, and Lesion Location Within the Nervous System

Dysarthria	Neuromotor Basis	Lesion Locale
Flaccid	Hypotonia and weakness	Lower motor neuron
Spastic	Spasticity and weakness	Bilateral upper motor neuron
Unilateral Upper Motor Neuron	Spasticity and weakness	Unilateral upper motor neuron
Ataxic	Incoordination	Cerebellum or cerebellar connections within CNS
Hypokinetic	Reduced movement and reduced range of motion	Basal ganglia or basal ganglia connections within CNS
Hyperkinetic	Extra and abnormal movements	Basal ganglia or basal ganglia connections within CNS

Source: Adapted from Duffy, J. (2005). Motor speech disorders: Substrates, differential diagnosis, and management (2nd ed.). St. Louis, MO: Elsevier-Mosby.

Hyperreflexia An excess of reflexes, overactive reflexes

Hypertonic An excess of muscle tone, a tight muscle tone

Hypokinetic A lack of appropriate level of movement

Hyporeflexia A lack of appropriate reflexes

Hypotonic A lack of appropriate muscle tone

Ipsilateral On the same side

Lesion An abnormal change in body tissue usually as a result of disease or trauma

Paralysis A total loss of movement

Paresis A partial or incomplete loss of movement (weakness)

Speech systems Systems supporting the production of speech, including the articulatory system, the resonatory system, the phonatory system, and the respiratory system

Unilateral On one side

Flaccid Dysarthria

Flaccid dysarthria results from the flaccid weakness or paralysis of musculature used to produce speech. Flaccid weakness and paralysis are created by a low muscle tone (hypotonia) and a weakness in the muscles. Flaccid dysarthria can affect articulation, resonance, phonation, or respiration individually or all together, depending on which nerves are damaged. In general, the articulation of those with flaccid dysarthria has a slurred quality resulting from weakness in the lips and/or tongue. The voice of those with flaccid dysarthria is often breathy and soft, and the resonance of these individuals can be hypernasal. Listed in Table 7-2 are common speech characteristics of flaccid dysarthria in rank order of prominence.

Anatomic Basis of Flaccid Dysarthria

The origin of flaccid dysarthria is damage to the lower motor neurons of the cranial nerves. A lower motor neuron (LMN) is the efferent component of a cranial or spinal nerve. The LMNs are also referred

Hypertonic An excess of muscle tone; an excessively tight muscle tone.

Hypokinetic A lack of appropriate level of movement; too little movement.

Hyporeflexia A lack of appropriate reflexes.

Hypotonic A lack of appropriate muscle tone; a loose muscle tone.

Ipsilateral To be on the same side.

Lesion An abnormal change in body tissue usually as a result of disease or trauma.

Paralysis A total loss of movement.

Paresis A partial or incomplete loss of movement (weakness).

Speech systems Systems that support the production of speech, including the articulatory system, the resonatory system, the phonatory system, and the respiratory system.

Unilateral To be on one side.

Flaccid dysarthria A motor speech disorder resulting from flaccid weakness or paralysis of musculature used to produce speech.

Lower motor neuron (LMN) The efferent component of a cranial or spinal nerve. Also known as the final common pathway.

Table 7-2 Deviant Speech Characteristics of Flaccid Dysarthria Listed in Order from Most Common to Least Common.

Deviant Speech Characteristic
Hypernasality
Imprecise consonants
Breathy voice
Monopitch
Nasal emission
Audible inspiration
Harsh voice
Short phrases
Monoloud

Source: Adapted from Darley, F., Aronson, A., Brown, J. (1969b). Differential diagnostic patterns of dysarthria. Journal of Speech and Hearing Research 12, 246–269.

to as the *final common pathway* (Darley et al., 1975). Duffy (2005) explains that the term *final common pathway* is used because all motor activity and planning that occurs in the CNS must, ultimately, be funneled through and activate the LMNs before the muscles can appropriately execute motor plans; hence, the LMNs are the final and common mediator of motor activity through which all motor plans must pass before reaching the muscles.

The LMNs of the cranial and spinal nerves each serve specific muscles of the body. The LMNs of the cranial nerves serve the head and neck musculature necessary for speech production and synapse with the upper motor neurons (efferent motor tracts in the CNS; discussed later) in the brain stem. After the LMNs synapse with the upper motor neurons the axons of the LMNs course out through the soft tissue of the body to serve specific muscles, dividing and subdividing to innervate individual muscle fibers.

Although this chapter is primarily concerned with the motor functions of the cranial nerves, readers must not forget that some cranial nerves have both afferent and efferent pathways and some have only one or the other. Also, the cranial nerves are paired nerves but sometimes they are discussed as a single nerve,

for instance, *the trigeminal* refers to both the right trigeminal nerve that works to innervate the muscles of mastication on the right side of the mandible and the left trigeminal nerve that innervates the muscles of mastication on the left side of the mandible.

When an LMN is damaged, the muscle fibers innervated by that LMN cannot be activated for movement. This occurs because the neural impulse responsible for activating the muscles cannot be transmitted along the damaged LMN to the muscle to cue muscle activation.

When an LMN is damaged, the neural impulses sent to the muscle cannot reach the muscle or are degraded and weak by the time they reach the muscle as a result of poor conduction along the damaged nerve. This results in an inability of the muscle to carry out or fully carry out the action designated by the motor plans. In other words, the muscle displays a weakness or paralysis. However, not only is the damaged LMN unable to activate muscles properly for volitional motor movement but the LMN is also unable to activate musculature for the reflexive impulses (e.g., the stretch reflex), which give muscles their appropriate tone. These reflexive impulses are among the extrapyramidal impulses transmitted along the upper motor neuron. Because of the inability of a damaged LMN to activate muscles to execute these involuntary impulses of muscle tone maintenance, muscles innervated by the damaged LMN have decreased tone. A muscle with too little tone is hypotonic or flaccid. Hence, damage to the LMNs produces weakness and flaccidity. The outcome of this weakness and flaccidity in the muscles of the articulators and speech structures is the motor speech disorder known as flaccid dysarthria.

Common Etiologies of Flaccid Dysarthria

Flaccid dysarthria is created by damage to the LMNs of the cranial nerves or to the connections between the LMNs and muscle fibers (the motor units).

Essentially, any etiology that damages the cranial nerves involved in speech can produce a flaccid dysarthria. Strokes that occur in the brain stem and damage the cranial nerve nuclei (the structures where cranial nerves synapse with the CNS) are a common cause of flaccid dysarthria. Flaccid dysarthria can occur alone or is often seen mixed with spastic dysarthria, such as in traumatic brain injuries where trauma damages the upper motor neurons within the brain stem as well as the cranial nerve nuclei associated with the brain stem. Other common etiologies of flaccid dysarthria are surgical trauma, tumor, toxins, mass effect, congenital syndromes, and disease.

Any infectious, autoimmune, or neurodegenerative disease that is capable of affecting the LMNs of the cranial nerves or the LMN's connections to muscles is capable of producing a flaccid dysarthria. Examples of well-known infectious diseases that affect the LMNs of the cranial nerves are poliomyelitis (polio), (see the video *Poliomyelitis* for a discussion of LMN damage following polio infection), HIV/AIDS (Kennedy, 1988; Nicholas et al., 2010), peripheral neuroborreliosis (a variant of Lyme disease; Zajkowska et al., 2010), and Hansen's disease (leprosy; Aridon et al., 2010; Ooi & Srinivasan, 2004). Certain autoimmune diseases can also strike the LMNs, including Guillain-Barré syndrome, myasthenia gravis, and Lambert-Eaten syndrome. Some degenerative diseases that affect the PNS and the LMNs within it include muscular dystrophy, amyotrophic lateral sclerosis (ALS), progressive bulbar palsy, and Kennedy's disease (Duffy, 2005).

The Flaccid Dysarthrias

The cranial nerves that are most important for speech are the trigeminal (cranial nerve V), the facial (VII), the vagus (X), and the hypoglossal (XII). Because dysarthria is a disorder of speech production, and because the cranial nerves innervate most of the musculature necessary for speech production, discussion of the flaccid dysarthrias is largely a discussion of the role of the cranial nerves and the speech problems that occur when the LMNs of these nerves are damaged.

Damage to the LMNs of the cranial nerves usually occurs where they synapse at the brain stem at the cranial nerve nuclei, but damage to the LMNs of the cranial nerves is possible anywhere along the nerves. Lesion to each cranial nerve involved in speech can create an individual and distinct flaccid dysarthria. Because of the possible manifestations of flaccid dysarthria, Duffy (2005) argues that flaccid dysarthria should be thought of not as a single disorder but as many individual dysarthrias, each with its own outcomes and implications for lesion localization.

Flaccid Dysarthria Arising from Trigeminal Nerve Damage

The trigeminal synapses with the CNS at the level of the pons. This large cranial nerve has three branches: the ophthalmic, the maxillary, and the mandibular. While the ophthalmic and the maxillary are sensory branches of the trigeminal, the mandibular branch fulfills an important motor function: the innervation of the muscles of the mandible. Successful volitional movement of the mandible is important for mastication of foods and is also very important for articulation.

The tongue rests on the floor of the oral cavity, which is created by the muscles slung between the right and left sides of the mandible. For appropriate articulation of lingua-alveolar and linguadental phonemes, the tongue has to be able to approximate and make sufficient contact with the alveolar ridge and the maxillary incisors. For labiodental phonemes, the bottom lip must be able to approximate the upper teeth. For bilabial phonemes, the bottom lip must approximate the upper lip. To accomplish these actions necessary for appropriate articulation, the mandible must be raised enough to bring the tongue and lower lip close enough to these other articulators. When the trigeminal is damaged, the ability to elevate the mandible for the articulatory actions described above can be compromised.

Lesion to only the right or left trigeminal weakens or disables only the corresponding side of the mandible, leaving the contralateral and undamaged side functional for mastication and articulation mostly intact. Nonetheless, some mild articulatory difficulties or slow rate of speech to compensate for articulatory difficulties are possible with a lesion along one side of the trigeminal. In a case of unilateral mandibular weakness, the mandible deviates toward the side of the damaged nerve and consequently weakened musculature when the mandible is fully lowered (opening the mouth wide open). Over time, the weakened musculature (primarily the masseter muscle) innervated by the damaged trigeminal might atrophy from disuse while the intact musculature on the contralateral side of the mandible strengthens as a result of more frequent and intense use. Upon palpation, the intact masseter might present as larger and more prominent on contraction than the contralateral weakened masseter muscle.

Bilateral damage to the trigeminal is a far more dire situation for mastication and speech than unilateral damage. If both the right and left trigeminal are damaged, both the right and left sides of the mandible will be weakened or paralyzed. The mandible might hang open and the patient might have difficulty closing her mouth to any degree. Upon examination, these individuals might be unable to raise their mandible appropriately for articulation or mastication purposes. Their speech is often heavily affected and possibly wholly unintelligible. Phonemes that might be difficult or impossible to produce with bilateral damage to the trigeminal are the lingua-alveolar, linguadental, labio-alveolar, and bilabial phonemes.

Flaccid Dysarthria Arising from Facial Nerve Damage

The facial nerve is a complex nerve with branches that serve both sensory and motor functions. The motor fibers of the facial nerve originate in the pons. They course out through the internal auditory meatus and then through a foramen of the skull to travel to and innervate the facial muscles. Upon reaching the soft tissue of the face just anterior to the ear, the facial nerve divides into the temporal, zygomatic, buccal, and mandibular branches. The temporal branch of the facial nerve innervates muscles around the eyes and movement of the forehead. These muscles are necessary for appropriate facial movement for expression. The zygomatic, buccal, and mandibular branches innervate the muscles of the lower face, which control the lips and compression of the cheeks.

Damage to the facial nerve creates deficits in the ability to move the muscles of the face. Most often, lesion to the facial nerve occurs along the nerve prior to the place where it divides into the temporal, zygomatic, buccal, and mandibular branches. Therefore, a unilateral lesion to the facial nerve usually decreases the motor function ipsilaterally in all those areas of the face innervated by the affected nerve and creates facial weakness or paralysis (generically known as a facial palsy) on the entire side of the face ipsilateral to the lesion while the motor function on the side of the face contralateral to the lesion is spared. This unilateral facial palsy manifests as facial asymmetry involving the affected lips, eyes, and forehead. The weakened side of the lips sag below the contralateral and unaffected side of the lips. Because of weak labial closure, these individuals often spill liquid out of the weakened side of their lips when drinking from a cup due to poor labial seal. Air also leaks out of the weak side of the lips when they attempt to inflate their cheeks. These individuals might have difficulty blinking the eye on the affected side of their face and can have ptosis (droopy eyelid) on the affected eyelid as well. When an individual with this facial weakness is asked to raise his eyebrows, he can move the eyebrow and wrinkle the forehead only on the unaffected side of the face while the affected eyebrow shows decreased range of motion. The affected side of the forehead remains smooth, whereas the unaffected side of the forehead is still wrinkled and creased as normal. Articulation and production of phonemes requiring strong labial seal, such as plosives, can be mildly impaired by unilateral damage to the facial nerve and the consequent unilateral labial weakness. This manifests in speech as a distortion of certain phonemes such as bilabial and labiodentals, which might be accompanied by a cheek flutter on the affected side of the body. However, functional articulation abilities are usually preserved because affected individuals learn to rely less on the weakened side of their lips and more on the unaffected side.

This pattern of facial weakness created by unilateral LMN lesion (lesion to the facial nerve) is a different pattern of facial weakness than that created by a unilateral upper motor neuron lesion. Recognition of these two profiles is important for localization of the lesion to the lower or upper motor neuron as well as to the right or left side of the body. (See the section titled "Unilateral Upper Motor Neuron Dysarthria" later in this chapter for a direct comparison of the two.)

Bilateral lesion to the facial nerve creates bilateral facial weakness. The effects of bilateral weakness of the lips on articulation are far worse than unilateral weakness. These individuals might be unable to bring the lips together at all, which might entirely remove the possibility of producing any bilabial or labiodental phonemes. Bilateral facial weakness, although more severe than unilateral facial weakness, can be more difficult to recognize because the affected individual's face remains symmetrical, lacking the hallmark asymmetry that makes unilateral weakness readily noticeable.

Flaccid Dysarthria Arising from Vagus Nerve Damage

The 10th cranial nerve, the vagus, is a large and complex nerve. The vagus courses through the head and neck prior to moving into the thorax. As it courses through the head and neck its branches innervate many important structures for speech.

Lesion to the Pharyngeal Plexus

After exiting the medulla, the first branch of the vagus important for speech is the pharyngeal plexus.

The pharyngeal plexus of the vagus innervates most of the muscles of the pharynx and velum (excluding the stylopharyngeus and the palatoglossus). These muscles are responsible for pharyngeal constriction and velar elevation and as such play an important role in resonance.

When the pharyngeal plexus of the vagus nerve is unilaterally damaged, weakness occurs on the ipsilateral side of the pharynx and the velum while leaving the motor function on the contralateral side intact. During oral motor evaluation, a visible result of the unilaterally weak velum is observable as a nonuniform or uncentered velum and uvula (**Figure 7-1A**). When the intact muscles on the unaffected side of the velum maintain normal muscle tone (tension), the weakened and hypotonic side of the velum is pulled toward the unaffected side. The most obvious result of this shift of the velum away from the weakened side is that the uvula is off center (Figure 7-1A).

The speech of a person with unilateral weakness of the velum as a result of unilateral damage to the pharyngeal plexus can have resonance issues because the individual has difficulty maintaining velopharyngeal closure during production of nonnasal phonemes. However, the velum might still partially perform its duty of sealing off the nasal cavity from the pharyngeal cavity during speech to some albeit a possibly lesser degree. This is because the unaffected side of the velum can still raise the velum for closure and pulls the weak side with it, though it may not be able to entirely seal off the nasal cavity during speech. As a result, resonance may be hypernasal, though usually not severely or profoundly hypernasal. As a result, articulation and intelligibility might be only mildly affected.

In contrast, bilateral damage to the right and left pharyngeal plexi presents a much worse outcome. If both the right and left pharyngeal plexi are damaged, flaccid weakness is displayed on both sides of the velum, severely limiting motor function. There is no intact side to perform any compensatory actions. A bilaterally weakened velum results in significant levels

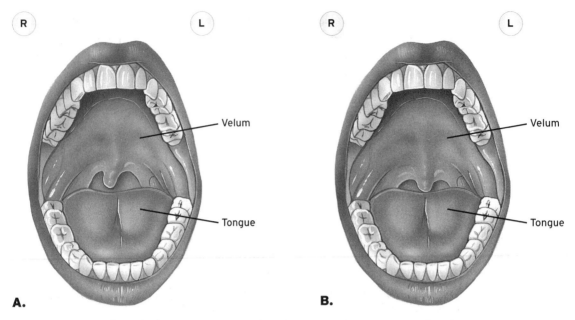

Figure 7-1 A. Left unilateral damage to the pharyngeal plexus resulting in asymmetry where the uvula is pulled to the right. B. Bilateral damage to the pharyngeal plexus resulting in a centered and low-hanging uvula.

of hypernasal resonance far above the level of hypernasality resulting from unilateral weakness of the velum. Upon observation, the bilaterally weakened uvula and the velum are centered because there is no unaffected side pulling it off center. This can make bilateral flaccid weakness of the velum less obvious. However, the bilaterally weakened velum, though still centered, hangs low and the uvula might rest on the back of the tongue (Figure 7-1B).

Lesion to the Superior Laryngeal Branch of the Vagus

The second branch of the vagus is the superior laryngeal branch, also known as the superior laryngeal nerve (SLN). The extrinsic branch of the SLN is responsible for innervating the cricothyroid muscle. The cricothyroid muscle functions as the primary tensor of the vocal folds. As such, its role in speech is to modulate the pitch of the voice.

Unilateral damage to the SLN paralyzes or weakens the ipsilateral side of the paired cricothyroid muscles. However, the right and left cricothyroid muscles

originate and insert into the same structures, the cricoid and thyroid cartilages. Therefore, if one side of the muscle is not functioning properly, the unaffected side can still work to tense the vocal folds. The unaffected contralateral cricothyroid muscle can compensate somewhat for the affected cricothyroid muscle, resulting in mild difficulties in voice modulation and a more monotone voice.

Bilateral damage to the SLN paralyzes or weakens both the right and left cricothyroid muscles, resulting in a significantly more monotone voice than unilateral damage to the SLN creates. In this case, as is usual, bilateral damage to a cranial nerve has far more devastating results than unilateral damage does.

Lesion to the Recurrent Laryngeal Branch of the Vagus

As the vagus continues initially past the larynx and passes inferiorly into the thorax, the right vagus nerve passes under the subclavian artery on the right and the left vagus passes under the aorta of the heart on the left. Both of these branches then immediately course superiorly to innervate all the intrinsic muscles of the larynx (except for the cricothyroid). Because the vagus here changes course and returns (or recurs) to the larynx, this branch of the vagus is referred to as the recurrent laryngeal branch, or the recurrent laryngeal nerve (RLN). Because the RLN is closely associated with the heart, it is common for this nerve to be damaged during open heart surgery. The intrinsic muscles of the larynx (excluding the cricothyroid) innervated by the RLN are responsible for the abduction and adduction of the vocal folds. Appropriate abduction and adduction of the vocal folds are essential for phonation. However, keep in mind that a person cannot breathe through adducted vocal folds—the vocal folds must be abducted for breathing, and one must breathe to live. Therefore, disruption of vocal fold abduction and adduction can have serious implications beyond phonation.

Damage to the right or left RLN results in paresis or paralysis of the ipsilateral vocal fold. This can make phonation breathy or hoarse. However, some phonation is usually possible because the intact and unaffected vocal fold can get close to approximating the weakened vocal fold. However, bilateral damage to both RLNs creates far more severe problems with phonation. With bilateral damage to the RLNs the vocal folds are often paralyzed at midline (not fully abducted or adducted) and are unable to approximate for appropriate phonation. Respiration can also be difficult with vocal folds stuck in their closed to midline positions. In mild cases, this results in an audible inspiratory stridor. In severe cases, the individual can require tracheotomy to reestablish the ability to breathe. ▶ (Find this scenario discussed in the video, *Surgical Trauma to the Vagus*.)

Flaccid Dysarthria Arising from Hypoglossal Nerve Damage

The 12th cranial nerve, the hypoglossal, originates at the medulla. Its fibers exit the medulla to course out through the skull and soft tissue to innervate all the intrinsic and extrinsic muscles of the tongue except the palatoglossus. The intrinsic muscles are responsible for fine motor movement of the tongue and the extrinsic are responsible for more gross motor movement of the tongue. As such, the hypoglossal performs a primary role of delivering plans of motor movement to the muscles of the tongue.

Damage to the hypoglossal creates lingual weakness (weakness of the tongue). Unilateral damage to the hypoglossal creates weakness on the side of the tongue ipsilateral to the lesion and can be observed during an oral mechanism evaluation when the affected individual protrudes the tongue. A tongue that is unilaterally weakened involuntarily deviates, upon protrusion, toward the weakened side. Articulation is mildly to moderately affected by unilateral lingual weakness and can manifest as noisiness from escaping air during production of lingual stops, lingual fricatives, and lingual affricates.

Bilateral damage to the hypoglossal manifests as bilateral lingual weakness. With bilateral weakness, the individual has overall difficulty protruding the tongue or producing any other lingual movement. Those with a bilaterally weakened tongue display reduced lingual range of motion on all tasks. Articulation is severely impaired because virtually every phoneme involving movement of the tongue is negatively affected by this weakness.

In addition to weakness, the affected muscle tissue displays signs of atrophy. Atrophy can be observed as the tongue appearing shrunken and wrinkled. Fasciculations, small, fast, and erratic visible contractions of muscle tissue, can also be present within the atrophied muscle. ▶ (See the video, *Tongue Fasciculations*.)

Confirmatory Signs of Flaccid Dysarthria

If damage to the LMN is localized to certain cranial nerves, hypotonia, muscle atrophy, and possibly fasciculations will be present within the affected structure. For instance, if the facial nerve is damaged, these signs can manifest and be observable within the facial musculature. However, if there is a systemic degradation of the LMNs throughout the entire PNS as a result of degenerative disease, hypotonia, muscle atrophy, and fasciculations can manifest in all muscles of the body and be observable in the limbs as well as structures associated with speech. Hyporeflexia, or a lack of reflexes that are normally present, is a strong confirmatory sign of LMN involvement. For instance, a weak or absent patellar reflex can confirm the presence of pathology at the level of the LMNs.

Spastic Dysarthria

Spasticity is the combined manifestation of hypertonia and **resistance to passive movement** within musculature. Spasticity of musculature creates a spastic weakness or paralysis that is different from the hypotonia and weakness characterizing flaccid paralysis.

Spastic dysarthria is a speech disorder that results from the manifestation of spasticity in muscles associated with speech production. Hallmark characteristics of spastic dysarthria are imprecise articulation, strained/strangled voice quality, excess and equal stress (Darley et al., 1969b; Duffy, 2005). Contrast this with flaccid dysarthria, which is most often characterized by imprecise articulation, hypernasality, and a breathy vocal quality. Table 7-3 lists common speech

Resistance to passive movement The body resisting movement of a body part by an outside force.

Spastic dysarthria A motor speech disorder resulting from spasticity of musculature used to produce speech.

Upper motor neurons (UMNs) Descending (efferent) tracts of axons that originate in the cerebral cortex and travel in the central nervous system to synapse with the lower motor neurons of the peripheral nervous system at the cranial and spinal nerve nuclei.

Table 7-3 Deviant Speech Characteristics of Spastic Dysarthria Listed in Order from Most Common to Least Common

Deviant Speech Characteristic
Imprecise consonants
Monopitch
Reduced stress
Harsh voice
Monoloud
Low pitch
Slow rate
Hypernasality
Strained-Strangled voice quality
Short phrases
Vowels distorted
Pitch breaks
Breathy voice
Excess and equal stress

Source: Adapted from Darley, F., Aronson, A., Brown, J. (1969b). Differential diagnostic patterns of dysarthria. Journal of Speech and Hearing Research 12, 246–269.

characteristics of spastic dysarthria in rank order of prominence.

Anatomic Basis of Spastic Dysarthria

The **upper motor neurons (UMNs)** are descending (efferent) tracts of axons that originate in the cerebral cortex and travel in the CNS to synapse with the LMNs of the PNS at the cranial and spinal nerve nuclei. The origin of spastic dysarthria is bilateral damage to the UMNs. Unilateral damage to the UMNs creates a far milder dysarthria called unilateral upper motor neuron dysarthria (UUMN dysarthria), discussed later in this chapter.

The UMNs are primarily divided into pyramidal and extrapyramidal tracks. Some speech-language pathologists and researchers such as Duffy (2005) use the term *direct activation pathway* (DAP) to refer to the pyramidal track and *indirect activation pathway* (IAP) to refer to the extrapyramidal track. The DAP is the axons of the UMNs that course from the primary motor cortices, premotor cortices, and supplementary motor cortices of the frontal lobes *directly* down into the brain stem and spinal cord to synapse with the LMNs. Most of the fibers of the DAP in each cerebral hemisphere travel inferiorly to the brain stem and then cross over one another (decussate) to the contralateral side of the CNS before innervating the cranial and spinal nerves (**Figure 7-2**). The DAP is involved in transmission of impulses of fine motor and volitional motor movement. The section of the DAP that serves the cranial nerves is the corticobulbar tract. The section of the DAP that serves

the spinal nerves is the corticospinal tract. Fibers of the corticobulbar tract decussate individually to innervate the LMNs of the cranial nerves, whereas most of the fibers of the corticospinal tract decussate together at the level of the medulla.

In contrast to the DAP, the connections and pathways of the IAP travel a far more *indirect* route between the primary motor cortices and the LMNs. The IAP originates in the cerebral cortex and has multiple and complex connections with extrapyramidal structures such as the basal ganglia, cerebellum, and the reticular formation, before coursing inferiorly through the CNS to synapse with the LMNs. The IAP is involved in the transmission of impulses associated with automatic functions. Some important extrapyramidal impulses transmitted along the IAP are impulses for

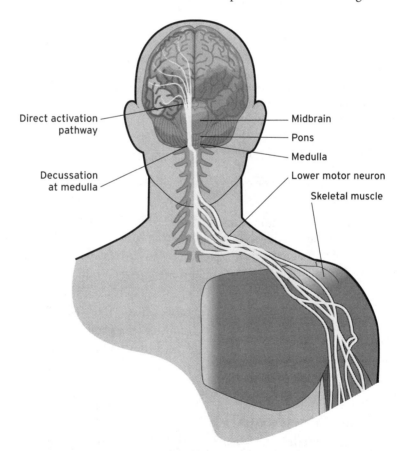

Direct activation pathway

Decussation at medulla

Midbrain

Pons

Medulla

Lower motor neuron

Skeletal muscle

Figure 7-2   **Decussation of direct activation pathway of the upper motor neuron and innervation of skeletal muscles by the lower motor neuron.**

Playing Piano

To illustrate the differences between the volitional pyramidal motor plans transmitted along the DAP and nonvolitional extrapyramidal motor plans transmitted along the IAP let us take the example of a person playing the piano. The impulses of fine motor movements of voluntary and skilled finger movement are generated in the pre, primary, and supplementary motor cortices of the cerebral hemispheres. These impulses are then transmitted from the major motor cortices along the DAP. The DAP transmits impulses of fine motor plans from the brain through the CNS to the LMNs. The LMNs then activate the muscles in the manner specified by these motor plans, which allows the person to play the keys in the necessary sequence, with the appropriate speed, and with the appropriate strength.

As the person plays the piano, muscles contract not just in the fingers but all over the body to keep appropriate tone and posture so that the person remains upright and appropriately positioned. These are the extrapyramidal impulses of tone maintenance and postural support, which are generated by the basal ganglia and then transmitted along the IAP. The IAP then delivers these impulses of muscle tone maintenance and postural support to the LMNs. The LMNs activate the muscles in the manner specified by the motor plans of tone maintenance and postural support.

Keep in mind that the LMNs work to activate muscles for DAP and IAP motor plans simultaneously so that a person can focus all thought on the movements of the fingers while still remaining sitting upright at the piano.

muscle tone regulation, reflex inhibition, and postural support. All these extrapyramidal signals transmitted by the IAP are generated and executed below the level of awareness.

When damage occurs to the UMNs, the DAP and IAP are most often simultaneously affected. Damage to the DAP weakens the transmission of volitional motor plans through the CNS to the LMNs, which

decreases activation of the LMNs. Decreased activation of the LMNs for volitional movement results in decreased muscle activation and muscle weakness. This weakness creates a deficit in the individual's ability to execute volitional motor plans, such as those fine motor plans associated with speech.

Damage to the IAP removes or weakens transmission of nonvolitional extrapyramidal impulses of muscle tone, muscle maintenance, postural support, and reflex inhibition. The lack of impulses of reflex inhibition generated by extrapyramidal structures creates a disinhibition of the stretch reflex. Deprived of certain inhibitory signals transmitted along the IAP, the stretch reflex becomes hyperactive (i.e., hyperreflexia) and instead of fulfilling its normal role of maintaining muscle position and appropriate muscle tone, it creates the situation where one's body actively resists passive movement of musculature as well as producing hypertone in affected musculature. This is how hyperreflexia creates the *resistance to movement* and hypertonia components of spasticity.

Confirmatory Signs of Spastic Dysarthria

In addition to differences in speech, bilateral UMN lesions produce confirmatory signs reflecting hypertonia and hyperreflexia. Spasticity in the limbs as well as articulators and speech systems is the most obvious. Also, in bilateral UMN syndromes, with the lack of efferent reflex inhibition signals, certain primitive or infantile reflexes that the body outgrows as it matures can be released. The Babinski reflex (also known as the plantar reflex) is normally seen in infants and is observed when a hard object such as a key or a pen strokes the outside of the sole of the infant's foot from heel to toe. (See the *Babinski Reflex* video for an example of an infant's positive Babinski sign.) Normally, infants display a positive Babinski sign after the sole of the foot is stroked, where the big toe extends and the four smaller toes splay out. After about the age of 2 years, this infantile response is replaced with the normal adult response, which is to clench the toes together and downward. A positive Babinski sign displayed by adults can be indicative of a UMN lesion along the corticospinal pathway of the DAP.

Some infantile oral reflexes also manifest with bilateral UMN disease. These include the rooting, suck, and snout reflexes. These are primitive reflexes that allow infants reflexively to position their head and mouth to find the nipple of a breast or bottle and suck when the nipple is appropriately positioned in the mouth. The rooting reflex occurs when a light stroking stimulus is applied to one side of an infant's mouth, and the infant responds by reaching the head and mouth toward the stimulus, as she would toward her mother's nipple. The snout reflex is when the lips pucker when given a light tap.

Common Etiologies of Spastic Dysarthria

The etiologies of spastic dysarthria include stroke, trauma, toxins, and any number of diseases that produce bilateral damage to the DAP and IAP pathways of the UMNs. Duffy (2005) states that spastic dysarthria seems to be most often encountered in the adult population primarily because of degenerative disorders, stroke and vascular problems, and trauma. In children, cerebral palsy and trauma are also common etiologies of spastic dysarthria. A degenerative disease that produces spastic dysarthria is primary lateral sclerosis (PLS), a variant of ALS. Unlike ALS, which affects both UMNs and LMNs and thereby produces a mixed spastic-flaccid dysarthria, PLS affects only the UMNs, leading to spastic dysarthria.

Lesion Effects

Unlike flaccid dysarthria, where LMN lesion effects can be seen affecting a single articulator or only one side of an articulator, bilateral lesion of the UMNs creates effects on both sides of the body and usually is not constrained to a single articulator or a single speech system. Physical manifestations of bilateral UMN lesions (bilateral spasticity) are seen on both sides of the body and therefore have a far greater impact on speech production than a unilateral UMN lesion does.

Unilateral Upper Motor Neuron Dysarthria

The same neuromotor basis underlying spastic dysarthria underlies unilateral upper motor neuron (UUMN) dysarthria, which is damage to the DAP and IAP of the UMN. However, **UUMN dysarthria** is the dysarthria that results from unilateral UMN damage (damage to either the left UMNs or right UMNs, but not both). This dysarthria is usually the result of stroke in a single cerebral hemisphere or on one side of the brain stem that damages the associated UMN tract. This dysarthria manifests as reduced strength and range of movement on one side of the lower face as well as possible concomitant hemiplegia or hemiparesis.

In UUMN dysarthria, the UMNs contralateral to the lesion are still operational, and because of this, UUMN dysarthria typically has a far less negative impact on speech than spastic dysarthria. This dysarthria usually presents with mild articulation difficulties resulting from unilateral labial and lingual weakness. Unilateral upper motor neuron dysarthria is also more transient and can resolve with no intervention within 3 weeks. Confirmatory signs of unilateral UMN lesions, such as the presence of abnormal or excessive reflexes or spasticity, can be present on the affected side of the body.

Unilateral upper motor neuron (UUMN) dysarthria The dysarthria that results from unilateral UMN damage.

This is the second dysarthria discussed in this chapter that can present with unilateral facial weakness. The first is flaccid dysarthria resulting from unilateral damage to the facial nerve. UUMN dysarthria, the second, results from unilateral UMN damage. Each of these dysarthrias creates a specific profile that is easily distinguished from one another. Individuals with flaccid dysarthria resulting from unilateral damage to the facial nerve display weakness in the upper and lower portions of the affected side of the face. In contrast, with UUMN dysarthria, facial weakness manifests primarily on the lower portion of the affected side of the face because the upper portion of the affected side of the face still receives motor plans from the ipsilateral cerebral hemisphere (the undamaged one) because of the bilateral innervation of the branches of the facial nerve that innervate the upper face.

Ataxic Dysarthria

The underlying motor characteristic of ataxic dysarthria is motor incoordination. **Ataxic dysarthria** is the dysarthria produced by the incoordination of the movements of the articulators, which produces a slushy or drunken-like speech quality. Darley, Aronson, and Brown (1969b) list the three most prominent characteristics of ataxic dysarthria as imprecise production of consonants, excess and equal stress, and irregular articulatory breakdowns. In pure ataxic dysarthria, weakness does not present and all oral and facial structures appear normal when at rest. Signs of ataxic dysarthria appear only during movement. Table 7-4 lists common characteristics of ataxic dysarthria.

> **Ataxic dysarthria** The dysarthria produced by the incoordination of the movements of the articulators, which produces a slushy or drunken-like speech quality.

Anatomic Basis of Ataxic Dysarthria

Ataxic dysarthria is the result of pathology of the cerebellum. The cerebellum is responsible for monitoring and correcting for errors in the timing, range,

Table 7-4 Deviant Speech Characteristics of Ataxic Dysarthria Listed in Order from Most Common to Least Common

Deviant Speech Characteristic
Imprecise consonants
Excess and equal stress
Irregular articulatory breakdowns
Vowels distorted
Harsh voice
Phonemes prolonged
Intervals prolonged
Monopitch
Monoloud
Slow rate

Source: Adapted from Darley, F., Aronson, A., Brown, J. (1969b). Differential diagnostic patterns of dysarthria. *Journal of Speech and Hearing Research 12,* 246–269.

force, and direction of motor movements (Darley et al., 1969b) that are present in the motor plan. When pathology decreases the appropriate functioning of the cerebellum, there arises incoordination that manifests as errors in the timing, range, force, and direction of movement. At the level of speech, the outcome of this incoordination in movement is a distinctive drunken-sounding dysarthria. The speech of a person with ataxic dysarthria is accurately described as sounding like the speech of someone who is drunk because when a person is intoxicated with alcohol, cerebellar functioning is decreased, thereby producing the same effects on speech as more permanent and degenerative cerebellar pathologies.

Etiologies of Ataxic Dysarthria

Any process that damages the cerebellum or its connections to the CNS can create ataxic dysarthria. Disease, stroke, trauma, and toxins are common etiologies. A few diseases associated with cerebellar degeneration are Friedreich's ataxia, multiple sclerosis, and multiple-systems atrophy (Shy-Drager syndrome). A single stroke to the midline structures of the cerebellum or bilateral strokes within the cerebellar hemispheres can also produce ataxic dysarthria. High forces of acceleration and deceleration as seen sometimes in closed head injuries damage the cerebellum, creating ataxic dysarthria.

Confirmatory Signs of Ataxic Dysarthria

The motor deficits produced by cerebellar pathology are usually not confined to speech production alone. Individuals with cerebellar pathology display many signs of decreased cerebellar functioning in addition to ataxic dysarthria. This constellation of signs is referred to as ataxia. Ataxia manifests as poorly controlled and poorly coordinated movement that is lacking in smoothness. Complex movements are often disintegrated and broken down and executed in their component parts.

Cerebellar diseases produce a distinctive gait disturbance referred to as ataxic gait. An ataxic gait is characterized by the feet spread more broadly apart than usual with irregular footsteps and a greater likelihood of falls. Titubation can present and is small and quick back-and-forth rhythmic movement of a body part. Similarly, nystagmus, which is a rapid back-and-forth motion of the eyes, can be observed. Dysmetria, which is the over- or undershooting of a movement of a body part while performing a volitional movement, such as reaching for an object, can also present.

Ataxia A set of deficits in the timing and coordination of body movements caused by pathology of the cerebellum.

Ataxic gait A type of gait characterized by the feet spread more broadly apart than usual accompanied by irregular footsteps and a greater likelihood of falls; associated with cerebellar pathology.

Titubation Involuntary, rapid, and small back-and-forth rhythmic movements of a body part.

Nystagmus Involuntary and rapid back-and-forth motion of the eyes.

Hypokinetic Dysarthria

Hypokinetic dysarthria is the dysarthria that results from pathology at the basal ganglia or its connections to other structures in the CNS. The underlying neuromotor basis of hypokinetic dysarthria is rigidity, reduced amounts of volitional movement, and a reduced range of motion present in the movement remaining. The movements of the structures of the speech system become erased or reduced in range of motion. The result is a monopitch, monoloud speech with reduced amounts of stress, imprecise consonants, and short bursts of rapid speech or articulation (Darley et al., 1969b). Voice production also becomes reduced in intensity. Table 7-5 lists speech characteristics of hypokinetic dysarthria in order of most common to least common. A hallmark characteristic of hypokinetic dysarthria is a variable and often above

Dysmetria The over- or undershooting of a body part while performing a volitional movement such as reaching for an object.

Hypokinetic dysarthria The dysarthria that results from pathology at the basal ganglia or its connections to other structures in the CNS.

Table 7-5 Deviant Speech Characteristics of Hypokinetic Dysarthria Listed in Order from Most Common to Least Common

Deviant Speech Characteristic
Monopitch
Reduced stress
Monoloud
Imprecise consonants
Inappropriate silences
Short rushes of speech
Harsh voice
Breathy voice
Low pitch
Variable rate of speech

Source: Adapted from Darley, F., Aronson, A., Brown, J. (1969b). Differential diagnostic patterns of dysarthria. Journal of Speech and Hearing Research 12, 246–269.

normal rate of speech. This is the one dysarthria in which rate of speech regularly increases. In hypokinetic dysarthria, speech can suddenly halt and then, once initiated, proceed in short and rapid bursts or become increasingly faster until articulation breaks down entirely. This quick and imprecise articulation is known as rapid-fire articulation.

Anatomic Basis of Hypokinetic Dysarthria

The anatomic origin of hypokinetic dysarthria is damage to structures of the basal ganglia, connections between structures of the basal ganglia, or connections between the basal ganglia and other CNS structures. The basic functions of the basal ganglia are to regulate muscle tone, control postural movements during skilled motor activities, assist in initiation of motor movement, and facilitate new motor learning. The basal ganglia also functions to dampen extraneous impulses of movement in motor plans that would manifest as extraneous or unnecessary movements. Through these functions, the basal ganglia provide a stable musculoskeletal system for the production of fine motor movements while ensuring smooth and appropriate fine motor movements for speech.

Given the responsibilities of the basal ganglia, it should come as no surprise that pathology to the basal ganglia creates rigid muscle tone, postural abnormalities, difficulties with initiating movement, deficits in the ability to learn new motor movements, and tremor at rest. Damage to the basal ganglia also results in the underdamping of motor plans, in which volitional motor plans become far reduced in force and range of motion, or the overdamping of motor plans, which allows the release and execution of excessive and involuntary movements (hyperkinesias). In hypokinetic dysarthria, the basal ganglia acts to underdamp motor plans, which creates the characteristic reduced amount of movement and reduced range of motion of volitional movements. However, with the application of the synthetic dopamine

replacement Levodopa, individuals with Parkinson's disease can modulate between states of hypokinesia, normality, and hyperkinesia, thereby possibly fluctuating between hypokinetic dysarthria and hyperkinetic dysarthria.

Etiologies of Hypokinetic Dysarthria

Any process that damages the basal ganglia or its connections to other CNS structures can create hypokinetic dysarthria. The most common etiology of basal ganglia pathology and resulting hypokinetic dysarthria is the degenerative condition Parkinson's disease. In Parkinson's disease, the basal ganglia cease to function appropriately because of a lack of the neurotransmitter dopamine. Dopamine is normally produced by a structure in the basal ganglia known as the substantia nigra, which is located in the midbrain section of the brain stem. Because the substantia nigra fails to produce dopamine for the body, symptoms of Parkinsonism begin to occur. Strokes and toxins can also damage the basal ganglia, thereby creating hypokinetic dysarthria. Repeated trauma to the head, as in the reoccurring concussions and mild traumatic brain injuries experienced most notably by athletes such as boxers and football players, creates problems with the functioning of the basal ganglia. Infectious disease such as AIDS, Creutzfeldt-Jakob disease, and syphilis also damage the basal ganglia and can also be etiologies of hypokinetic dysarthria.

Parkinson's Disease and Parkinsonism

Hypokinetic dysarthria is the iconic dysarthria of Parkinson's disease. However, the damage to the basal ganglia seen in Parkinson's disease that creates hypokinetic dysarthria also creates a spectrum of nonspeech motor symptoms that reflect basal ganglia damage. These motor changes include the following:

- Stooped posture with a lack of arm swing while walking

- Festination of gait, a shuffling gait of short and often quickening footsteps that seem to be an effort to retain balance
- Hypomimia, a reduced amount of movement in the face, creating a distinctive masked appearance and lack of facial expression
- Bradykinesia, an inability or difficulty initiating movement
- Akinesia, a freezing or immobility, a complete lack of movement
- Hypokinesia, a reduced amount of movement
- Micrographia, a progression from normal handwriting to abnormally diminutive handwriting

Cognitive changes are also present in Parkinson's disease.

Because damage to the basal ganglia produces the signs of Parkinson's disease, and because there can be more than one cause of damage to the basal ganglia, other conditions can present with these symptoms. When signs of basal ganglia dysfunction are present resulting from etiologies other than Parkinson's disease, they are referred to as Parkinsonian signs, or as Parkinsonism, despite their lack of direct association with Parkinson's disease. Any of the non-Parkinson's etiologies of hypokinetic dysarthria mentioned above can produce Parkinsonian signs. It is important to note that the presence of Parkinsonism does not necessarily imply that the degenerative disease process of Parkinson's disease is causing the damage that is producing these symptoms. See the video, *Parkinson's Disease Caregiver and Advocate* for a discussion of Parkinson's disease and the video, *Multiple Systems Atrophy Parkinsonism* to hear an interview with an individual with many of the symptoms discussed.

Hyperkinetic Dysarthria

Hyperkinetic dysarthria is created by the presence of hyperkinesias (extra and involuntary movements) that interfere with speech production. As hyperkinetic dysarthria is caused by the presence of extra movements that interfere with speech, it is often the easiest dysarthria to identify. There is a wide variety of hyperkinesias, ranging from the very quick to the very slow, regular to irregular, and the very small to the very large. Following is a list of important forms of hyperkinesias, or dyskinesias, that can result in a hyperkinetic dysarthria:

- **Athetosis**: An involuntary slow writhing movement
- **Ballism**: Bilateral, involuntary, irregular, possibly wild or violent movement of extremities
- **Chorea**: Involuntary and quick dance-like movements of the feet, hands, extremities, and head and neck (The term *chorea* is derived from *choros*, the Greek word for dance.)
- **Dystonia**: An involuntary slow, irregular, often painful, twisting of extremities and body that manifests as abnormal and involuntary posturing of the body
- **Hemiballism**: Unilateral, involuntary, irregular, possibly wild or violent movement of extremities

Festination A progressive speeding up of a repetitive movement often displayed in various forms by individuals with Parkinson's disease.

Hyperkinesia Extra and involuntary movement of the body or body parts. Also known as dyskinesia.

Hyperkinetic dysarthria The dysarthria created by the presence of hyperkinesias that interfere with speech production.

Athetosis An involuntary slow, writhing movement.

Ballism Bilateral, involuntary, irregular, possibly wild or violent flinging of extremities. A hyperkinesia.

Chorea Involuntary and quick dance-like movements of the feet, hands, extremities, and head and neck. *Chorea* is derived from *choros*, the Greek word for dance.

Dystonia An involuntary slow, irregular, often painful twisting of extremities and body parts that often manifests as abnormal and involuntary posturing of the body. A hyperkinesia.

Hemiballism Unilateral, involuntary, irregular, possibly wild or violent flinging of extremities. A hyperkinesia.

- **Spasm**: An involuntary and sudden muscle contraction
- **Tic**: An involuntary quick, repetitive, and stereotyped movement
- **Tremor**: An involuntary, rhythmic, and quick movement usually occurring three to five times per second

The impact hyperkinesias have on production of speech varies with the type and severity and body location of the hyperkinesias. For example, an infrequent tic of the lips might not affect speech at all, whereas a frequent spasm of the laryngeal muscles upon phonation affects speech a great deal. Darley, Aronson, and Brown (1969b) identify some common speech characteristics of individuals with dystonia-related hyperkinetic dysarthria as imprecise consonants, distorted vowels, harsh voice, irregular articulatory breakdowns, and a strained-strangled voice quality. These same authors identify common aspects of chorea-related hyperkinetic dysarthria as imprecise consonants, variable rate of speech, monopitch, and harsh voice.

Spasm An involuntary and sudden muscle contraction.

Tic An involuntary, quick, repetitive, and stereotyped movement. A hyperkinesia.

Tremor An involuntary, rhythmic, and quick movement usually occurring three to five times per second.

Anatomic Basis of Hyperkinetic Dysarthria

Extraneous or unwanted movements of the body can be produced in many different ways. The etiology of hyperkinesias and hyperkinetic dysarthria usually involves damage or pathology of the extrapyramidal structures such as the basal ganglia and the cerebellum, which are responsible for refining motor plans and inhibiting or removing hyperkinesias from the motor plans. They might also be produced by damage to the IAP, which transmits these extrapyramidal impulses.

Etiologies of Hyperkinetic Dysarthria

Etiologies of hyperkinetic dysarthria are varied, complex, and include stroke, trauma, tumor, mass effect, infectious or degenerative disease, congenital conditions, and exposure to toxins. A thorough discussion of all these hyperkinesias and their etiologies is beyond the scope of this chapter. That said, here follows a discussion of a handful of notable diseases and conditions that produce hyperkinesias that affect speech production, thereby creating hyperkinetic dysarthria.

Sydenham's chorea is a complication following childhood infection of rheumatic fever, which causes choreic movements of the extremities as well as choreic movements of the head and neck and possibly facial grimacing. Sydenham's chorea occurs after the onset of acute rheumatic fever. The exact pathogenesis of Sydenham's chorea is unknown but is thought to be an autoimmune reaction of the body to rheumatic fever that damages the basal ganglia (Cardoso, 2011). Although remission of this chorea usually occurs spontaneously within 8 months of onset, it can persist in some individuals (Cardoso, 2011).

Huntington's chorea (also known as Huntington's disease) is a terminal and progressive disease producing dementia and abnormal motor signs. This disease is inherited and caused by an autosomal-dominant mutant gene (Chua & Chiu, 2005). Practically speaking, *autosomal dominant* means that a child of a parent with the Huntington's gene has a 50% chance of inheriting the disease. Huntington's chorea is caused by atrophy of parts of the basal ganglia, which produces the involuntary choreic movements associated with the disorder (Bamford, Caine, Kido, Cox, & Shoulson, 1995; Bamford, Caine, Kido, Plassche, & Shoulson, 1989). The hyperkinesias associated with Huntington's disease begin in milder forms but increase in severity over time to become disabling. Atrophy also occurs in other areas of the brain such as the frontal lobes. Atrophy of the frontal lobes presents as personality changes and cognitive decline.

Tourette syndrome is a disorder involving the presence of vocal or motor tics. Tourette syndrome presents during early childhood, mostly affects males, has no effect on life span, and often involves tics of the head and face. The exact etiology of Tourette syndrome is unknown but is thought to have a genetic component that affects the basal ganglia. Vocal tics include such behaviors as spitting, coughing, throat clearing, grunting, and echolalia or coprolalia. Echolalia and copralalia are complex vocal tics involving the compulsive production of entire words or utterances. Echolalia is the compulsive repetition of someone else's utterances. Copralalia is the compulsive, repetitive production of swear words. Echolalic and copralalic words and utterances do not reflect the thoughts or intentions of the speaker but are simply a motor manifestation of Tourette syndrome. Although copralalia is possibly the most well-known feature of Tourette syndrome, it is a relatively rare manifestation of the disorder. Most cases of Tourette syndrome are mild and the presence and severity of tics tend to climax at 10 years of age and from there decrease (Leckman et al., 1998).

Spasmodic dysphonia is a disorder of extra movement present at the level of the vocal folds. The three types of spasmodic dysphonia are adductor, abductor, and mixed. The abductor type involves the vocal folds involuntarily and randomly pulling apart during phonation. This creates an intermittently breathy or aphonic voice quality. In contrast, adductor spasmodic dysphonia causes random and involuntary hyperadduction during phonation, which creates an intermittently harsh or strained, strangled voice quality. Mixed spasmodic dysphonia is the combination of both the adductor and abductor types. Beware the similarities of the words *spastic* and *spasmodic*.

Echolalia The compulsive repetition of someone else's utterances.

Copralalia The compulsive and repetitive production of swear words.

Mixed dysarthria A simultaneous manifestation of more than one type of dysarthria.

Note that *spasmodic* dysphonia is caused by the presence of extra and involuntary movements of the vocal folds, making it a hyperkinetic dysarthria, not a *spastic* dysarthria.

Mixed Dysarthrias

Damage to the human nervous system can occur in an endless variety of ways and can produce any combination of the dysarthrias. Thus, the term mixed dysarthria is used to describe a manifestation of two or more dysarthrias in a single individual. In fact, mixed dysarthria is encountered clinically far more often than any other individual dysarthria type (Duffy, 2005).

Although any combination of dysarthrias is possible, certain combinations manifest with certain diseases or types of trauma:

- *Amyotrophic lateral sclerosis (ALS):* Caused by demyelination of the UMNs and LMNs. ALS presents with a mixed flaccid-spastic dysarthria.
- *Multiple sclerosis (MS):* Caused by demyelination within the CNS. MS can present with virtually any neurologic sign, making it difficult to establish a diagnosis of MS initially. Individuals with MS can present with any CNS-based dysarthria, but spastic-ataxic is a common mixture (Merson & Rolnick, 1998). A distinguishing sign of MS is possible waxing and waning of the presence of dysarthria. When this occurs, it is known as paroxysmal dysarthria (Blanco, Compta, Graus, & Saiz, 2008). ▶ See the video, *Living with Multiple Sclerosis* for a discussion with a person living with multiple sclerosis.
- *Friedreich's ataxia:* Primarily a cerebellar disorder manifesting in speech as ataxic dysarthria, but Friedreich's ataxia can also present with concomitant spasticity, which creates a mixed spastic-ataxic dysarthria.
- *Traumatic brain injury (TBI):* Trauma to the nervous system can occur in so many ways that

any dysarthria or combination of dysarthrias potentially is created. However, in motor vehicle accidents involving high speed or force the UMNs are often damaged as a result of coup-contrecoup injuries or diffuse axonal shearing. The cranial nerve nuclei of the LMNs in the brain stem often suffer damage as the brain is twisted or warped inside the skull during the accident. The cerebellum also is likely to suffer damage in a coup-contrecoup scenario. Therefore, the combination of flaccid, spastic, and ataxic dysarthrias commonly presents in motor vehicle–related TBIs. However, other dysarthrias can be present as well depending on the site and severity of damage.

- *Brain stem stroke:* Many important neurologic structures are located in the brain stem within a very small space. Even a small lesion to the brain stem has potential to damage many important structures. For instance, a stroke to the pons of the brain stem is likely to damage UMNs that pass through the brain stem. This same stroke might also damage the cranial nerve nuclei in the pons. In this scenario, a spastic-flaccid dysarthria would occur. However, cerebellar connections to the CNS are also located in the pons. It is possible that a single stroke at the pons could damage the connections between the cerebellum and the CNS, which would limit cerebellar input to ongoing motor activity and create an ataxic dysarthria as well. The pons is the only place in the nervous system where a single stroke can create a mixture of three different dysarthrias: flaccid-spastic-ataxic (Duffy, 2005). ▶ See the video, *Brain Stem Stroke* to hear an individual with this condition discuss the onset of his stroke and deficits following.

Restorative strategy A therapy strategy that has the goal of restoring lost function by reducing the severity of the underlying deficits.

Compensatory strategy A therapy strategy that has the goal of restoring lost function by compensating for underlying deficits.

Management of the Dysarthrias

Treatment of the dysarthrias first must ensure that the affected individual possesses some form of functional communication so that the individual can communicate to meet basic wants and needs. Functional communication in the short term can involve the use of some other modality of communication, such as writing or some form of augmentative or alternative communication (AAC).

When it is appropriate to begin to target improvement of speech production, many different treatment approaches are available. **Restorative strategies** reduce the severity of dysarthria by restoring lost motor abilities. **Compensatory strategies** reduce the impact of the dysarthria on speech by providing alternate methods of communication while not actually reducing the severity of the underlying neuromotor deficits. Which management approaches are used varies from individual to individual based on the patient's motor speech deficits, medical status, and communicative needs. This section discusses only a few therapy approaches for illustrative purposes. For a more thorough review of therapy strategies, see Duffy (2005).

Restorative Strategies

The goal of restorative strategies is to restore normal motor function by reducing the underlying pathologic neuromotor condition that is creating the dysarthria (e.g., weakness, spasticity, incoordination). Reduction of the underlying pathology thereby reduces the severity of the dysarthria. Although there is some overlap in the neuromotor bases of the dysarthrias, there is also a great deal of differentiation. As a result, restorative strategies that are appropriate for one type of dysarthria can be wholly inappropriate for another type of dysarthria. For instance, relaxation techniques (discussed later) are appropriate for reducing spasticity in spastic dysarthria but are useless in treatment of flaccid dysarthria, where the muscles are already too relaxed. Great care must be taken to apply restorative strategies correctly to their appropriate neuromotor targets.

Strengthening Exercises

For individuals with the underlying neuromotor characteristic of weakness as a component of their dysarthria, speech-language pathologists often attempt to strengthen weakened muscles to improve respiration, resonance, voice, and articulation. Weakness manifests in flaccid, spastic, and hypokinetic dysarthrias. Resistive breathing exercises are used to strengthen muscles of inspiration to increase breath support for speech. Devices such as the PFlex or The Breather are small, portable devices that provide a graded resistance to inspiration, thereby over time increasing the user's ability to take in more air for respiration and speech (Sobush & Dunning, 1989). Resistance training for the velum can be accomplished using a CPAP (continuous positive airway pressure) machine. A CPAP machine (**Figure 7-3**) pushes a steady stream of air into the nose to keep the velum open. These machines are often worn by individuals at night to reduce snoring or sleep apnea. The pressure provided by CPAP to hold the velum open can function as a form of resistance so that a person exercises the velum against this resistance while speaking. Over time, the muscles of the velum can be strengthened to produce more appropriate velopharyngeal closure for less hypernasality (Kuehn, 1997).

Strengthening exercises for voice usually involve attempts at increasing the strength of the muscles of vocal fold adduction. These exercises to increase phonation might include such tasks as attempts at repetitive completions of hard glottal stops. However, for those with spastic dysarthria the problem is one of hyperadduction, not hypoadduction, so exercises to increase adduction are inappropriate.

Strengthening exercises to improve articulation are a controversial subject. Many speech-language

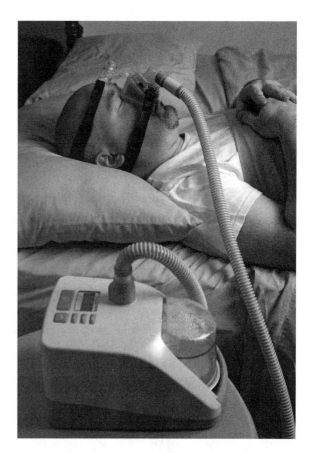

Figure 7-3   A CPAP machine.
Source: © Amy Walters/ShutterStock, Inc.

pathologists use oral motor exercises (nonspeech oral motor exercises) to strengthen weakened articulators such as the mandible, lips, and tongue. These exercises can include but are not limited to protrusion/retraction/lateralization of the tongue with or without resistance provided by a tongue blade, protraction/retraction of the tongue with or without resistance provided by a tongue blade, and the opening/closing of the mandible with or without resistance provided by the speech-language pathologist using a hand to resist the movement of the mandible. Although strengthening these structures is appropriate at times, the tongue and lips actually require very little of their overall strength (10–30%) for normal articulation (Barlow & Abbs, 1983). Also, to maximize the positive impact of nonspeech oral motor exercise on speech production, the exercise must be executed using the appropriate exercise principles, including the following:

- *Repetition:* Exercises must be executed with an appropriate number of repetitions (Kays & Robbins, 2007).
- *Intensity:* Exercises need to have a graded increase in difficulty (resistance) over time so that the muscles being exercised are worked hard enough to cause the muscle to strengthen.
- *Task specific:* Strength, endurance, or mobility gained during one activity is greatest for that one activity. These gains might not generalize to other activities that do not resemble the original exercise. Therefore, exercises to improve speech must be task specific, meaning that to improve an articulator's strength during speech production, the strengthening exercise needs to resemble speech production as closely as possible or be conducted as a component of actual speech production.

The use of CPAP to target hypernasality is a wonderful example of a task-specific exercise. The working of the velum against the CPAP machine occurs as the speaker is actually producing speech. An exercise that is not task specific to speech is retracting/protruding the tongue with the purpose of increasing strength of the tongue for production of certain phonemes. The less task specific an exercise is, the less likely gains made during the exercise will generalize to speech production. However, there are those individuals who will benefit from the use of the nonspeech oral motor tasks, but application of these exercises should be conducted carefully and using the exercise principles listed above to maximize their impact.

Relaxation Techniques

For individuals with hypertone, rigidity, or spasticity, progressive relaxation of the body or of affected musculature can allow a more appropriate production of voice or articulation that generalizes to sentences and spontaneous speech in drill-type therapy. One relaxation technique is the jaw shaking exercise, in which the individual loosens up the mandibular muscles by wagging the head back and forth with the mouth hanging open (Froeschels, 1943). Rosenbek and LaPointe (1978) liken this activity to the action a puppy takes while shaking stuffing out of a sack. Laryngeal massage and massage of the neck can also be used to relax hyperactive muscles and increase appropriate phonation.

Stretching Exercises

In stretching exercises, a limb or articulator is moved through its full range of movement. Slow stretching of the limbs is used in physical therapy to reduce spasticity by inhibiting the stretch reflex. This reduction in spasticity creates a greater range of motion for the affected body part. In contrast to slow stretches, quick stretches can be employed with hypotonic muscles to stimulate the stretch reflex and thereby increase muscle tone.

Stretching exercises can be active, meaning that patients stretch their own body parts using the muscles intrinsic to that particular body part (e.g., extending an arm or rolling the head). Or stretching exercises can be passive, meaning that an external force (e.g., an apparatus or the speech-language pathologist) moves the body part in question.

Most stretching exercises used in speech-language pathology are slow stretches of the lips and tongue (Clark, 2003). These are usually active stretches, though at times speech-language pathologists will hold the tongue with gauze and stretch it passively. The muscles of the lips and tongue lack the typical pattern of the stretch reflex that limbs and other body parts have. Therefore, the use of slow, passive stretches to reduce spasticity in these structures is questionable. Clark (2003) suggests that because the muscles of mastication do display stretch reflexes, stretching techniques are more appropriate to use on these muscles.

Medical Management

Medical management of dysarthria involves pharmacological treatment or surgical intervention. As elucidated in this chapter, medical conditions (disease, trauma, stroke, etc.) are usually the etiology of the dysarthrias. Often, pharmacological or surgical treatment of these medical conditions results in the remediation or effective treatment of the underlying etiology of the dysarthria. In this fashion, medical treatment can lessen or fully remediate the dysarthrias. An example of common pharmacological treatment of a dysarthria is the administration of Levodopa to those with Parkinson's disease. Because hypokinetic dysarthria is often present in Parkinson's disease, the administration of Levodopa relieves for a time the motor symptoms of Parkinson's disease, including hypokinetic dysarthria.

Surgical intervention is an option for certain dysarthric problems, though surgery should be undertaken only after exhausting all other less-invasive options. As previously mentioned, difficulties adducting the vocal folds for phonation can result from damage to the vagus nerve. A surgical option for improving vocal fold adduction includes the injection of a biocompatible gel into the paralyzed vocal fold to lend it more bulk, thereby bringing it to rest closer to midline so that the contralateral and intact vocal fold can approximate it for phonation. For those with hypernasal resonance resulting from dysarthria, pharyngeal flap surgery can be warranted. There are different forms of this surgery, but the procedure generally repositions existing pharyngeal tissue to reduce the size of the velopharyngeal opening, thereby reducing hypernasality by more appropriately controlling the escape of air through the nasal cavity during the production of nonnasal phonemes.

Compensatory Strategies

As mentioned previously, compensatory strategies for the treatment of the dysarthrias facilitate communication despite the presence of the dysarthria. Compensatory strategies can be categorized as speech and nonspeech strategies. **Speech compensatory strategies** are techniques that increase intelligibility of the speaker and reduce the impact of dysarthria on speech while not directly targeting the pathologic neuromotor condition producing the dysarthria (i.e., the weakness, spasticity, incoordination). **Nonspeech compensatory strategies** entirely bypass speech production to focus on improving overall communication. They also do not directly target reduction of the underlying neuromotor deficits that create dysarthria (as restorative therapy does) or reduction of the impact that dysarthria has on speech (as speech compensatory strategies do).

> **Speech compensatory strategy** A compensatory technique that increases intelligibility of the speaker and reduces the impact of dysarthria on speech while not directly targeting the pathologic neuromotor condition producing the dysarthria.
>
> **Nonspeech compensatory strategy** A compensatory strategy that entirely bypasses speech production to focus on improving overall communication.

Speech Compensatory Strategies

Many different speech compensatory strategies are used to target the wide range of speech difficulties produced by the dysarthrias. If an individual has inappropriate breath support for speech, the speech-language pathologist will teach that individual methods for best using the breath support available to produce speech. Examples include teaching the individual to take more breaths during the production of an utterance and teaching the patient to initiate speech at the very beginning of expiration to maximize breath support for speech. If hypernasality is a problem, possible speech compensatory strategies are to occlude the nares (pinch the nostrils shut) during speech or to increase the degree to which the speaker's mouth opens during speech, thereby allowing more air and sound to pass through the oral cavity, increasing oral resonance, and decreasing the inappropriate nasal resonance. If an individual's intelligibility is compromised by dysarthria, the speech-language pathologist might attempt to improve intelligibility by teaching the individual to slow or increase rate of speech or by teaching the speaker to exaggerate articulation to better approximate normal articulation. If the individual has phonatory difficulties that affect the intensity of phonation during speech, then correct positioning of the head or increasing effort can help to increase loudness.

A particularly notable therapy strategy is the Lee Silverman Voice Treatment (LSVT). The Lee Silverman Voice Treatment was developed by Ramig and colleagues to target the reduced amplitude of motor movement that is the underlying feature of hypokinetic dysarthria associated with Parkinson's disease. Hypokinetic dysarthria associated with Parkinson's disease manifests as a quiet and breathy voice. The goals of LSVT are to increase vocal fold adduction and intensity of voice while also reducing level of monotone of the affected individual's voice. LSVT is notable among the motor speech literature for its use of principles of motor learning and a substantial amount of evidence supporting its use (Ramig, Countryman, O'Brian, Hoehn, M., & Thompson, 1996; Ramig, Countryman, Thompson, Horri, 1995;, Ramig, Sapir, Countryman, Pawlas, O'Brian, Hoehn, et al., 2001; Ramig, Sapir, Fox, Countryman, 2001).

LSVT is used to teach individuals with Parkinson's disease to increase vocal effort and loudness by increasing vocal fold adduction and subglottal air pressure through exercises. These individuals are then taught to apply this increased effort learned in exercises to increase loudness of voice in conversation. This important transition is embodied in the LSVT mantra of *Think Loud*, which is the cue used to remind patients to expend what they may perceive to be an abnormally high level of effort on phonation and speech in order to approximate normal levels of loudness.

Oftentimes, individuals participating in this therapy may feel like they are shouting and may be hesitant

to employ the therapy techniques. In this scenario it has to be displayed to the individuals that although they may feel like they are shouting, the motor output reaching the muscles and being executed is increasing the intensity of their voice to simply an appropriate level of loudness for conversation. This may be demonstrated to the patient using biofeedback techniques as well as audio or video recording (Ramig, Pawlas, Countryman, 1995).

At times, prosthetic devices are used to help those with dysarthria compensate for their speech deficits. Abdominal binders, corsets, and certain types of vests can be used to constrain the abdomen and support respiration for phonation. Duffy (2005) highlights the importance of seeking medical approval before using any binding techniques because these devices can restrict inspiration. Portable amplification devices worn on the body can be used to increase loudness of those with weak voices.

A common prosthetic device used to manage hypernasality, most often occurring in those with flaccid dysarthria, is the palatal lift. Palatal lifts resemble the retainers worn after braces. The palatal portion of the lift connects to rear molars while the lift portion of the prosthesis extends back toward the velum. The lift portion rests against the dysfunctional velum and raises the velum toward the posterior pharyngeal wall to control air that is escaping through the velopharyngeal port, thereby reducing hypernasality during speech. The use of palatal lifts is counterindicated in individuals with impaired cognition, uncontrollable or hyperactive gag reflex or spasticity, and those with no dentition.

Nonspeech Compensatory Strategies

Speakers with severe dysarthria who have the necessary cognitive and motor skills intact might be able to use nonspeech compensatory strategies such as AAC devices as an alternative to speech. Low-tech examples are communication boards or alphabet boards, and high-tech speech production devices are the Vanguard Plus and Vantage Lite made by Prentke Romich, and DynaVox's Maestro and DynaWrite.

If a speaker does not require total replacement of speech for effective communication, then AAC devices or strategies can be used simply to augment speech. For example, a patient can use an alphabet board to spell out any words or phonemes he cannot produce intelligibly in speech. Another use of alphabet boards is to introduce a topic of conversation to the listener, which enables the listener to interpret the speech of the individual with dysarthria more accurately. The use of gestures as an augmentative strategy can also effectively facilitate listener comprehension.

Other nonspeech compensatory strategies can be employed to increase the comprehensibility of dysarthric speech while not necessarily increasing the intelligibility of articulation. Examples of these strategies that speakers with dysarthria can use are monitoring the faces of listeners to confirm that they comprehend what is being said and teaching the speaker with dysarthria to gain the attention of the listener before beginning to speak (Duffy, 2005).

Some strategies listeners can use to comprehend dysarthric speech better are maintaining eye contact with the speaker, asking for clarification, listening actively and attentively, maximizing their own visual and hearing acuity using glasses and hearing aides, and modifying the environment for best communication by reducing background noise and distractions (Duffy, 2005).

Main Points

- The dysarthrias are neurologic speech disorders resulting from abnormal strength, speed, range, steadiness, tone, or accuracy of movements required for the appropriate production of speech.
- If a speech-language pathologist can discern the differences between the dysarthrias, the therapist can use that information to localize the lesion causing the dysarthria in the nervous system.
- There are six different dysarthrias: flaccid, spastic, unilateral upper motor neuron, ataxic, hypokinetic, and hyperkinetic. In addition, mixed dysarthrias present with signs and symptoms of two or more dysarthrias.
- Flaccid dysarthria results from flaccid weakness or paralysis of the musculature used to produce speech. Flaccid dysarthria is caused by damage to the lower motor neurons, which are the efferent components of cranial and spinal nerves. Flaccid dysarthria can affect articulation, resonance, voice production, and respiration.

Flaccid dysarthria can be caused by infection, autoimmune/degenerative diseases, surgical trauma, tumor, toxins, mass effects, congenital syndromes, and brain stem stroke to the cranial nerve nuclei.

- Flaccid dysarthrias display a range of deficits depending on lesion location:
  - Unilateral trigeminal nerve damage might weaken or disable the corresponding side of the mandible, whereas the contralateral side of the mandible is still functional. In the case of unilateral damage to the trigeminal nerve, the mandible deviates toward the weakened side when the mouth is opened. Unilateral mandibular weakness may result in mild articulatory difficulties or slow rates of speech.
  - Bilateral trigeminal nerve damage can weaken or paralyze both the right and left sides of the mandible. The mandible might hang open and the affected individual can

have great difficulty closing it. This results in unintelligible speech with articulatory difficulties for lingua-alveolar, linguadental, labioalveolar, and bilabial phonemes.

- Unilateral facial nerve damage usually creates weakness or paralysis on the entire side of the face ipsilateral to the lesion. This can result in mild articulatory distortion of bilabial and labiodental phonemes, though functional abilities are preserved. Facial asymmetry is present. The patient's smile deviates away from the weakened side of the face.
- Bilateral facial nerve damage creates bilateral facial weakness. Bilateral facial weakness might be more difficult to recognize than unilateral weakness because the face remains symmetrical. Bilateral damage results in difficulty bringing the lips together entirely, including the inability to produce bilabial or labiodental phonemes.

- Flaccid dysarthrias resulting from lesion to the vagus nerve have the following characteristics:
  - Unilateral damage to right or left pharyngeal plexus creates weakness on the ipsilateral side of the pharynx and velum with contralateral function intact. This results in resonance difficulties and mild articulatory and intelligibility difficulties. The velum and/or uvula is nonuniform and off center. The uvula is pulled away from the weakened side of the velum.
  - Bilateral damage to the pharyngeal plexus creates weakness on the right and left sides of the velum. This results in hypernasal resonance. The bilaterally weakened uvula and velum are centered, though they might hang low and rest on the back of the tongue.
  - Unilateral damage to the extrinsic branch of the superior laryngeal nerve can weaken or paralyze one side of the paired cricothyroid muscles. The unaffected contralateral cricothyroid muscle can compensate for the affected cricothyroid muscle a great deal. This

lesion can lead to mild difficulties in voice modulation with a monotone voice.
  - Bilateral damage to the extrinsic branch of the superior laryngeal nerve is the result of a lesion to both the right and left sides of the superior laryngeal nerve that can paralyze or weaken both the right and left cricothyroid muscles. This results in a far more monotone voice than a unilateral lesion does.
  - Unilateral damage to the recurrent laryngeal nerve can cause paresis or paralysis of the ipsilateral vocal fold, which results in a breathy or hoarse voice. Some phonation is usually possible because the intact vocal fold can begin to approximate the weakened vocal fold.
  - Bilateral damage to the recurrent laryngeal nerve causes weakness or paralysis of both vocal folds. This can result in the inability to adduct the vocal folds for phonation or even abduct the vocal folds for respiration.
  - Unilateral hypoglossal nerve damage causes unilateral weakness on the side of the tongue that is ipsilateral to the lesion. On protrusion, the tongue deviates toward the weakened side. This results in mild or moderately affected articulation because of noise created around the weakened side of the tongue during lingual stops, lingual fricatives, and lingual affricates.
  - Bilateral hypoglossal nerve damage causes bilateral lingual weakness. This results in severely impaired articulation because every phoneme involving tongue movement is affected.

- Spastic dysarthria results from spasticity in the muscles associated with speech production. Spasticity is a combination of hypertonia and resistance to passive movement in the muscles. Spastic dysarthria is caused by bilateral damage to the upper motor neurons (UMNs), which are the descending efferent nerves within the CNS that synapse with LMNs of the PNS. Hallmark characteristics of spastic dysarthria include imprecise articulation, strained/strangled voice quality, excess and equal stress. Spastic dysarthria can be caused by stroke, trauma, toxins, diseases, and cerebral palsy.

- The upper motor neurons are divided into two tracts: pyramidal and extrapyramidal.

- The pyramidal tract, also called the direct activation pathway (DAP), is the UMN pathway that transmits impulses of fine motor and volitional motor movement. Damage to the DAP weakens the transmission of volitional motor plans, which creates a deficit in the ability to execute volitional motor plans such as the fine motor plans associated with speech.

- The extrapyramidal tract, also called the indirect activation pathway (IAP), is the pathway of the UMNs that transmits impulses associated with automatic functions that are executed below the level of awareness such as muscle tone regulation, reflex inhibition, and postural support. Damage to the IAP removes or weakens the transmission of muscle tone, muscle maintenance, postural support, and reflex inhibition. This disinhibits the stretch reflex, which causes it to become hyperactive and leads affected musculature to become hypertonic and resistant to passive movement.

- Unilateral upper motor neuron (UUMN) dysarthria results from the same neuromotor basis that underlies spastic dysarthria but is created by unilateral damage to the UMNs, not bilateral damage as in spastic dysarthria. UUMN dysarthria is usually caused by unilateral stroke.

- UUMN dysarthria causes facial weakness on primarily the lower portion of the affected side of the face. The upper portion of the affected side still receives motor plans along the facial nerve from the ipsilateral cerebral hemisphere as a result of bilateral innervation of the facial nerve. UUMN dysarthria results in mild articulation difficulties caused by unilateral labial and lingual weakness.

- Ataxic dysarthria results from the incoordination of articulator movements caused by pathology of the cerebellum. This incoordination results in slurred speech and errors in timing, range, and direction of movement of the articulators. Ataxic dysarthria can be caused by disease, strokes, trauma, or toxins.

- Hypokinetic dysarthria results from a pathology at the basal ganglia, which is responsible for regulating muscle tone, controlling postural movements, assisting in initiation of motor movement, and facilitating new motor learning. Lesion to the basal ganglia results in rigid muscle tone, postural abnormalities, difficulties initiating movement, deficits in the ability to learn new motor movement, and tremors at rest. Underdamping of motor plans reduces force and range of motion in volitional motor plans, and overdamping of motor plans allows the release and execution of excessive and extraneous movements. Hypokinetic dysarthria is known primarily as the dysarthria of Parkinson's disease but can also be caused by strokes, toxins, repeated head trauma, and infectious diseases.

- The etiologies of hyperkinesias and hyperkinetic dysarthria usually involve damage to extrapyramidal structures such as the basal ganglia and the cerebellum, which are responsible for refining motor plans and inhibiting or removing hyperkinesias from the motor plans. Hyperkinesias and hyperkinetic dysarthria can also be produced by damage to the IAP, which transmits extrapyramidal impulses. Hyperkinetic dysarthria can be caused by stroke, trauma, tumor, mass effects, infectious diseases, degenerative diseases, congenital conditions, and toxins.

- Mixed dysarthria is a manifestation of two or more dysarthrias in a single individual.

- Appropriate management of the dysarthrias first ensures that the affected individual has functional communication to meet basic wants and needs before targeting improvement of speech production.

- Restorative strategies reduce the severity of the dysarthria by restoring lost motor abilities.
- Compensatory strategies reduce the impact of the dysarthria on speech or communication while not seeking to reduce the underlying neuromotor deficits.

- Speech compensatory strategies increase intelligibility of the speaker and reduce the impact of dysarthria on speech while not directly targeting the pathologic neuromotor condition producing the dysarthria.
- Nonspeech compensatory strategies entirely bypass speech production to focus on improving overall communication.

Review Questions

1. List the six major types of dysarthria.
2. Why is lesion localization important to the speech-language pathologist?
3. How do unilateral and bilateral trigeminal nerve damage affect speech differently from each another?
4. How do unilateral and bilateral facial nerve damage affect speech differently from each another?
5. How do unilateral and bilateral vagus nerve damage to the pharyngeal plexus affect speech differently from each another?
6. How do unilateral and bilateral vagus nerve damage to the extrinsic branch of the superior laryngeal nerve affect speech differently from each another?
7. How do unilateral and bilateral vagus nerve damage to the recurrent laryngeal nerve affect speech differently from each another?
8. Explain the function of the recurrent laryngeal nerve and why is it called *recurrent*.
9. How do unilateral and bilateral hypoglossal nerve damage affect speech differently from each another?
10. Why does a lesion to the UMN produce spasticity?
11. In UUMN dysarthria, explain why the lower portion of the face contralateral to the lesion is more weakened than the upper portion of the face contralateral to the lesion.
12. In flaccid dysarthria as a result of unilateral lesion to the facial nerve, explain why this condition (in contrast to UUMN dysarthria) produces weakness equally across the entire affected side of the face.
13. What is the lesion site for ataxic dysarthria and why does a lesion at this location produce the speech qualities associated with ataxic dysarthria?
14. What are the speech characteristics of hypokinetic dysarthria?
15. What are two common profiles of mixed dysarthria and what conditions create these profiles?
16. Where in the CNS can a single small lesion create a mixed dysarthria with three dysarthrias present?
17. Strengthening exercises might be appropriate for which dysarthrias? Explain your rationale.
18. List and explain the exercise principles of strengthening exercises necessary to maximize positive impact on speech.
19. Why are relaxation techniques contraindicated for those with flaccid dysarthria? For which dysarthria(s) are relaxation techniques appropriate?
20. Give an example of a speech compensatory strategy and a nonspeech compensatory strategy.

References

1. Aridon, P., Ragonese, P., Mazzola, M., Terruso, V., Palermo, A., D'Amelio, M., & Savettieri, G. (2010). Leprosy: Report of a case with severe peripheral neuropathy. *Neurological Science, 31*, 75–77.

2. Bamford, K., Caine, E., Kido, D., Cox, C., & Shoulson, I. (1995). A prospective evaluation of cognitive decline in early Huntington's disease: Functional and radiographic correlates. *Neurology, 45*, 1867–1873.

3. Bamford, K., Caine, E., Kido, D., Plassche, W., & Shoulson, I. (1989). Clinical pathologic correlation in Huntington's disease: A neuropsychological and computer tomography study. *Neurology, 39*, 796–801.

4. Barlow, S., & Abbs, J. (1983). Force transducters for the evaluation of labial, lingual, and mandibular function in dysarthria. *Journal of Speech, Language, and Hearing Research, 26*, 616.

5. Blanco, Y., Compta, Y., Graus, F., & Saiz, A. (2008). Midbrain lesions and paroxysmal dysarthria in multiple sclerosis. *Multiple Sclerosis, 14*, 694–697.

6. Cardoso, F. (2011). Sydenham's chorea. *Handbook of Clinical Neurology, 100*, 221–229.

7. Chua, P., & Chiu, E. (2005). Huntington's disease. In A. Burns, J. O'Brien, & D. Ames (Eds.), *Dementia* (3rd ed., pp. 754–762). London, England: Hodder Arnold.

8. Clark, H. (2003). Neuromuscular treatments for speech and swallowing: A tutorial. *American Journal of Speech-Language Pathology, 12*, 400–415.

9. Darley, F., Aronson, A., & Brown, J. (1969a). Clusters of deviant speech dimensions in the dysarthrias. *Journal of Speech and Hearing Research, 12*, 462–496.

10. Darley, F., Aronson, A., & Brown, J. (1969b). Differential diagnostic patterns of dysarthria. *Journal of Speech and Hearing Research, 12*, 246–269.

11. Darley, F., Aronson, A., & Brown, J. (1975). *Motor speech disorders*. Philadelphia, PA: W. B. Saunders.

12. Duffy, J. (2005). *Motor speech disorders: Substrates, differential diagnosis, and management* (2nd ed.). St. Louis, MO: Mosby.

13. Froeschels, E. (1943). A contribution to the pathology and therapy of dysarthria due to certain cerebral lesions. *Journal of Speech Disorders, 8*, 301.

14. Kays, S., & Robbins, J. (2007). Framing oral motor exercise in principles of neural plasticity. *Neurophysiology and Neurogenic Speech and Language Disorders, 17*(4), 11–17.

15. Kennedy, P. (1988). Neurological complications of human immunodeficiency virus infection. *Postgraduate Medical Journal, 64*, 180–187.

16. Kent, R., Wiesmer, G., Kent, J., & Rosenbek, J. (1989). Toward phonetic intelligibility testing in dysarthria. *Journal of Speech and Hearing Disorders, 54*(4), 482–499.

17. Kuehn, D. P. (1997). The development of a new technique for treating hypernasality: CPAP. *American Journal of Speech-Language Pathology, 6*, 5–8.

18. Leckman, J., Zhang, H., Vitale, A., Lahnin, F., Lynch, K., Bondi, C., … Peterson, B. (1998). Course of tic severity in Tourette syndrome: The first two decades. *Pediatrics, 102*(1), 14–19.

19. Merson, R., & Rolnick, M. (1998). Speech-language pathology and dysphagia in multiple sclerosis. *Physical Medicine and Rehabilitation Clinics of North America, 9*(3), 631–641.

20. Nicholas, P., Voss, J., Wantland, D., Lindgren, T., Huang, E., Holzemer, W., & Bain, C. (2010). Prevalence, self-care behaviors, and self-care activities for peripheral neuropathy symptoms of HIV/AIDS. *Nursing and Health Science, 12*, 119–126.

21. Ooi, W., & Srinivasan, J. (2004). Leprosy and the peripheral nervous system: Basic and clinical aspects. *Muscle and Nerve, 30*, 393–403.

22. Ramig, L., Countryman, S, O'Brian, C., Hoehn, M., Thompson, I. (1996). Intensive speech treatment for patients with Parkinson disease: Short and long term comparison of two techniques. Neurology, 47, 1496-1504.

23. Ramig, L., Countryman, S., Thompson, L., Horri, Y. (1995). A comparison of two forms of intensive voice treatment for Parkinson disease. Journal of Speech and Hearing Research, 38, 1232-1251.

24. Ramig, L., Pawlas, A., Countryman, S. (1995). The Lee Silverman Voice Treatment. Iowa City, IA: National Center for Voice and Speech.

25. Ramig, L., Sapir, S., Countryman, S., Pawlas, A., O'Brian, C., Hoehn, M, et al. (2001). Intensive voice treatment (LSVT) for individuals with Parkinson's disease: A 2 year follow-up. Journal of Neurology, Neurosurgery, and Psychiatry, 71(4), 493-499.

26. Rosenbek, J., & LaPointe, L. (1978). The dysarthrias: Description, diagnosis, and treatment. In D. Johns (Ed.), *Clinical management of neurogenic communicative*

disorders. (pp. 251–310). Boston, MA: Little, Brown and Company.

27. Sobush, D., & Dunning, M. (1989). Providing resistive breathing exercise to the inspiratory muscles using the PFLEX device. *Physical Therapy, 66*(4), 542–544.

28. Zajkowska, J., Kulakowska, A., Tarasiuk, J., Pancewicz, S., Drozdowski, W., & Lekarski, P. (2010). Peripheral neuropathies in Lyme borreliosis. *Organ Polskiego Towarzystwa Lekarskiego, 29*, 115–118.

Chapter 8

Traumatic Brain Injury

▶ *Where this icon appears, visit http://go.jblearning.com/ManascoCWS to view the corresponding video.*

Whereas the disorders stemming from stroke and degenerative diseases overwhelmingly occur among the older demographic, traumatic brain injury is a common source of speech, language, and cognitive problems among all age groups, from infants to older adults. No matter the speech-language pathologist's work setting, from nursing home to school, acute care center to children's hospital, knowledge of traumatic brain injury, how it occurs, how to recognize it, and how to address it in therapy is imperative.

The word **trauma** is used to describe serious and potentially life-threatening levels of physical injury. A traumatic brain injury (TBI) is damage to the brain that results from an external and usually forceful event. This definition excludes damage to the brain resulting from disease, stroke, or surgery. Severity of a TBI can range from a concussion that causes a transient amnesia and changes in consciousness to a more severe TBI that leads to coma or death.

Trauma Serious and potentially life-threatening levels of physical injury.

It is estimated that approximately 1.4 million individuals experience a TBI each year in the United States and more than 57 million people worldwide live with the effects of TBI (Faul, Xu, Wald, & Coronado, 2010; Kimbler, Murphy, & Dhandapani, 2011). Kimbler, Murphy, and Dhandapani (2011) note that TBI is more common than AIDS, breast cancer, multiple sclerosis, and spinal cord injury combined. The most common causes of TBI are falls, motor vehicle and traffic accidents, incidents of a person being struck by an object, sports accidents, and violent assaults (Faul et al., 2010).

The most at risk populations include children younger than age 4 years, individuals older than 75 years, and adolescent males. Male children 4 years and younger experience the highest rates of TBI (Faul et al., 2010). To some degree these statistics can be accounted for by TBI from fall injuries. TBI resulting from falls are most common in very young children but are also common among older adults. Adolescent males from 15 to 19 years of age are most likely to acquire a TBI as a result of motor vehicle accidents or assault (Faul et al., 2010). Typically, males are far more likely to experience TBI than females are because males are more likely to engage in high-risk activities and behaviors. This is especially true in the adolescent male population. Adolescent females are less likely to engage in high-risk activities by themselves. However, it is not uncommon for a young woman to acquire a TBI as a result of association with adolescent males. A common example is young adolescent women riding in cars or on motorcycles driven by young males who, because of the adolescent males' reckless driving behaviors, end up in a vehicle accident and suffer from a TBI. Other risk factors are the use of alcohol as well as recreational drugs (Ylvisaker, Szekeres, & Feeney, 2008). Also, individuals with lower socioeconomic status (SES) are more likely to experience TBI than those with higher SES. Individuals who have previously experienced a TBI are three times more likely to experience additional TBI (Annegers, Grabow, Kurland, & Laws, 1980).

Law enforcement and military personnel are also at great risk for TBI. These are high-risk professions in which individuals are often victims of assault and/or are involved in traffic-related accidents. In fact, following the recent U.S. foreign wars, waves of soldiers have returned home with diagnosed and undiagnosed TBI. Deficits following TBI are many, complex, varied, and are typically a function of the areas of the brain that were damaged and to what extent. Traumatic brain injuries are usually divided into two primary forms: closed head injuries and open head injuries (Figure 8-1).

Closed Head Traumatic Brain Injuries

Forms of trauma causing damage to the brain that do not break an individual's skull open and penetrate the cerebral meninges surrounding the brain are categorized as closed head injuries. In closed head TBI, the skull remains intact. There are two primary categorizations of closed head TBI: acceleration-deceleration injuries and impact-based injuries (Brookshire, 2007)

Closed head injury A subcategory of traumatic brain injury in which an individual's skull is not broken open.

(Figure 8-1). Depending on the circumstances of the trauma, these two forms of closed head injury can occur singly or in combination.

Acceleration-Deceleration Closed Head Injury

In modern society, people often find themselves (and their brains) moving at very high speeds through space. We move at speeds that, though seemingly normal to us, are breakneck levels for our brains should anything go wrong. We move quickly from one place to another in cars and on motorcycles and bicycles. We move very quickly skateboarding, snowboarding, running a football, dribbling a soccer ball, and in a variety of other activities. We also move very fast toward the ground if we trip and fall.

Acceleration-deceleration closed head injuries occur when a person's body, and therefore the brain, is moving very fast through space (acceleration) and then comes to a very abrupt halt (deceleration) that is sudden enough to cause the brain as a result of inertia to slam into and bounce around the inside of the skull with damaging levels of force (Brookshire, 2007). Consequently, closed head injuries are seen often in motor vehicle and traffic accidents where vehicles collide and suddenly change from great speeds to less speeds, as when a fast-moving car hits a stationary object. Acceleration-deceleration injuries can also occur when a still car is hit by a moving vehicle.

A typical profile of damage to the brain in acceleration-deceleration closed head TBIs is coup-contrecoup (see Figure 8-2). *Coup* is pronounced "coo" and is the

Acceleration-deceleration closed head injury Damage to the brain created by the external forces that act on the brain when it is moving through space very quickly or coming to an abrupt halt.

Coup-contrecoup A pattern of brain damage that occurs when, due to external forces, the brain bounces back and forth inside the skull causing damage at the sites of impact.

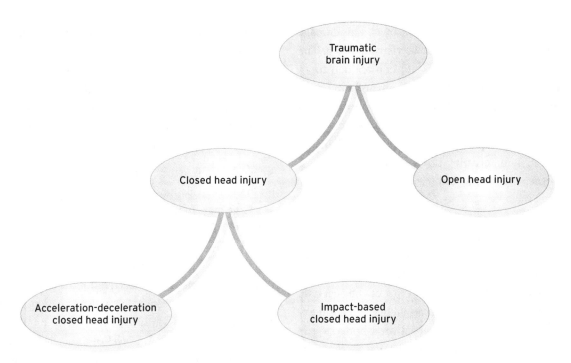

Figure 8-1   Types and subtypes of TBI.

French word for a severe hit or impact. For example, in a standard car wreck an individual in a motor vehicle collides head-on with an immovable object.

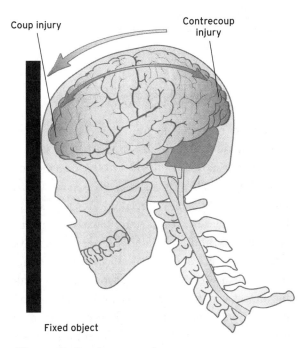

Figure 8-2   Coup-contrecoup.

Directly after the car is stopped by the immovable object, the inertial forces propel the driver's head to first impact the steering wheel or dashboard. As the driver's head moves from a high rate of speed through space to suddenly stopping by hitting the steering wheel or dashboard, the brain is pressed by deceleration forces against the inside front of the skull. The passenger's head then rebounds or ricochets backward to hit the neckrest with a lower, though still damaging level of inertial force. At this point, the posterior of the brain impacts the interior rear of the skull. The first impact of the brain against the inside front of the skull is coup damage. The contrecoup injury occurs as a result of the secondary impact of the brain hitting the inside back of the skull. In this example, the coup injury produces focalized damage to the most anterior-inferior portions of the frontal lobes and temporal lobes. This damage usually results in personality changes, motor deficits, memory deficits, expressive-receptive language deficits, and deficits in attention and higher-level cognition. In contrast, the contrecoup injury produces more generalized damage to the posterior part of the brain, the occipital lobes, and the vision areas. This damage results in visual deficits such as visual agnosia. The coup-contrecoup damage is not constrained to an anterior-posterior profile in the brain and can occur, depending on forces involved, in any one area and its opposite area of the brain. The back-and-forth action of the coup-contrecoup profile also damages the brain stem, creating possible deficits in arousal and other autonomic functions.

The brain can also be damaged by high levels of G-force not associated with impact. The *G* in **G-force** stands for *gravitational* but the term *G-force* also refers to the amount of force exerted on an object by acceleration forces. The lift out of the seat as a roller-coaster rockets down an incline is a good example of G-force being exerted on a body as it is pulled speedily away from where it was. In the military, jet pilots feel G-force as they are pushed back into their seat as the jet flies through space. If the G-force is too high for too long, the pilot will pass out as blood is forced away from the brain. If the G-force continues to increase (as can happen if a jet enters a tailspin), the pilot's brain will eventually be warped and pushed with damaging force against the inside of the skull, causing brain trauma and even death. The trauma from this warping effect breaks delicate connections between neurons and also between blood vessels in the brain. This type of damage does not usually occur in a single focal area of the brain but is generalized across large areas of the brain exposed to the damaging forces involved. When neuronal connections are pulled apart in this way, micro

G-force   The amount of stress being applied to a body by acceleration forces.

Diffuse axonal shearing   The breaking of neuronal connections that occurs across large areas of the brain and is seen commonly in closed head traumatic brain injury.

Impact-based TBI   A form of closed head injury in which a moving object impacts the head forcing the skull inward on the brain producing focal damage to the area of the brain compressed.

lesions are created across large areas of the brain. This form of damage is known as **diffuse axonal shearing**. Diffuse axonal shearing is often seen in traffic accidents. When a vehicle enters a high-speed spin in the midst of a collision, the rotational forces (G-force) exerted on passengers in the vehicle can be high enough to cause this form of damage.

In acceleration–deceleration closed head TBIs, the brain stem can also suffer damage. Think of the brain as a large mass of tissue sitting atop a relatively small and delicate brain stem. The brain is not made to be pulled away from the brain stem or twisted on top of it by G-force, so the brain stem often suffers great damage in acceleration–deceleration injuries when this occurs. The reticular formation, an important structure housed within the brain stem, regulates the sleep–wake cycle and level of arousal. In other words, the reticular formation enables an individual to stay awake and fall asleep and switch normally between these two states. When the reticular formation is damaged, the body has problems regulating its level of arousal, resulting in coma or vegetative states. Indeed, comas and vegetative states are commonly seen in individuals who have experienced acceleration–deceleration closed head TBIs.

Impact-Based Closed Head Traumatic Brain Injury

Traumatic injury to the brain that occurs as a result of an individual's head being struck by a moving object is an **impact-based TBI**. When a moving object impacts a head, the skull is pressed inward on the brain. As the skull is forced inward at the site of the impact, it exerts compressive forces on that area of the brain (Brookshire, 2007). These compressive forces can bruise and tear the surface of the brain, producing focal damage localized to the area beneath the impact. This focal damage is unlike acceleration–deceleration damage, which results in diffuse damage across large areas of the brain. Violent assault is a common cause of impact-based TBI.

Open Head Traumatic Brain Injury

In contrast to closed head TBI, in which the skull is not opened, in **open head TBI** an object penetrates the skull into the brain. A common cause of open head TBI is ballistic trauma, such as when a projectile (a bullet or piece of shrapnel) passes through the skull and into brain. Although often associated with assault, open head TBI can also occur as a result of a fall in which the individual's head impacts an object sharp enough to penetrate the skull.

> **Open head TBI** A form of TBI in which the skull is broken open and the brain is penetrated.

The degree of injury to the brain produced by an open head TBI is dictated by the location and extent of the damage. For example, as a bullet passes through the head, it tears apart the tissue of the brain and surrounding blood vessels and admits foreign matter into the wound such as bullet fragments, pieces of skull, and hair. Nonsterile foreign objects such as these carry bacteria into the brain and can cause infection. Because of the risk of infection, this foreign matter must be removed.

Open head TBI produces focal lesions at the point of penetration into the brain, unlike acceleration–deceleration closed head TBI, which causes damage over larger areas of the brain. As open head TBI can damage a single area of the brain, leaving large areas of the brain intact, open head injury can result in more specific deficits in the absence of the global deficits seen in acceleration–deceleration TBI. The classic example of an open head injury is the case of Phineas Gage, who, despite the fact that a metal rod was shot through his frontal lobes, walked away from the injury, remained conscious, and thereafter displayed the specific deficits of memory loss, lack of social inhibition and executive function that are now known to arise from damage to the frontal lobe. In contrast, in a standard acceleration–deceleration

Clinical Note

Modern Ammunition

During World War II, a great many soldiers survived gunshot wounds to the head because the bullets remained intact and passed cleanly through the body. In fact, much of what we now know about how the brain works is a result of the careful study and documentation of the cognitive and language deficits displayed by soldiers of World War II who were shot in the head and survived (Russell & Espir, 1961).

Most modern ammunition is not designed to pass neatly and cleanly through flesh, as bullets did in the past, but to create as much damage as possible to the body as they pass through. Most modern bullets do this by rapidly expanding and distorting in shape as they impact a body. The distortion is accomplished by a variety of means, one of which is placing soft lead on the tips of the bullet that buckles and mushrooms into an erratic and more detrimental shape on impact. In handgun ammunition, this effect is also achieved by hollow-tipped bullets.

The expansion and distortion of a bullet gives it more surface area and a more irregular shape that causes it to follow a more irregular trajectory through the body and create more collateral damage to tissues surrounding the wound. Modern ammunition creates extensive trauma to the body that would not have been seen in most gunshot wounds of the past. Because of the increased trauma, survival of a gunshot wound to the head is far more rare now than in the past. However, smaller-caliber handgun ammunition and sometimes more solid practice rounds of the larger-caliber bullets at times still pass cleanly through the head, thereby increasing the victim's chances of survival.

TBI, the individual might immediately become unconscious, perhaps progress into a coma, and over the course of weeks or months might awaken from the coma into a state of confusion and suffer deficits of motor and cognitive functions. A flow chart delineating the types and subtypes of TBI covered so far is provided in Figure 8-2.

Secondary Mechanisms of Damage in Traumatic Brain Injury

Primary mechanisms of damage to the brain in traumatic brain injury are the acceleration–deceleration forces that produce coup-contrecoup injuries, the rotational forces that produce diffuse axonal shearing, the compression forces present in impact-based TBI, and the violent penetration of a foreign object into brain tissue. However, in all these scenarios, the initial sources of damage can be followed by any number of consequent, secondary mechanisms of injury.

Intracranial pressure is the amount of pressure present within the skull and therefore the amount of pressure exerted on the brain. When intracranial pressure rises above normal it is called increased intracranial pressure. Increased intracranial pressure is a major risk following any damage to the brain. If intracranial pressure becomes higher than blood pressure, the heart will have difficulty pushing blood into the brain. Then, hypoxia or anoxia occurs, causing brain damage or death if not treated quickly.

When damage to the brain occurs, multiple possible mechanisms create heightened and dangerous levels of intracranial pressure. Cerebral edema is the swelling of brain tissue and can occur following trauma to the brain. This expansive swelling of brain tissue increases intracranial pressure.

At times, damage to the brain disrupts the cerebrospinal fluid (CSF) system, which nourishes the brain. Following disruption, the brain might become unable to reabsorb old cerebrospinal fluid while it still produces fresh cerebrospinal fluid in the lateral ventricles. This process is known as traumatic hydrocephalus and can raise intracranial pressure to a life-threatening level. This condition is usually treated by the placement of a CSF shunt, a device placed into a lateral ventricle that drains off excess cerebrospinal fluid, thereby keeping intracranial pressure normal. A CSF shunt is surgically placed under the skin of the patient and has a tube traveling under the skin from the brain out of the skull to drain excess fluid to a more appropriate place in the body, like the urinary system.

As a result of warping or movement of the brain within the skull, hemorrhaging (bleeding) of blood vessels is likely to occur. Traumatic hemorrhage is bleeding as a result of trauma. Traumatic hemorrhages are usually intracerebral, subdural, or epidural. If a traumatic hemorrhage occurs within the brain, it is an intracerebral hemorrhage. If the traumatic hemorrhage occurs between the dura mater and the arachnoid mater, it is a subdural hemorrhage. If the bleed occurs between the dura mater and the skull, the term epidural hemorrhage is applied.

Hematomas are a threat associated with traumatic hemorrhage. A hematoma is the gathering of blood outside a blood vessel following a hemorrhage. Stretching and trauma to blood vessels in and around

---

Increased intracranial pressure A raised level of pressure within the skull above the normal and healthy level.

Cerebral edema The swelling of brain tissue.

Traumatic hydrocephalus A disruption of the brain's ability to reabsorb excess cerebrospinal fluid that is caused by a traumatic event and leads to a life-threatening increase in intracranial pressure.

Traumatic hemorrhage Bleeding as a result of trauma.

Subdural hemorrhage A hemorrhage that occurs between the dura mater and the arachnoid mater, usually of traumatic origin.

Epidural hemorrhage A hemorrhage that occurs between the dura mater and the skull, usually of traumatic origin.

Hematoma The gathering of blood outside a blood vessel following a hemorrhage.

Subdural hematoma A hematoma that occurs when veins between the dura mater and the brain are broken and bleed out between the dura mater and brain.

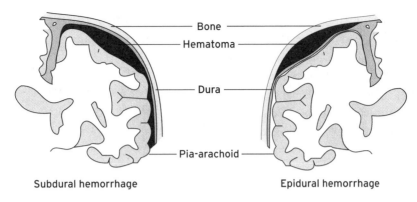

Figure 8-3 **Comparative locations of subdural and epidural hematomas.**

the brain during TBI makes hematoma a common threat. A subdural hematoma occurs when veins between the dura mater and the brain are broken and then bleed out between the dura mater and brain. The blood pooling between the dura mater and the brain can cause an increase in intracranial pressure and compress brain tissue. Epidural hematoma occurs when a blood vessel bursts between the dura mater and the skull and can cause increased intracranial pressure. (See Figure 8-3.)

Seizures are also a known and common consequence of TBI. Seizures occurring consequent to TBI (i.e., post onset, or after the onset, of TBI) are known as post-traumatic epilepsy (PTE; Agrawal, Timothy, Pandit, & Manju, 2006). These seizures cause additional damage to the brain and significantly and negatively affect prognosis for recovery of lost functions. It is not uncommon that a severe PTE seizure sets back the rehabilitation of an individual with a TBI by days or weeks. Post-traumatic epilepsy is most common following open head TBI such as gunshot wounds or military-type open head TBI. In fact, 50% of those with open (penetrating) head wounds experience some degree of PTE (Annegers et al., 1998). The strongest risk factors for seizure activity following TBI include the severity of the damage to the brain, contusions, and subdural hematomas (Annegers et al., 1998).

Special Topics in Traumatic Brain Injury

Two other specific and important profiles of traumatic brain injury, interestingly, are common forms of TBI experienced by the physically weakest among us—infants younger than age 2 years—and the physically strongest among us—athletes, soldiers, and military personnel.

Shaken Baby Syndrome

Although this text focuses on adult neurogenic communication disorders, this chapter must cover one of the most common and devastating forms of traumatic brain injury, shaken baby syndrome. Traumatic brain injury is one of the most common causes of death in children, and physical abuse is the leading cause of these TBIs (American Academy of Pediatrics, 2001). In fact, Bruce and

Epidural hematoma A hematoma that occurs when a blood vessel bursts between the dura mater and the skull.

Post-traumatic epilepsy Seizures that occur as a result of a traumatic brain injury.

Shaken baby syndrome A profile of traumatic brain injury seen in infants and small children most often caused by physical abuse, usually a shaking of the child, by the caregiver.

Zimmerman (1989) document that 80% of deaths from TBI in children younger than 2 years were non-accidental (i.e., intentional). Usually, in such young children abuse takes the form of a caregiver hitting or violently shaking an infant. The usual trigger for abuse of an infant is the infant's crying. The violence of the shaking action by the adult is often recognized by observers as obviously dangerous and likely to cause death to the child (American Academy of Pediatrics, 2001). The violent shaking of an infant results in an identifiable profile of injuries and deficits known as shaken baby syndrome.

The sources of damage to the child's brain in shaken baby syndrome are the strong rotational and acceleration–deceleration forces imposed on it by the intensity of the back-and-forth shaking. Mortality rates in shaken infants are high. Severe physical, visual, and cognitive disabilities are often present in those who survive. Multiple mechanisms of damage to a child's brain occur as a result of being shaken. Diffuse axonal shearing is often a component of the injuries. Also, the capillaries of the pia mater surrounding the brains of infants are very fragile and any significant level of rotational or acceleration–deceleration forces is likely to break blood vessels open, resulting in subdural hematoma, which can cause intracranial pressure to rise, limiting blood flow into the brain and posing significant risk of death to the child. Localized contusions to a child's brain are also likely to occur as a result of the shaken child's brain impacting irregular or jagged areas on the inside of the cranium. An additional threat secondary to any other form of brain damage is cerebral edema, or swelling of the brain. Like a hematoma, cerebral edema also raises intracranial pressure. If intracranial pressure rises above the arterial blood pressure, the heart cannot force more blood into the brain and the subsequent lack of oxygen can lead to coma or death.

Signs and symptoms of shaken baby syndrome vary widely as a function of the severity of the damage imposed. However, the American Academy of Pediatrics (2001) lists these common symptoms of shaken baby syndrome:

- Vomiting
- Difficulty feeding (poor suck/swallow)
- Lethargy
- Altered consciousness (comatose state)
- Irritability
- Retinal hemorrhages
- Impaired tracking of eyes
- Seizures
- Lack of smile and vocalizations
- Respiratory difficulties

Usually, other signs of abuse are present such as bruises, broken bones, or a history of or evidence of past injuries. Shaken baby syndrome at times is misdiagnosed by medical doctors because the caregiver might not know the baby was shaken or the caregiver is the abuser who will not readily admit to the abuse.

In addition to medical treatment, these children also need physical, occupational, visual, and speech therapy as they recover, grow, and develop. Although the speech-language pathologist probably plays no part in the emergency medical treatment of shaken infants, the speech-language pathologist working in pediatrics and early pediatrics must be able to recognize the signs of this syndrome to make the quick and appropriate referrals for the well-being of the child. Survival of these children depends on timely recognition of the abuse and immediate medical attention. The role of the speech-language pathologist in shaken baby syndrome usually depends on the age of the injured child and the extent and nature of the injuries and deficits. However, in the medical setting the speech-language pathologist will probably focus on treating the acquired feeding or swallowing problems of shaken infants in the neonatal intensive care unit (NICU). Once these children reach school age, the school speech-language pathologist can treat these children for articulation difficulties, language problems, and cognitive problems resulting from being shaken as an infant. For more information on shaken baby syndrome, visit the website of the National Center on Shaken Baby Syndrome at www.dontshake.org.

Military Traumatic Brain Injury

A Brief History

Injuries to the brain produced in modern wars have contributed to scientific and medical understanding of the brain. In World War I and World War II, the penetrating or open head wound as a result of gunshot to the head was the most common form of traumatic brain injury. During World War I, large numbers of soldiers shot in the head initially survived these open head traumatic brain injuries. However, medical knowledge of how to manage these injuries successfully did not exist at the time, and these soldiers often suffered meningitis and chronic cerebral abscesses (Russel & Espir, 1961). However, lessons were taken from battlefield treatment of these World War I soldiers. Medical treatment progressed a great deal from the knowledge gained from the treatment of soldiers in World War I. As a result, during World War II debridement techniques were used to remove bone fragments, foreign debris, and irreparably damaged brain tissue from the injured brain that otherwise would have been left inside the wounded soldier's head, possibly to cause immediate and future problems (Russel & Espir, 1961). Alongside these techniques, the then-recent advent of antibiotics increased World War II soldiers' chances of survival of gunshot wounds to the head (Russel & Espir, 1961). The survival of these men in large numbers paved the way for large-scale systematic studies of the deficits and disorders produced by head wounds. This research following World War II by individuals such as Luria (1947), Russel and Espir (1961), and Schiller (1947) documents the impact and result of damage by ballistic trauma to parts of the brain that were perhaps only rarely damaged in isolation by stroke. In this way, medical science learned a great deal about the

functioning of the brain. The results of these studies form much of the knowledge on left hemisphere and right hemisphere syndromes presented in this text.

Mechanisms of Traumatic Brain Injury in Current Military Conflicts

The modern-day traumatic brain injuries that military personnel most often experience are not the result of gunshot wounds to the head but of damage resulting from exposure to explosions. Makeshift bombs, known as improvised explosive devices (IEDs), have been the primary weapon of choice by enemy combatants and insurgents in recent American wars in Iraq and Afghanistan. More often than not, these devices are planted on roadways to explode when run over by military vehicles or on footpaths to explode when tread upon.

When a person is exposed to a bomb blast, a series of tissue-damaging events quickly unfolds. The different mechanisms of injury delivered by a bomb blast are referred to as primary, secondary, tertiary, and quaternary levels of damage (Centers for Disease Control and Prevention [CDC], 2011). The term **polytrauma** is used to describe the various types of trauma experienced by soldiers following exposure to an IED blast. When these soldiers exposed to IED blasts return home for rehabilitation services, they display many language and cognitive deficits that a speech-language pathologist can address. It is therefore worthy of the time of the student of speech-language pathology to examine the mechanisms of damage to the brain induced by exposure to IED explosions.

> **Polytrauma** A profile of traumatic injury resulting from many different types of trauma.

The primary level is the most immediate impact of an IED explosion and is the direct result of the shock wave created by the explosion. A shock wave occurs when the rapidly combusting matter of the explosive device causes air pressure to rise dramatically above normal atmospheric pressure levels. This wave of intense heat and compression emanates from the explosive device and is followed by a reactionary wave of decompressed air molecules that reduces air pressure far below normal levels. It is these tremendous shifts in pressure caused by the explosion that make the shock wave such a destructive force to those positioned nearby. Trauma induced by exposure to intense levels of pressure changes following an explosion is termed barotrauma (Roth, 2007).

When a shock wave hits the human body, it compresses the body tissues and moves through the body, compressing and releasing the tissues as it travels through the body. On a molecular level, body tissue is first compressed by the shock wave and then pulled apart by the reactionary wave. Parts of the body most susceptible to barotrauma are the brain, eyes, and air- and fluid-filled organs of the abdomen.

Although barotrauma can be devastating to the body, it can also produce less severe results such as concussion or mild TBI. Soldiers who are exposed to an IED explosion and who experience concussion or mild TBI with no physical sign of trauma are likely to walk away from the explosion, possibly staying in combat. In fact, in recent wars the first attempts by the U.S. military to screen for mild cognitive deficits following TBI were thwarted by the soldiers memorizing the answers to the screening procedure, knowing that if they responded correctly, they would be allowed to stay in combat. In this way, many soldiers accrued multiple TBIs from repeated exposure to IED explosions.

Barotrauma Trauma induced by exposure to intense levels of pressure changes following an explosion.

In addition to the shock wave, explosions usually create flying debris and bomb fragments (CDC, 2011). When these bomb fragments or debris hit soldiers and bystanders this is known as the secondary level of blast trauma.

The tertiary level of blast trauma results from the physical displacement of the body when impacted by the force of the wind associated with the shock wave. Often, soldiers and bystanders are knocked off their feet or thrown into nearby structures by the shock wave. These individuals might suffer further trauma to the body or the brain as a result of the impact with the ground or an object. Closed or open head traumatic brain injuries might occur on the tertiary level.

The quaternary level of blast trauma is any trauma created by the blast that is not attributable to primary, secondary, or tertiary mechanisms. Examples of quaternary trauma are difficulties breathing following inhalation of the toxic gases, smoke, or dust of an explosion and burns to the body sustained as a result of the blast (CDC, 2011; Roth, 2007).

Sports-Related TBI

Another population of individuals at risk for closed head TBI is athletes. Athletes' risk of TBI has been well known for decades but has recently taken the media spotlight because of the chronic and neurodegenerative Alzheimer's and Parkinson's-like conditions known as chronic traumatic encephalopathy, which are being experienced by certain retired professional American football players. Chronic traumatic encephalopathy is a degenerative disease of the brain caused by repeated head trauma, such as repeated concussions in sports or repeated exposure to IED blasts in soldiers. It manifests as dementia, confusion, memory loss, headache, depression, and excessive aggression within months or years of brain damage. Recent attention has been directed to chronic traumatic encephalopathy as a result of a trend of suicide among retired National Football League players who were known to be affected by the disease.

Chronic traumatic encephalopathy A degenerative disease of the brain caused by repeated head trauma such as repeated concussions in sports or repeated exposure to IED blasts in soldiers that manifests within months or years of brain damage as dementia, confusion, memory loss, headache, depression, and excessive aggression.

Although athletes of all kinds are at risk, athletes involved in contact sports such as American football, wrestling, soccer, hockey, and boxing are at highest risk. Even adolescent athletes are at risk for TBI. Female athletes, especially adolescent females, are at higher risk for TBI than males because they have less muscle mass in the neck to stabilize the head and reduce sudden movements of the head during impact (Grady, 2010).

The typical sports-related TBI is known as mild TBI or a concussion. Concussion is traditionally defined as a period of confusion following impact to the head with no loss of consciousness. However, the modern and general consensus is that concussion is a "complex pathophysiological process affecting the brain, induced by traumatic biomechanical forces" (Grady, 2010). Immediate and acute symptoms of concussion are confusion, loss of self-awareness, and possible loss of consciousness (Kimbler et al., 2011).

Concussion A pathologic and traumatic event affecting the brain that creates a state of confusion, often with no loss of consciousness.

Athletes are also at risk for multiple concussions because acute symptoms might go unrecognized or their significance is unknown to players and coaches. Because there may be no loss of consciousness, players and coaches often misjudge the head injury as nonharmful and players are sent back into play, possibly to suffer additional concussions before the brain and body can heal from the first trauma. The long-term effects of repeated concussions are more severe and include impulsiveness, depression, irritability, chronic headache, dizziness, and vertigo (DeKosky, Ikonomovic, & Gandy, 2010).

Baseline cognitive testing for athletes of all kinds prior to the playing season is becoming standard as researchers and clinicians attempt to track and prevent the immediate and long-term effects of sports-related concussion and address these deficits appropriately.

Deficits Following Traumatic Brain Injury

The type and severity of deficits that arise from traumatic brain injury are determined by the areas of the brain that are damaged and the severity of damage. Diffuse damage to the brain produces generalized deficits in most skill areas. In contrast, focal lesions might create deficits constrained to certain abilities while leaving the holistic function of the brain intact.

A General Picture of TBI

Before discussing actual deficits, let us take a moment to imagine how a person with TBI presents following the trauma and hospital admittance. Of course, no two people with TBI will present exactly alike. Nonetheless, useful generalizations can be made.

Individuals with TBI are usually unconscious, minimally conscious, or, at best, very confused and disoriented directly after their trauma. They will be in a hospital bed, perhaps hooked to a ventilator that breathes for them. They might have undergone tracheotomy where a hole was cut into the trachea below the larynx through which a mechanical ventilator delivers air to the lungs for respiration. If they did not require tracheotomy, the tube for the ventilator passes orally through the mouth into the larynx.

Many TBI patients require immediate brain surgery to resolve secondary issues such as hemorrhage or increased intracranial pressure, so their heads are shaved. A nasogastric (NG) feeding tube might pass through the nose, the pharynx, and into the esophagus to deliver hydration and nutrition to the body while the person remains unconscious or unable to eat or drink. An NG tube is usually a short-term fix whereas a percutaneous endoscopic gastrostomy (PEG) feeding tube might be placed for longer-term purposes (longer than a week). A PEG tube enters the abdomen and delivers nutrition and hydration straight into the stomach.

Because high intracranial pressure following trauma to the brain is often an issue, a cerebral spinal fluid (CSF) shunt may have been placed in the brain. A **craniotomy** is a surgery to remove part of the skull to allow the brain to swell without incurring damage from being crushed by pressure within the skull. Craniotomies are also commonly performed if the threat of increased intracranial pressure is considered life threatening.

Craniotomy A surgery to remove part of the skull to allow the brain to swell without the brain incurring damage from increased pressure within the skull.

Even if arousable, doctors may keep the individual with TBI intentionally unconscious or in what is known as a medically induced coma to better manage them medically, allow the body and brain to heal, and spare the patient extreme pain. Given that many causes of TBI are violent assault or traffic accidents, there is a good chance that these individuals will have any number of other serious medical problems concurrent to brain trauma.

As TBI patients recover from coma or a vegetative state, they can exhibit severe cognitive and language deficits leading to confusion, disorientation, and aggression. They will probably spend a great part of the day sleeping and might be restrained in their bed to keep them from injuring themselves. Once patients' cognitive skills begin to return and their levels of confusion, agitation, and disorientation decline to more natural levels, their skills reemerge from the cognitive fog they have been experiencing.

The speech of patients with TBI is usually characterized by any number of dysarthrias. Patients with TBI tend to show impulsivity and a lack of awareness of their deficits. Speech-language pathologists can start to rehabilitate cognition and language by using strategies and therapies often used in other populations, such as those with aphasia, right hemisphere deficits, and dementia. However, patient fatigue is an issue in patients with TBI. Patients at all recovery levels of TBI are highly susceptible to fatigue, and the therapist must monitor level of patient fatigue carefully.

Successful rehabilitation of patients with TBI returns them as closely as possible to pretrauma ability levels and continues to work to reintegrate them into society. Social pragmatic deficits as well as higher-level executive functioning deficits often significantly impair patients' performance in the long term and inhibit their successful reintegration into society.

Motor Deficits Following Traumatic Brain Injury

Motor deficits are common following any injury to the brain. The primary areas of the brain dedicated to motor function are within the frontal lobes. Therefore, damage to the frontal lobes often results in problems moving the body. Diffuse bilateral damage to the upper motor neurons (UMNs) in the frontal lobes creates spastic bilateral paralysis or paresis in the body whereas unilateral traumatic damage to the UMNs in a single frontal lobe creates a contralateral hemiplegia similar to that seen in stroke patients. Individuals with TBI often have severe gross and fine motor deficits. They might have abnormal muscle tone, and possible damage to the cerebellum, which will create ataxia causing incoordination of movements and impaired balance.

Particular motor deficits of concern to the speech-language pathologist are deficits in the planning or execution of movements involved in the production of speech (motor speech disorders) and swallowing (dysphagia). Motor speech disorders that can present with TBI are apraxia of speech and the dysarthrias. Possible types of dysarthria present in TBI are spastic, flaccid, ataxic, hypokinetic dysarthrias, or some combination of these four.

Cognitive Deficits Following Traumatic Brain Injury

Following TBI, individuals display a host of specific deficits in the realm of cognition. It is common for those with TBI to spend time following the trauma in a coma or a decreased state of arousal when little or no cognition is possible. However, even when patients with TBI regain a level of arousal at which they can take in and process information from the environment, they usually display many, if not all, of the cognitive (and language) deficits associated with right and left hemisphere damage. For instance, these individuals display deficits in the areas of orientation to self, orientation to place and time, sustained attention, selective attention, alternating attention, divided attention, working memory, short-term memory, long-term memory, problem solving, inferencing, and they can also experience personality changes.

Individuals who experience posterior trauma to the brain are likely to have visual processing deficits that make it difficult for them to understand what they are seeing. Patients with TBI might also display impulsivity in their behaviors, emotional lability (inappropriate emotional responses), periods of aggression or agitation, or a lack of motivation. Also, they are typically unaware of their deficits, which can lead them to be noncompliant during therapy or passive and unengaged in rehabilitation. Furthermore, because of depressed cognitive skills they tend to apply their impaired judgment to themselves and severely underestimate their deficit levels. The two issues of decreased arousal (coma/vegetative state) and personality changes are worthy of further examination in the following subsections.

Altered States of Consciousness: Coma and Vegetative State

A coma is a period of unconsciousness lasting more than 6 hours during which the unconscious individual cannot be awakened and is unresponsive to sensory stimuli. Comas are common following TBI. The duration of the coma is a known prognostic variable. Prognoses of individuals who experience shorter comas are more positive for recovery than those of patients who experience deeper and longer altered states of consciousness (Macniven, 1994).

Awakening from a coma is usually a slow process that occurs over days or weeks. The individual might become minimally arousable and might respond to some stimuli such as touch, pain, or sound but still does not reach full consciousness or awareness of the surroundings. These individuals might direct their eyes toward bright or moving objects. They might move their heads toward a sound source and even display a normal sleep/wake cycle. However, they can be entirely lacking in cognition. A condition in which a person is minimally responsive to stimuli but lacking consciousness and cognition is known as a **vegetative state**. If a vegetative state continues longer than 4 weeks, it is labeled a **persistent vegetative state**. The likelihood of fully awaking from a vegetative state decreases the longer the patient remains in the vegetative state. Approximately 3% of those with severe head injuries display a persistent vegetative state 1 year post trauma (Braakman, Jennet, & Minderhoud, 1988).

> **Coma**   A period of unconsciousness lasting more than 6 hours during which the unconscious individual cannot be awakened and is unresponsive to sensory stimuli.
>
> **Vegetative state**   A condition in which a person is minimally responsive to stimuli but lacking consciousness and cognition.
>
> **Persistent vegetative state**   A vegetative state lasting longer than 4 weeks.

Those who do recover from coma and vegetative states often display an amnesia following the trauma referred to as **post-traumatic amnesia**. Post-traumatic amnesia is a usual consequence of significant injury to the brain and typically presents as a combination of both retrograde and anterograde memory losses. This condition creates an inability to take on new memories (anterograde amnesia) to the extent that most individuals recovering from TBI usually cannot remember a large part of their hospital stay or rehabilitation following the trauma. The longer the duration of post-traumatic amnesia, the less positive the prognosis for recovery (Bond, 1976; Katz, 1992). Usually, post-traumatic amnesia has a retrograde component that destroys recently acquired memory, often up until days, weeks, or months before the trauma. Katz (1992) studied patients with closed head injury and found that post-traumatic amnesia that lasts longer than 2 weeks is associated with a better recovery whereas post-traumatic amnesia that lasts 12 weeks or longer is associated with far lower levels of recovery.

Post-traumatic amnesia Memory loss following trauma to the brain that is usually a combination of retrograde and anterograde amnesia.

Personality Changes

Many common forms of TBI result in damage to the frontal lobes. As discussed earlier, the frontal lobes play a role in personality and personal preferences as well as the inhibition of inappropriate social behaviors. As a result of frontal lobe damage, individuals with TBI often display dramatic personality changes resulting from loss of social inhibition. These individuals might make inappropriate sexual advances toward others or say inappropriate things at inappropriate times. They can be far less aware of or attentive to usual social and cultural conventions. Inappropriate social behavior often diminishes as recovery from the TBI progresses. However, more subtle changes can also occur as a result of frontal lobe damage such as changes in food and music preferences.

Language Deficits Following Traumatic Brain Injury

Language losses as a result of TBI occur often and are determined by the location and extent of damage to the brain. Language deficits such as anomia and aphasia following closed head injuries are often present but can be dwarfed by deficits in arousal and cognition. Individuals with generalized damage across large portions of the brain usually display some level of receptive and expressive language deficit. In open head TBI with focal damage, the individual might have more specific language deficits. In speech-language therapy, once patients recover language abilities, rehabilitation must then focus on training the appropriate use of those language abilities as these individuals struggle to regain their former lives.

Assessment of Traumatic Brain Injury

The type of assessment used with individuals with TBI varies according to the patient's age, educational level, and severity of deficits. For instance, the procedures for evaluating a severely affected patient in an altered state of consciousness are wholly different from procedures used to evaluate a patient with mild TBI perhaps with only a few higher-level deficits.

Because most TBI patients begin therapy with deep cognitive deficits, a formal interview or opportunity to observe connected speech might not be possible. In this scenario, the patient's background and medical history must be taken from medical records, charts, and interviews with the family and any rehabilitation or medical professionals who have been interacting with the patient.

Memory Assessment

As mentioned, individuals with TBI can display deficits in working memory, short-term memory, long-term memory, or any subcategory of these.

The speech-language pathologist can assess long-term memory during the interview by posing biographical questions to patients regarding personal history, such as asking them where they grew up, who is in their family, what their profession is, and to describe significant family events. A caveat here is that the speech-language pathologist must know the correct answers to these questions before asking the patient or there is no way to judge whether the patient is providing accurate, inaccurate, or even confabulatory answers. Having family members or caregivers present during the patient interview addresses this concern because they can confirm the patient's answers.

Many tests of visual memory require the patient to draw from memory the visual stimuli presented earlier. However, because of the motor deficits often present in TBI that inhibit drawing, speech-language pathologists often rely on simple presentation of objects or pictures, then request patients to identify from a field of pictures or objects which were presented. The fifth edition of the Benton Visual Retention Test (Benton, 2003) is a formal test of visual memory that is appropriate to use in populations with brain damage and dementia. It accounts for possible concomitant perceptual deficits that can co-occur in these populations.

Immediate recall of auditory information is tested by presenting an unrelated string of words and asking the patient to repeat them. A test of short-term memory for auditory information is presenting an unrelated string of words followed by a distracter task (such as asking one or two simple unrelated questions), and then returning to the primary task asking the patient to remember the words presented. An additional task to test short-term recall of auditory information is reciting a detail-heavy paragraph or story to the patient, and then asking the patient to recall as many details as possible. Purer versions of this task are free recall tasks in which the speech-language pathologist recites multiple words or numbers and asks the patient to recall as many words or numbers as possible.

Assessment of Level of Arousal
Coma Scales

Deficits in arousal are generally assessed with coma scales. These are simple categorical scales that assign a person a number that indicates his or her level of arousal based on the presence of certain behaviors and response to stimuli. The most commonly used

scales for adults are the Glascow Coma Scale and the Ranchos Los Amigos Levels of Cognitive Functioning Coma Scale (Hagen, 1981). The Adelaide Coma Scale is used in pediatrics.

- *Glasgow Coma Scale* (*GCS*; Teasdale & Jennett, 1974): The GCS is a 15-point scale that rates patients on parameters of eye opening, motor response, and verbal response. The GCS classifies patients with TBI as mild (scores of 13–15), moderate (scores of 11–12), or severe (scores of 8 and below). (See Table 8-1.)
- *Ranchos Los Amigos Levels of Cognitive Functioning* (Hagen, 1981): The Ranchos Los Amigos

Table 8-1   Glasgow Coma Scale

Eye Opening	
Spontaneous	4
To sound	3
To pain	2
None	1
Best Verbal Response	
Oriented	5
Confused conversation	4
Inappropriate words	3
Incomprehensible sounds	2
None	1
Best Motor Response	
Obeys commands	6
Localizes pain	5
Withdrawal	4
Abnormal flexion	3
Extension	2
None	1
Total Score	3-15

Source: Adapted from *The Lancet*, Vol. 304, Graham Teasdale and Bryan Jennett, "Assessment of Coma and Impaired Consciousness," p. 81-84, 1974, Elsevier, with adjustments reflecting current medical practice.

Levels of Cognitive Functioning scale categorizes patients on an eight-level scale. Patients are scored on responsiveness, orientation, purposeful activity, self-regulation, memory, spontaneity, and independence. Levels of severity range from no response to purposeful and appropriate.

- *Adelaide Coma Scale (ACS):* Adult coma scales are usually inappropriate for children because they take into account verbal and motor responses that are not present during various stages of childhood (Westbrook, 1997). The ACS is a version of the GCS adapted for use in the pediatric population and takes into account a child's age and developmental level. The ACS is designed to be applied to infants too young to speak.

Assessment of Orientation

When patients with TBI begin to demonstrate an increased level of alertness and responsiveness to their environment they usually display high levels of confusion, agitation, and disorientation. As they progress further in recovery, confusion is reduced and they can begin to reorient themselves to their surroundings (Ylvisaker et al., 2008). Orientation is evaluated as a component of most standard cognitive assessments such as the Mini Mental State Examination (Folstein, Folstein, & McHugh, 1975). Orientation to person, place, and time is usually assessed simply by asking patients simple questions such as the following:

- What is your name?
- What is your age?
- Where are you?
- What city are we in?
- What happened to you? (Why are you here?)
- What time is it?
- What day is it? What month is it? What year is it?
- Who is president of the United States?

When assessing for orientation it is important to remove clocks, calendars, and any other external indicator that the patient can use as a cue. However, it does provide valuable insight if the patient does look at the clock, calendar, or out the window for indications of time and place.

Assessment of Agitation and Aggression

As patients with TBI recover from coma and vegetative state, their motor skills might return faster than their cognitive skills, creating the problematic situation of a motorically intact patient who is severely disoriented, confused, and possibly agitated. These patients generally have a disregard for safety and often require some level of physical restraint to keep them unharmed in their bed and to keep them from hurting anyone else. Confused and agitated patients might be unable to walk but still insist on standing and trying to walk. When medical professionals and staff try to restrain them they can become agitated and aggressive and might attempt any conceivable form of physical or verbal assault.

Many assessment scales and tests measure level of agitation in the overall evaluation of the patient. However, the Agitated Behavior Scale (ABS; Bogner, Corrigan, Stange, & Rabold, 1999) is designed specifically to assess level of agitation and track over time changes in agitation in patients with TBI. Brookshire (2007) suggests the use of the Overt Aggression Scale (Yudofsky et al., 1986) to assess the presence of aggression in the absence of agitation. The Overt Aggression Scale measures verbal aggression and physical aggression against others, oneself, and objects.

Assessment of Communication/ Language/Cognition

Evaluation of communication, language, and cognitive deficits in TBI can use the same types of assessment methods as used for aphasia, right hemisphere disorders, and dementia. A caveat is that often the communication deficits displayed by those with TBI are the result of their underlying cognitive deficits and not language deficits; hence, the assessment of cognition in TBI should not be neglected.

Formal Tests for Traumatic Brain Injury

At times, the speech-language pathologist might prefer to apply a formal assessment for deficits associated with TBI. When testing an individual with TBI for any length of time, the speech-language pathologist must carefully monitor the patient's level of fatigue. Patients with TBI usually have significant issues with fatigue that must be worked around in therapy. Following are formal assessments of deficits associated with TBI:

- Burns Brief Inventory of Communication and Cognition (Burns, 1997)
- Brief Test of Head Injury (Helm-Estabrooks & Hotz, 1991)
- Cognitive-Linguistic Quick Test (CLQT; Helm-Estabrooks, 2001)
- Scales of Cognitive Ability for Traumatic Brain Injury (SCATBI; Adamovich & Henderson, 1992)
- Ross Information Processing Assessment (2nd ed., RIPA-2; Ross-Swain, 1996)

Therapy for Traumatic Brain Injury

Goals for the treatment of the patient with TBI reflect the patient's deficits as identified in assessment. The therapies used to target deficits depend on the severity level and level of impact on functioning of the deficits as well as the patient's overall prognosis and stage of recovery. Therapy for TBI often begins by treating low-level cognitive deficits and slowly

working up to remediate higher-level deficits. Over the course of rehabilitation, therapy procedures and tasks vary as the therapist constantly alters and fine tunes therapy to the meet the changing needs of the patient.

Therapy for Decreased Level of Arousal

Sensory Stimulation Therapy

Sensory stimulation therapy, also known as coma stimulation therapy, is used in the hope of increasing level of arousal in a patient in a coma or vegetative state. Gerber (2005) defines sensory stimulation therapy as attempting to heighten arousal when arousal is limited or nonexistent. Davis and White (1995) state that sensory stimulation therapy targets the stimulation of all senses in a structured fashion to increase awareness and decrease the long-term effects of coma and vegetative state.

Although studies support the use of sensory stimulation therapy (Hall, MacDonald, & Young, 1992; Kater, 1989; Mitchell, Bradley, Welch, & Britton, 1990), other researchers argue that there is too little evidence to support this type of therapy (Baker, 1988; Helwick, 1994; Lombardi, Taricco, De Tant, Telaro & Liberati, 2002). Sensory stimulation sessions typically occur daily and might involve stimulation of only one sensory modality or all five (Lombardi et al., 2002). Nonetheless, many speech-language pathologists as well as nurses currently practice coma stimulation. Selected sensory stimulation strategies are as follows:

- *Visual stimulation:* Visual stimulation is the presentation of visual stimuli to engage attention and encourage the patient to track the stimulus with the eyes. An example is moving large and brightly colored objects across the patient's field of vision.
- *Auditory stimulation:* Auditory stimulation is the presentation of auditory stimuli to arouse the patient. Talking to patients, greeting them

by name, and asking yes or no questions are considered auditory stimulation. Sometimes auditory stimulation is paired with other stimulation methods (e.g., "Keep your eyes on me, I'm moving the ball" or "I'm going to touch your arm now with this cold washcloth").

- *Oral stimulation:* Oral stimulation is stimulation to the lips or mouth. Brushing teeth and cleaning the oral cavity with flavored swabs are oral stimulation techniques meant to cue a response or raise the arousal level of a patient in a minimally conscious state.
- *Olfactory stimulation:* The use of fragrances with personal meaning such as perfumes or the smell of favorite foods is olfactory stimulation.
- *Cutaneous stimulation:* Cutaneous or tactile stimulation is the systematic stimulation of an individual's skin such as light brushing or application of warm or cold objects.
- *Gustatory stimulation:* Stimulation to the sense of taste is called gustatory stimulation. Typically this is accomplished using flavored swabs. A caveat is to avoid anything that the patient might aspirate, if risk of aspiration is present.

Therapy for Attention Deficits

Therapy strategies for attention deficits accompanying TBI mirror the therapy for attention deficits present in right and left hemisphere disorders.

Therapy for Problem-Solving Deficits

The particular tasks used to address problem-solving deficits in TBI are dictated by the capabilities and deficits of the patient. Paper-and-pencil tasks available in worksheet-style therapy books are used. They usually involve problem-solving tasks ranging from simple math problems and short word problems to visual stimuli such as line drawings that present a problematic or dangerous situation that must be resolved. Functional problem-solving tasks can be used

to target the patient's deficits in activities of daily living. For example, counting change, balancing a checkbook, navigating the hospital hallways to find the cafeteria, and tasks such as calling a friend or loved one on the phone or checking email accounts are all functional problem-solving tasks.

Therapy for Memory Deficits

Presented below are selected strategies for targeting working memory. Following this section on working memory, approaches for the treatment of memory deficits are grouped into restorative memory approaches and internal and external memory strategies.

Recommendations for Targeting Working Memory

Following is a list of strategies to address deficits in working memory (modified from Parente & Herrman, 2003):

1. *Be sure instructions and utterances are produced as succinctly (shortly) as possible.* For instance, consider these instructions given to a patient: "I'm going to show you some pictures. After I show them to you, I want you to tell me what is in the picture." These simple instructions are 24 words long, which might be far too many words to be held for processing in the working memory of an individual with brain damage. In contrast, these instructions can be replaced with much shorter directions simply by presenting the picture and asking, "What is this?" The second way conveys the same functional meaning and is only three words long. The shortened form of the instructions is far more likely to be understood by the patient with brain damage.

2. *Use functional tasks to target memory deficits in the context of activities of daily living.* For example, instead of using workbook or drill activities to target working memory, use functional tasks more likely to generalize to other activities, such

as working with money (making change, basic calculations for purchases) or even working in the kitchen following recipes.

3. *Avoid speaking fast.* Speak at a slower rate to give the patient more time to process what you are saying.

4. *Emphasize important words or phrases to bring the individual's attention to the most important parts of the utterance.*

5. *Increase automaticity of response.* Any action that can be overlearned to the point where the target response is given automatically can be used to reduce reliance on working memory.

6. *Break down complex tasks into individual components.* Once the patient has learned the individual components, reintegrate the individual parts into a whole to execute a complex task. For example, to call someone on the phone the patient must find the phone, know how to use it, recall the phone number, dial the number, and greet the answering party appropriately when the call is answered. This is a complex task for someone with significant cognitive deficits. Yet the single complex action of *calling a friend* can be reduced to component parts; for example, the patient can begin by practicing finding the phone until the patient's knowledge of where to find the phone is overlearned and automatic. Then, the patient individually practices picking up the receiver, recalling the phone number, dialing a number, and providing a greeting. When the patient succeeds with all these individual actions, the individual components can be put together so that the patient can successfully complete the single complex action of *calling a friend*. In this way, reliance on working memory is minimized, increasing the odds of success.

Restorative Memory Approaches

Restorative memory approaches do not allow the patient to compensate for deficits using external devices (external memory strategies) or cognitive methods and devices (internal memory strategies). Restorative memory strategies work to rehabilitate memory abilities.

Spaced retrieval training is a strategy that involves presenting information to the patient and cueing the patient to recall the information over increasingly longer intervals of time, effectively stretching his or her memory ability.

Internal Memory Strategies

Internal memory strategies are cognitive acts that can increase the likelihood of retaining information over the short and long terms. Unimpaired individuals usually use these techniques, and individuals with TBI can also use them to compensate for memory deficits. Selected internal memory strategies include the following:

- *Rehearsal training* (Parente & Herrman, 2003). Training patients to repeat (rehearse) information to themselves that they need to remember increases the likelihood of the patients retaining the information. The speech-language pathologist establishes the number of rehearsals required for the patient to recall information successfully, and then therapy establishes the independent use of these rehearsals in the patient's everyday life.

- *Mnemonics.* A method of consciously converting information into a format that the brain can more easily remember and retain.

- *Imaging and visual associations.* Training the patient to create a visual image of the information to be recalled increases the likelihood of retaining that information. If a patient is given multiple details to remember, these details can be combined into a single mental image. Use of humor or absurdity in this strategy often increases success. For instance, when asking a patient to remember *cup*, *baseball*, and *dog*, the speech-language pathologist can encourage the patient to create a single visual image of a dog running to catch a baseball with a cup. The image can be further strengthened by suggesting the patient visually imagine his own favorite dog in this scenario.

- *Verbal chaining* (Brookshire, 2007). Information can be strung together in a narrative to increase the likelihood of effective recall. For example, the three details in the previous example, *cup, baseball,* and *dog,* can be cached with a narrative such as, "The *baseball*-catching *dog* sipped from the *cup*"; then, the details might be more easily recalled.

External Memory Strategies

Whereas internal memory strategies are cognitive acts an individual uses to compensate for memory deficits, external strategies or memory aids are material devices used to allow for compensation of memory deficits. These strategies can be low tech, such as the use of checklists, calendars, schedules, memory books, diaries, memo pads, watch alarms, or high-tech devices such as the use of smartphones and computers. An example of external memory strategies to target long-term memory deficits are an audio recording reciting the patient's personal details and a life history video, which does the same thing in video format, that are presented to the patient.

Therapy for Orientation Deficits

Reorientation to self, person, and place following TBI is accomplished by repetitively exposing the patient to relevant facts. Other than this, restorative strategies to increase orientation mirror strategies mentioned earlier for increasing long-term memory (i.e., repetitively presenting information to the patient by audio or video recording to increase retention of the information).

Compensatory strategies to increase orientation rely on external devices that increase awareness to self, place, and time. Examples include posting a calendar or clock in the patient's room (and directing the patient's to the object often) to assist in keeping the patient oriented to date and time. Also, posting family photos around the room can help facilitate orientation to self and stimulate long-term memories.

Main Points

- Trauma is serious or potentially life-threatening levels of physical injury.
- Traumatic brain injury (TBI) is damage to the brain that occurs as a result of an external and usually forceful event. TBI does not include damage to the brain resulting from disease, stroke, or surgery.
- TBIs can be caused by falls, motor vehicle and traffic accidents, incidents of a person being struck by an object, sports accidents, and violent assaults.
- Individuals most at risk for TBI are those who are younger than age 4 years, older than age 75 years, adolescent males, alcohol and recreational drug users, those from lower socioeconomic status, and law enforcement and military personnel. Also, individuals who have experienced past TBI are more likely to experience additional TBI.
- Forms of trauma causing damage to the brain that do not break an individual's skull open and penetrate the cerebral meninges surrounding the brain are categorized as closed head injuries.
  - Acceleration–deceleration closed head injuries occur when a person's body is moving very fast through space and then comes to a very abrupt halt sudden enough to cause the person's brain to slam into and bounce

around with damaging levels of force the inside of the skull.

- Coup-contrecoup is a two-step profile of damage from an acceleration–deceleration-style closed head injury. The coup portion of the damage occurs when a person's head is slung forward to hit an object. The head comes to an abrupt halt and causes the frontal lobes of the brain to impact the anterior inside of the skull. The contrecoup portion of this damage profile occurs when the head ricochets backward from the initial impact and the head makes a second impact and damages another portion of the brain (usually brain stem, cerebellum, and occipital lobes).
- Diffuse axonal shearing occurs when neuronal connections are broken and create micro lesions across large areas of the brain as a result of the brain being warped inside the skull by high levels of G-force.
- Impact-based TBI is injury to the brain that occurs as a result of an individual's head being impacted by a moving object. This can result in the skull being forced inward at the site of impact, which exerts compressive forces to the area of the brain beneath the site of impact. These compressive forces bruise and tear the surface of the brain, which results in focal damage to the brain at the site of impact.

- Open head traumatic brain injury is injury that penetrates the skull into the brain.
- Secondary mechanisms of damage in TBI include the following:
  - Increased intracranial pressure is when the amount of intracranial pressure (pressure within the skull that is exerted on the brain) rises above normal.
  - Cerebral edema is the swelling of brain tissue that occurs following trauma to the brain. This can cause increased intracranial pressure.
  - Traumatic hydrocephalus is when the brain is unable to reabsorb excess cerebrospinal fluid yet continues producing more cerebrospinal fluid, thereby leading to increased intracranial pressure.
- Traumatic hemorrhage is bleeding of blood vessels as a result of trauma.
  - Intracerebral hemorrhage is a traumatic hemorrhage within the brain itself.
  - Subdural hemorrhage is a hemorrhage that occurs between the dura mater and the arachnoid mater.
  - Epidural hemorrhage is a hemorrhage that occurs between the dura mater and the skull.
- A hematoma is the gathering of blood outside of a blood vessel following a hemorrhage.
  - Subdural hematoma occurs when veins between the dura mater and the brain are broken and bleed out between the dura mater and the brain.
  - Epidural hematoma occurs when a blood vessel bursts between the dura mater and the skull and bleeds out to create a pool of blood between the dura mater and the skull.
  - Subdural and epidural hematomas can both lead to life-threatening increases in intracranial pressure.
- Post-traumatic epilepsy is a seizure condition that occurs consequent to a TBI.
- Shaken baby syndrome is a common cause of traumatic brain injury and death in children. The abuse is the physical violence of a caregiver shaking the child. The brain damage resulting from the shaking of the child is caused by the rotational and acceleration–deceleration forces imposed on the child's brain that likely create diffuse axonal shearing, cerebral edema, and traumatic hemorrhages with hematoma.
- The signature traumatic brain injury experienced by military personnel in modern warfare is the blast-induced trauma caused by exposure to an improvised explosive device (IED).
- Polytrauma describes the multiple causes of trauma experienced by soldiers following exposure to an IED blast.

- Primary-level damage is the result of the shock wave created by the IED explosion. Trauma following exposure to intense levels of pressure following an explosion is barotrauma. Barotrauma can affect the brain, eyes, and air-filled or fluid-filled organs of the abdomen.
- Secondary-level damage is the result of flying debris and bomb fragments.
- Tertiary-level damage is the result of physical displacement of the body when impacted by the force of the wind associated with the shock wave. This can cause open or closed head TBIs and further trauma to the body and brain.
- Quaternary-level damage is any trauma created by the blast that is not attributable to primary, secondary, or tertiary mechanisms. This includes inhalation of toxic gases, smoke, or dust and any burns sustained to the body.
- Sports-related traumatic brain injuries are closed head TBIs experienced by athletes. Athletes at high risk are those involved in contact sports such as American football, wrestling, soccer, hockey, and boxing.
  - Chronic trauma encephalopathy is a degenerative disease of the brain caused by repeated head trauma (such as repeated concussions in sports or repeated exposure to IED blasts) that manifests as dementia, confusion, memory loss, headache, depression, and excessive aggression within months or years of brain damage.
  - Concussion is a "complex pathophysiological process affecting the brain, induced by traumatic biomechanical forces" (Grady, 2010). Athletes are at risk for suffering multiple concussions because their symptoms might be unrecognized or the symptoms' significance might be unknown.
- Damage to the frontal lobes often results in motor deficits. Diffuse bilateral damage to the UMNs within the frontal lobes creates spastic bilateral paralysis or paresis in the body whereas unilateral traumatic damage to the UMNs within a single frontal lobe creates spastic contralateral hemiplegia similar to that often seen in stroke patients. Damage to the cerebellum can create ataxia.
  - Swallowing disorders and motor speech disorders such as spastic dysarthria, flaccid dysarthria, ataxic dysarthria, or some combination of the three might be present in individuals who have sustained a TBI.
- Cognitive deficits following a TBI can be impaired arousal, orientation, attention, memory, problem-solving abilities, inferencing, and personality changes. Those with TBI can also display impulsivity, emotional lability, lack of motivation, and underestimation of their deficits.
  - A coma is a period of unconsciousness lasting more than 6 hours during which the unconscious individual cannot be awakened and is unresponsive to sensory stimuli.
  - A vegetative state is when a person is minimally responsive to stimuli but lacking consciousness and condition.
  - A persistent vegetative state is when a vegetative state continues longer than 4 weeks.
  - Post-traumatic amnesia is a combination of retrograde and anterograde memory losses that present in individuals following TBI.
- Personality changes often occur following a TBI and can result in inappropriate sexual advances, inappropriate statements at inappropriate times, loss of awareness of social and cultural conventions, and milder alterations such as changes in food and music preference.
- Language deficits following closed head TBI are often present and can be dwarfed by deficits in arousal or cognition. Individuals with generalized damage across large portions of the brain usually display some level of receptive

and expressive language deficit. In open head TBI with focal damage, it is possible to have more specific language deficits in the context of far fewer cognitive deficits than is seen in closed head TBI.

- Assessment of deficits resulting from a TBI varies depending on the individual's age, educational level, and severity of deficits.
- Long-term memory is often assessed through biographical questions posed to the patient during the interview portion of the evaluation. Visual memory is assessed through drawing a previously presented stimulus or the Benton Visual Retention Test.
- Immediate recall of auditory information is assessed by presenting an unrelated string of words for repetition.
- Short-term recall of auditory information is assessed by presenting an unrelated string of words followed by a distractor task or reciting a detail-heavy paragraph and asking the individual to recall as many details as possible.
- Level of arousal is assessed through coma scales, which are categorical scales in which the patient is assigned a number that indicates level of arousal based on the presence or absence of certain behaviors or responses to stimuli.
- Orientation to person, place, and time is assessed by asking the individual simple questions regarding orientation.
- Agitation is assessed using the Agitated Behavior Scale, which determines the level of agitation and tracks changes in agitation over time. The Overt Aggression Scale assesses the presence of verbal or physical aggression toward others, oneself, or objects.
- Evaluation for communication, language, and cognitive deficits mirrors those procedures used to assess aphasia and right hemisphere disorders.
- Formal tests for TBI might be preferred, though the individual's level of fatigue must be monitored.

- Goals for the treatment of the patient with TBI reflect the person's deficits identified in assessment. The therapies used to target the deficits of the TBI patient depend on the deficits themselves (i.e., severity level, impact on functioning) as well as the patient's overall prognosis and stage of recovery.
- Decreased levels of arousal can be targeted through sensory stimulation therapy, which includes visual stimulation, auditory stimulation, oral stimulation, olfactory stimulation, cutaneous stimulation, and gustatory stimulation.
- Therapy strategies for attention deficits seen in TBI mirror the therapy for the same deficits in right hemisphere disorders and left hemisphere disorders.
- The particular tasks used to address problem-solving deficits in traumatic TBI are dictated by the capabilities and deficits of the patient.
- Working memory deficits can be targeted by using instructions and utterances that are short, using functional tasks in the context of activities of daily living, avoiding speaking fast, emphasizing important words or phrases, increasing automaticity of responses, and breaking down complex tasks into individual components.
- Restorative memory approaches do not allow the patient to compensate for deficits using external devices (external memory strategies) or cognitive methods and devices (internal memory strategies).
- Spaced retrieval training involves presenting information and cueing the patient to recall the information over increasingly greater intervals of time.
- Internal memory strategies are cognitive acts that increase the likelihood of retaining information over the short term and long term to compensate for memory deficits.
- External memory strategies are material devices used to allow compensation for memory deficits.

Review Questions

1. What is a traumatic brain injury?
2. Who are the populations most at risk for sustaining a TBI?
3. How are closed head injuries and open head injuries different?
4. How do acceleration–deceleration injuries cause brain damage?
5. What are the two forms of damage that can occur from an acceleration–deceleration injury?
6. How does an impact-based TBI cause brain damage?
7. List and explain six possible secondary mechanisms of damage following TBI.
8. How does shaken baby syndrome cause brain damage or death?
9. What are the major symptoms of shaken baby syndrome?
10. List and describe the four levels of damage that can cause trauma to a soldier or person exposed to an IED blast.
11. Why are individuals with sports-related injuries at risk for suffering multiple concussions?
12. Explain how a person acquires chronic traumatic encephalopathy.
13. What are three cognitive deficits that can occur with a TBI?
14. What are the differences among a coma, vegetative state, and persistent vegetative state?
15. How might level of arousal be tested?
16. List major areas of deficit often encountered in TBI.
17. List three formal tests used to assess individuals with TBI.
18. How might a speech-language pathologist treat decreased levels of arousal and problem-solving deficits?
19. How are external memory strategies, internal memory strategies, and restorative memory approaches different from one another?
20. Provide and explain examples of external and internal memory strategies.

References

1. Adamovich, B., & Henderson, J. (1992). *Scales of cognitive ability for traumatic brain injury*. Austin, TX: Pro-Ed.
2. Agrawal, A., Timothy, J., Pandit, L., & Manju, M. (2006). Post-traumatic epilepsy: An overview. *Clinical Neurology and Neurosurgery, 108*, 433–439.
3. American Academy of Pediatrics. (2001). Shaken baby syndrome: Rotational cranial injuries—technical report. *Pediatrics, 108*(1), 206–210.
4. Annegers, J., Grabow, J., Kurland, L., & Laws, E. (1980). The incidence, causes, and secular trends of head trauma in Olmsted County, Minnesota, 1935–1974. *Neurology, 30*, 912–919.
5. Annegers, J., Hauser, W., Coan, S., & Rocca, W. A. (1998). A population-based study of seizures after traumatic brain injuries. *New England Journal of Medicine, 338*(1), 20–24.
6. Baker, J. (1988). Explaining coma arousal therapy. *Australian Nurses Journal, 17*(11), 8–11.
7. Benton, A. (2003). *Benton Visual Retention Test* (5th ed.). San Antonio, TX: Psychological Corporation.
8. Bogner, J., Corrigan, J., Stange, M., & Rabold, D. (1999). Reliability of the agitated behavior scale. *Journal of Head Trauma Rehabilitation, 14*, 91–96.
9. Bond, M. (1976). Assessment of the psychological outcome of severe head injury. *Acta Neurochirurgica, 34*, 57–70.
10. Braakman, R., Jennet, W., & Minderhoud, J. (1988). Prognosis of the post-traumatic vegetative state. *Acta Neurochirurgica, 95*, 49–52.
11. Brookshire, R. (2007). *Introduction to neurogenic communication disorders* (7th ed.). St. Louis, MO: Mosby Elsevier.
12. Bruce, D., & Zimmerman, R. (1989). Shaken impact syndrome. *Pediatric Annals, 18*, 482–494.
13. Burns, M. (1997). *Burns Brief Inventory of Communication and Cognition*. Upper Saddle River, NJ: Pearson.

14. Centers for Disease Control and Prevention. (2011). Explosions and Blast Injuries: A Primer for Clinicians. Retrieved from http://www.bt.cdc.gov/masscasualties/pdf/explosions blast-injuries.pdf

15. Davis, A., & White, J. (1995). Innovative sensory input for the comatose brain-injured patient. *Psychosocial and Environmental Considerations in Critical Care*, 351–361.

16. Dekosky, S., Ikonomovic, M., & Gandy, S. (2010). Traumatic brain injury: Football, warfare, and long-term effects. *New England Journal of Medicine, 363*(14), 1293–1296.

17. Faul, M., Xu, L., Wald, M., & Coronado, V. (2010). *Traumatic brain injury in the United States: Emergency department visits, hospitalizations, and deaths*. Atlanta, GA: Centers for Disease Control and Prevention, National Center for Injury Prevention and Control.

18. Folstein, M., Folstein, S., & McHugh, P. (1975). "Mini-Mental State." A practical method for grading the cognitive state of patients for the clinician. *Journal of Psychiatric Research, 12*(3), 189–198.

19. Gerber, C. (2005). Understanding and managing coma stimulation: Are we doing everything we can? *Critical Care Nurse Quarterly, 28*(2), 94–110.

20. Grady, M. (2010). Concussion in the adolescent athlete. *Current Problems in Pediatric and Adolescent Health Care, 40*, 154–169.

21. Hagen, C. (1981). Language disorders secondary to closed head injuries. *Topics in Language Disorders, 1*, 73–87.

22. Hall, M., MacDonald, S., & Young, G. (1992). The effectiveness of directed multisensory stimulation vs. nondirected stimulation in comatose CHI patients: Pilot study of a single subject design. *Brain Injury, 6*, 435–445.

23. Helm-Estabrooks, N. (2001). *Cognitive Linguistic Quick Scale*. San Antonio, TX: Psychological Corporation.

24. Helm-Estabrooks, N., & Hotz, G. (1991). *Brief Test of Head Injury*. Austin, TX: Pro-Ed.

25. Helwick, L. (1994). Stimulation programs for coma patients. *Critical Care Nurse, 14*(4), 47–52.

26. Kater, D. (1989). Response of head injured patients to sensory stimulation. *Western Journal of Nursing Research, 11*(1), 20–33.

27. Katz, D. (1992). Recovery following severe head injuries. *Journal of Head Trauma Rehabilitation, 7*, 1–15.

28. Kimbler, D., Murphy, M., & Dhandapani, K. (2011). Concussion and the adolescent athlete. *Journal of Neuroscience Nursing, 43*(6), 286–290.

29. Lombardi, F., Taricco, M., DeTant, A., Telaro, E., & Liberati, A. (2002). Sensory stimulation of brain-injured individuals in coma or vegetative state: Results of a Cochrane systematic review. *Clinical Rehabilitation, 16*(5), 464–472.

30. Luria, A. (1947). *Traumatic aphasia: Its syndromes, psychopathology, and treatment*. Moscow, Russia: Academy of Medical Sciences.

31. Macniven, E. (1994). Factors affecting head injury rehabilitation outcome: Premorbid and clinican parameters. In M. A. Finlayson & S. H. Garner (Eds.), *Brain injury rehabilitation: Clinical considerations*. Baltimore, MD: Williams & Wilkins.

32. Mitchell, S., Bradley, V., Welch, J., & Britton, P. (1990). Coma arousal procedure: A therapeutic intervention in the treatment of head injury. *Brain Injury, 4*(3), 273–279.

33. Parente, R., & Herrman, D. (2003). *Retraining cognition: Techniques and applications* (3rd ed.). Austin, TX: Pro-Ed.

34. Parente, R., Kolakowski-Haynor, S., Krug, K., & Wilk, C. (1999). Retraining working memory after traumatic brain injury. *NeuroRehabilitation, 13*, 157–163.

35. Ross-Swain, D. (1996). *Ross Information Processing Assessment* (2nd ed.). Austin, TX: Pro-Ed.

36. Roth, C. (2007). Mechanisms and sequelae of blast injuries. *Perspectives on Neurophysiology and Neurogenic Speech and Language Disorders. 17*(3), 20–24.

37. Russell, R., & Espir, M. (1961). *Traumatic aphasia: A study of war wounds of the brain*. New York, NY. Oxford University Press.

38. Schiller, F. (1947). Aphasia studied in patients with missile wounds. *Journal of Neurology, Neurosurgery, and Psychiatry, 10*, 183.

39. Teasdale, G., & Jennet, B. (1974). Assessment of coma and impaired consciousness. *Lancet, 13*(2), 81–84.

40. Westbrook, A. (1997). The use of a pediatric coma scale for monitoring infants and young children with head injuries. *Nursing in Critical Care, 2*(2), 72–75.

41. Ylvisaker, M., Szekeres, S., & Feeney, T. (2008). Communication disorders associated with traumatic brain injury. In R. Chapey (Ed.), *Language intervention strategies in aphasia and related neurogenic communication disorders* (5th ed.). Baltimore, MD: Lippincott Williams & Wilkins.

42. Yudofsky, S., Silver, S., Jackson, W., Endicott, J., & Williams, D. (1986). The Overt Aggression Scale for the objective rating of verbal and physical aggression. *American Journal of Psychiatry, 143*, 35–39.

Chapter 9

Dementia

Where this icon appears, visit http://go.jblearning.com/ManascoCWS to view the corresponding video.

Dementia is one of the most common syndromes that a speech-language pathologist encounters when working outside of the pediatric population. The disease processes that cause the cognitive losses associated with dementia also usually create language deficits and eventually speech and swallowing deficits. Every major area of concern of the speech-language pathologist is impacted by dementia and the diseases that create dementia. Knowing disease profiles and being able to anticipate the oncoming deficits created by these diseases as they progress are essential to the effective management of deficits created by dementia.

Defining Dementia

Dementia is an acquired global loss of brain function with a slow insidious onset caused by a variety of diseases. The Latin basis for the term *dementia* is *de*, meaning "out of," and *mens*, meaning "one's mind." Though primarily associated with memory loss, dementia is a syndrome. A syndrome is a collection of possible symptoms, not a single deficit. Cummings (1984) defines dementia as follows:

> An acquired persistent compromise in intellectual function with impairments in at least three of the following spheres of mental activity: language, memory, visuospatial skills, personality, and cognition. It is distinguished from acute confusional states in the persistence of the intellectual deficits; it is differentiated from mental retardation in that the intellectual deficiencies are acquired rather than congenital in nature.

However, the most widely used definition of dementia comes from the fourth edition of the *Diagnostic and Statistical Manual of Mental Disorders* (*DSM-IV*) of the American Psychiatric Association. *DSM-IV* describes dementia as memory loss plus deficits in at least one of the following areas:

- Verbal expression or verbal and written receptive language skills
- Recognition and identification of objects
- Ability to execute motor activities (assuming normal motor skills, normal sensory function, and comprehension of the task)
- Abstract thinking, judgment, and execution of complex tasks.

DSM-IV also stipulates that these deficits must affect the individual's ability to execute activities of daily living (ADLs).

> **Dementia** A condition of memory loss plus deficits in at least one other of the following areas: verbal expression or auditory and written receptive language skills, recognition and identification of objects, ability to execute motor activities, abstract thinking, judgment, and execution of complex tasks.

It is important to note that dementia is not a disease itself but rather a symptom of disease or pathology. Multiple diseases, conditions, and pathologies produce dementia, many of which are discussed here. By far, the most common etiology of dementia is Alzheimer's disease, which accounts for 60–80% of all cases (Alzheimer's Association, 2011). Vascular dementia, mixed dementia, Lewy body disease, Parkinson's disease, and frontotemporal dementia are also common etiologies of dementia (Alzheimer's Association, 2011; Mathers & Leonardi, 2000).

It is estimated that 24.3 million people in the world today live with dementia, with 4.6 million new cases each year (Ferri et al., 2005). In fact, it is estimated that every 7 seconds someone develops dementia (Ferri et al., 2005). In the undeveloped world, people generally do not live long enough to develop high rates of dementia. However, as countries develop and their people cease dying from other causes such as infectious disease and starvation, the rates of dementia rise sharply. Since the early 1990s, China has seen a doubling of the prevalence of Alzheimer's disease alongside its rapid development (Mathers & Leonardi, 2000). In the developed world, dementia is on the rise as well. In the United States, this is the result of a rapidly expanding demographic of aging baby boomers. Present estimates suggest that approximately 5.4 million people in the United States have Alzheimer's disease and that it is the sixth leading cause of death (Xu, Kochanek, Sherry, Murphy, & Tejada-Vera, 2010).

Delirium and Mild Cognitive Impairment

Dementia is clinically different from *delirium*. Whereas dementia produces changes in cognition that usually have a slow onset, do not vary much throughout the course of a day, and are usually the result of very dire changes in the brain, delirium is described in the *DSM-IV* as a sudden disturbance in consciousness or a change in cognitive ability that fluctuates through the course of a day and where the onset is usually the result of a general medical condition (such as a urinary tract infection, which is known to cause delirium).

Early signs of dementia often manifest as subtle cognitive changes that usually go undiagnosed. However, if these changes are diagnosed, they are usually labeled as mild cognitive impairment. The changes associated with mild cognitive impairment are significant enough not to be within the spectrum of changes associated with normal aging but not severe enough to significantly affect the daily lives of affected individuals. Those with mild cognitive impairment experience decreased abilities to concentrate, decreased word finding abilities, decreased short-term memory, and difficulty following detail-heavy conversations or writings. Typically, mild cognitive impairment progresses into Alzheimer's disease or another type of dementia that produces this condition, though some individuals do not progress further into cognitive decline and might even recover, depending on the pathologic process causing these changes.

> **Delirium** A sudden disturbance in consciousness or a change in cognitive ability that fluctuates through the course of a day with an onset that is a result of a general medical condition.
>
> **Mild cognitive impairment** Subtle cognitive changes that are often prediagnostic signs of dementia and usually manifest as decreased ability to concentrate, decreased word finding abilities, decreased short-term memory, and difficulty following detail-heavy conversations or writings.

Communication Deficits Resulting from Cognitive Deficits

As stated by the American Speech-Language-Hearing Association, in dementia the role of the speech-language pathologist is the assessment and treatment of cognitive and communication deficits, as well as the training and counseling of caregivers (American Speech-Language-Hearing Association [ASHA], 2005). A frequent question is, "If dementia is primarily cognitive deficits and not speech or language deficits, why do speech-language pathologists have to bother with cognition?" The answer is that speech-language pathologists are ultimately concerned, not merely with language, but with communication. Communication and cognition cannot be separated as neatly as one may expect. Effective communication arises in no small part from intact cognitive abilities. Therefore, problems in communication likely arise when cognitive abilities are disrupted. Here is a simple example to illustrate this point:

> A person with dementia has severe attention and memory deficits. This person has trouble paying attention to what is being said to him and, even when he pays attention to the speech of others, he cannot remember what has just been said. If he cannot attend to what is being said or remember a conversation, how can he respond appropriately? He cannot. Therefore, communication suffers directly from his cognitive deficits of attention and memory. To restore appropriate communication, the therapist must first address his cognition. Only when attention and/or memory skills have been improved or his losses in these areas compensated for in some way, will he be able to communicate.

Normal Changes with Age

Early changes in cognition and language caused by dementia often go unnoticed or undiagnosed because many similar changes occur with normal aging. However, the normal cognitive changes that occur with age are not significant enough to affect a person's performance of activities of daily living (ADLs).

Language abilities tend to remain resilient with age with one primary exception: a slight decrease in word finding abilities. As any adult older than age 50 years can attest, the amount of time it takes to retrieve names or certain words increases with age. Because significant word finding difficulties are an early sign of dementia, these normal changes in word finding ability (or perceptions of what are normal changes in word finding ability associated with age) often mask the insidious onset of dementia.

Sustained attention abilities remain mostly intact in normal aging, but selective attention skills decrease slightly (Plude & Doussard-Roosevelt, 1989). In daily life, this is reflected by older adults having greater difficulty ignoring competing stimuli to focus on a task. Divided attention skills remain intact on simple tasks during normal aging, but for more complex tasks, multitasking skills decrease (Verghese, Buschke, Viola, Katz, & Hall, 2002). Reaction time is also slowed in older adults. This is seen in research when older adults are required to provide certain responses to incoming stimuli (Kramer, Humphrey, Larish, Logan, & Strayer, 1994).

In normal aging, mild changes in memory are also documented. Episodic and short-term memory are reduced in older adults, resulting in older adults having greater difficulty remembering specific details such as when and where certain events were experienced (Craik, 2000). Long-term memory and procedural memory remain intact so that, although an older person might be able to store fewer details in short-term memory, memory for procedures (such as brushing teeth or driving a car) remains undamaged as does general long-term memory of details from life experiences.

Etiologies of Dementia

Although there are many possible etiologies of dementia, progressive diseases and terminal illnesses are the most common. Progressive and terminal dementing diseases can be divided into cortical, subcortical, and mixed categories based grossly on the areas of the brain that they affect the most. The cortical dementias are created primarily by degeneration of the cerebral cortex. In contrast, the subcortical dementias are caused primarily by degeneration of subcortical structures. The mixed dementias are the result of pathologic changes to the cortex and subcortex.

Cortical Dementias

Alzheimer's Disease

By far, the most common etiology of dementia is Alzheimer's disease. Dementia is so often the result of Alzheimer's disease that many a layperson assumes that the symptoms of dementia and Alzheimer's disease are one and the same.

Alzheimer's disease is the sixth most common cause of death in the United States and developed world (Alzheimer's Association, 2011). It is distinguished by the iconic memory deficits that usually hail the onset of the disease. Alzheimer's is a progressive and fatal disease. There are no known treatments to stop or even slow the progression of the disease. ▶ See the video, *Living with Alzheimer's Disease* for a presentation given by an individual with Alzheimer's disease and his caregiver regarding their firsthand experiences with the disease.

Neuropathology

Alzheimer's disease gained its name from the German scientist Alois Alzheimer. In 1906, Alois Alzheimer autopsied the brain of a former patient who displayed odd behaviors and a profound short-term memory loss. When he looked at brain tissue samples under a microscope, Alzheimer found pathologic anomalies in the brain that would eventually be described as neurofibrillary tangles, amyloid plaques, and granulovacuolar degeneration.

Neurofibrils are delicate threadlike structures coursing through the cytoplasm of neurons usually between dendrites or from a dendrite to a neuron. Neurofibrils normally serve a structural function. Neurofibrillary tangles are abnormal clumps of neurofibrils that are not broken down appropriately by the cell and that begin to occupy large amounts of space within a neuron, eventually rendering the cell dysfunctional (Figure 9-1).

Amyloid plaques are abnormal and pathologic deposits of the protein amyloid (Figure 9-2). These plaques reduce the ability of neurons to function. Although neurofibrillary tangles and amyloid plaques are signatures of Alzheimer's disease, these pathologic changes in brain tissue can often be found in the brains of individuals suffering from non-Alzheimer's-type

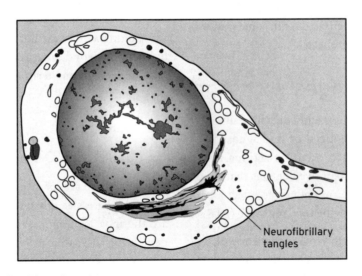

Figure 9-1 Neurofibrillary tangles.

Amyloid plaque   Granulovacuolar degeneration

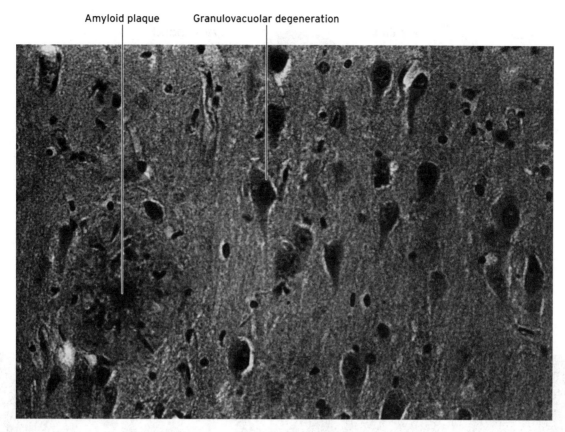

Figure 9-2   Granulovacuolar degeneration and amyloid plaque.

dementias (Figure 3-6), though the locations and numbers might vary.

A third change that takes place in the brains of those with Alzheimer's disease is granulovacuolar degeneration (Figure 9-2). Granulovacuolar degeneration is the formation of abnormal membranous sacks of fluid containing granules within the cytoplasm of certain neurons. The neurons of the hippocampus are inordinately affected by these structures, accounting, at least partially, for the short-term memory loss in individuals with Alzheimer's (**Figure 9-3**).

Ultimately, these individual pathologic changes at the tissue level in the brain either contribute to or are concomitant with the progressive decrease in the amount of brain tissue in the later stages of Alzheimer's (Figure 9-3). This overall change is known

as general neuronal atrophy and can be seen easily by the naked eye in autopsied brains as the shrinkage of gyri of the cortex (Figure 9-3). This is especially visible around the hippocampus, as is a widening of the cerebral ventricles. As the brain of the individual affected with Alzheimer's atrophies, the volume and weight of the brain decline. All these changes work together to inhibit normal functioning of neurons, which disrupts the brain's ability to function appropriately to produce normal thought processes.

Historically, Alzheimer's disease has been diagnosed using observation of the symptoms of the resultant dementia. For ultimate confirmation that the dementia in question was the result of Alzheimer's disease, an autopsy of the brain was required to verify the presence of signature amyloid plaques

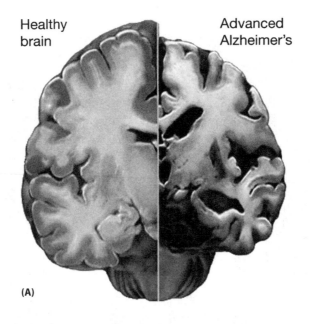

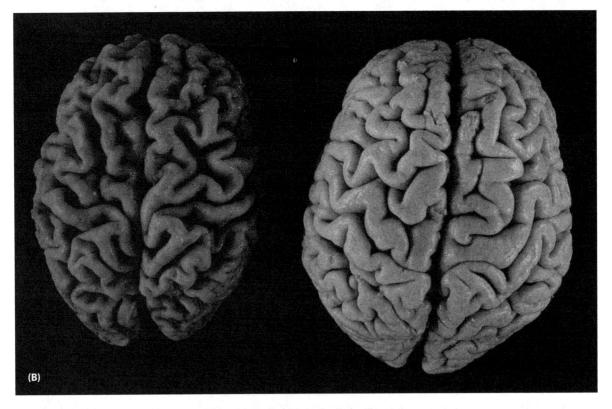

Figure 9-3 General atrophy of the brain in Alzheimer's disease.

and neurofibrillary tangles. Because the clinical presentation of Alzheimer's disease often mirrors other forms of dementias with different neuropathologies, having an actual diagnosis of Alzheimer's disease has historically been somewhat problematic because the patient had to die before the disease process creating the dementia could be truly confirmed.

However, in 2004 and 2005, researchers at the University of Pittsburgh developed a fairly noninvasive test for Alzheimer's disease using a combination of a radioactive compound and modern imaging technology (Klunk et al., 2004; Klunk et al., 2006). The diagnostic test uses a compound, known as Pittsburgh B compound, or simply PiB, that is injected into the bloodstream. Once PiB travels to the brain, it binds with amyloid deposits in the brain, and, when the brain is scanned using positron emission tomography, it makes visible to researchers if and where amyloid deposits are located. This allows researchers to actually view the pattern of amyloid buildup in the brains of living individuals. This diagnostic tool holds high promise for allowing for the optimal treatment of Alzheimer's disease through early and accurate diagnosing of the disease.

Risk Factors

Certain factors increase an individual's likelihood of developing Alzheimer's disease:

- Women are more likely than men to develop Alzheimer's disease. This might be explained in part by women living longer and therefore having more opportunity to develop the disease with age.
- A family history of individuals who developed Alzheimer's disease also increases the risk of developing the disease.
- A history of depression increases the risk of Alzheimer's disease.
- Past head trauma increases the likelihood of developing Alzheimer's disease.

- Individuals with less education are at higher risk for developing Alzheimer's disease than are those with higher levels of education.

Disease Progression

There are a few different methods of categorizing stages of Alzheimer's disease. This text divides the disease into early, mid, and late stages. This is the model used most widely clinically and is most meaningful in clinical discussions among professionals and with caregivers.

Onset for Alzheimer's disease most often occurs after the age of 65 years. When this disease presents before the age of 65, it is known as early-onset Alzheimer's. Although Alzheimer's is most often associated with older adults, it does at times present in individuals between the ages of 30 and 40 years. Nonetheless, early onset of Alzheimer's disease usually occurs in individuals in the age range of 50 to 60 years. Once diagnosed with Alzheimer's disease, an individual's average life span is 10 years.

The pathologic changes that lead to Alzheimer's disease usually begin many years before an actual diagnosis is made. The disease has a gradual and insidious onset and cognitive deterioration begins slowly (Collie & Maruff, 2000; Grober, Lipton, Hall, & Crystal, 2000). Often, early signs of the disease are mistaken for changes associated with normal aging. However, there usually comes a point during the early stage when caregivers or the affected individual realizes that something is wrong. Family members and those affected by Alzheimer's commonly report that the affected individual became uncharacteristically lost or confused and was unable to navigate very familiar territory in the car or find his or her way home.

During the early stage of Alzheimer's disease, the affected individual retains normal motor functioning and can still talk and walk and get about with no difficulty. The Alzheimer's Association (2011) reports that, on average, the early stage of Alzheimer's lasts approximately 2 years after diagnosis. The first indication of Alzheimer's disease is usually a loss of short-term memory. This manifests first in small matters, such as losing a purse or keys, forgetting the reason for going to the store, or repeatedly telling the same story or asking the same questions. Word finding difficulties also appear at this stage and manifest as a greater use of general terminology such as *thing*, *it*, *stuff* in place of more specific nouns. Also, difficulties with comprehension of verbal language appear and the person with Alzheimer's often misses or forgets the point of what is said. Personality changes may also present and often are the first truly noticeable problematic change that leads affected individuals or caregivers to suspect something is truly awry.

The middle stage of the disease can often last from 4 to 10 years after diagnosis. During the middle stage, the affected individual begins suffering from more debilitating symptoms that have a significant negative impact on ADLs and increase the individual's reliance on others. Intermittent periods of disorientation or consistent disorientation arise at this point in the disease progression. Memory and attention deficits continue to worsen and are displayed by the affected individual showing little or no short-term memory. More dramatic personality changes can occur, such as uncharacteristic difficulty dealing with frustration and anger. Visuospatial difficulties appear, causing problems with processing visual information. Visuoconstructive deficits also appear and can seriously inhibit ADLs. Examples include difficulty dressing oneself or performing some task as simple as making a sandwich. Expressive language deficits worsen as wording finding deficits grow. Memory deficits also begin to inhibit appropriate communication. Motor function remains mostly intact; therefore, speech is not affected or is affected little at this stage. Expression might be disfluent because of word finding deficits. A restless sense of wanderlust (desire to wander) can also arise during this stage. The combination of intact motor skills with wanderlust, disorientation, and confusion often leads to the iconic and dangerous wandering of these individuals. Bladder incontinence presents as a problem during this stage as do sleep disturbances. Also common is sundowner syndrome. The term *sundowner* comes to us as slang from the nursing homes in which those with mid and late-stage Alzheimer's disease often reside. Oftentimes individuals during the middle stage of this disease or other dementia may present as only mildly impaired during the daytime but then their cognitive and emotional state changes for the worse at nighttime, once the sun has set, and leads these individuals to present with far greater disorientation, confusion, and behavioral difficulties. Hence, the term *sundowner* is used to refer to someone whose abilities decline or whose behavior worsens toward nightfall.

During the late stage of Alzheimer's disease, individuals lose motor function and become nonambulatory, bedridden, incontinent, and unresponsive. Memory and cognitive deficits become profound, thereby severely affecting ability to carry out ADLs. Expressive language is often fluent but empty and nonsensical. Affected individuals might progress to muteness. With lost motor and cognitive function, the ability to eat (masticate and swallow safely) is also lost (dysphagia), and these individuals often die from aspiration pneumonia, anorexia, or other medical complications. Table 9-1 lists symptoms according to stage of disease.

Frontotemporal Dementia

Frontotemporal dementia is a category of degenerative diseases that are associated with the degeneration of the frontal and temporal lobes. Study and recognition of these disorders began in the late 1800s when the physician Arnold Pick identified the clinical syndrome that then became known as Pick's disease. Confusion then arose in the medical community when variant forms of the syndrome were recognized and a variety of labels came into existence. The broader category of frontotemporal

Table 9-1 Possible Symptoms of the Early, Mid, and Late Stages of Alzheimer's Disease

Symptoms of Early-Stage Alzheimer's
Short-term memory loss
Word finding deficits (anomia)
Receptive language deficits
Personality changes

Symptoms of Midstage Alzheimer's
Disorientation
Short-term memory loss continues to worsen
Attention deficits
More dramatic personality changes
Visuospatial deficits
Visuoconstructive deficits
Expressive language deficits
Wanderlust
General confusion
Bladder incontinence
Sleep disturbances
Sundowner syndrome

Symptoms of Late-Stage Alzheimer's
Lack of motor function
Bedridden
Incontinence
Unresponsiveness
Severe to profound memory deficits
Severe to profound cognitive deficits
Fluent but empty speech
Mutism
Dysphagia

dementia was created that includes Pick's disease and certain language variants. These language variants of frontotemporal dementia, which present primarily with loss of language, include the primary progressive aphasias: progressive nonfluent aphasia and semantic dementia.

Pick's Disease

Pick's disease is a dementia resulting from progressive degeneration of the frontal and temporal lobes. Given that Pick's disease is known to affect the frontal and temporal lobes, the changes presented by the affected individuals reflect damage to those areas of the brain. This disease presents with early behavioral abnormalities, changes in personality, antisocial and often inappropriate behavior, as well as memory loss (Dickson, 2001). Early behavioral abnormalities are a primary hallmark of Pick's disease. Affected individuals often present a lack of social inhibition and say things inappropriate to social situations. They have very poor judgment and can show a general apathy regarding their disease and behaviors. Because the frontal lobes and temporal lobes house the primary language areas (in the left hemisphere), language difficulties can become very pronounced. These deficits in cognition, language, and difficulties with behavior make appropriate assessment of the affected individual difficult or impossible.

Pick's disease affects women more than men, with an average age of onset between 50 years and 70 years. However, Pick's disease can present as early in life as age 20 or 30 years. The typical life span of an individual affected with Pick's disease is from 2 to 10 years after diagnosis. This disease is far rarer than Alzheimer's and as such often goes undiagnosed or is misdiagnosed.

Neuropathology

The neuropathologic changes that occur in the brain that are closely identified with the clinical syndrome of Pick's disease are abnormal spherical accumulations of the protein tau in neurons known as Pick bodies and ballooned neurons. Pick bodies are named after Arnold Pick, who identified this neuropathologic feature. Pick bodies proliferate in the frontal and temporal lobes. Over the progression of the disease, general atrophy can be observed in the frontal and temporal lobes with magnetic resonance imaging (MRI). This atrophy presents as the shrinking of the frontal and temporal lobes while the posterior areas of the brain remain intact. Amid the proliferation of Pick bodies, the brains of individuals affected with Pick's disease have no amyloid plaques or neurofibrillary tangles, as seen in Alzheimer's disease (Dickson, 2001).

Disease Progression

Pick's disease is a progressive terminal illness. It is differentiated from Alzheimer's disease early in its progression by the notable behavioral, emotional, and personality changes that occur as a result of frontal lobe degeneration. These early behavioral, emotional, and personality changes in the absence of significant language deficits are also used to differentiate Pick's disease from progressive nonfluent aphasia and semantic dementia, which present primarily as changes in modalities of language. Once again, this is in contrast to Alzheimer's disease, in which general language abilities are usually present until near the end stage of the disease. As Pick's disease progresses, cognition deteriorates. Though affected individuals do not show memory impairment at the beginning of Pick's disease, all cognitive functions become profoundly impaired as the affected individual slowly succumbs to the disease. Those with Pick's disease ultimately die mute and often from aspiration pneumonia or other medical complications.

Subcortical Dementias

Huntington's Disease

Once known as Huntington's chorea, Huntington's disease is a progressive terminal illness characterized by distinctive involuntary erratic body movements. Rates of this disease are approximately 4–10 cases per 100,000 individuals (Ross & Tabrizi, 2011).

Huntington's disease is a hereditary disorder whose onset can occur any time from infancy onward, although the average age of onset is between 40 and 50 years. This is an autosomal-dominant disorder, which means that a child with one parent carrying the chromosomal mutation that causes Huntington's disease has a 50% chance of inheriting the disease, and male and female children are equally at risk.

The symptoms of Huntington's disease are created by the progressive deterioration of the basal ganglia (striatum), frontal lobes, and temporal lobes (Bates, Harper, & Jones, 2002). Although the distinct, slow, choreic movements of the disease are the best-known manifestation, Huntington's disease also presents with changes in personality, cognition, and language as well as emotional problems such as depression, apathy, irritability/aggression, and anxiety (Rickards et al., 2011). Suicidal thoughts or tendencies are also common among those with Huntington's disease. Because it is a hereditary disorder, there is often a known family history of this disease, which makes accurate identification easier. Also, genetic testing can be performed on those at risk to determine whether they have the disease or whether they will develop the disease. The typical life span of an affected individual with Huntington's disease is approximately 20 years after diagnosis (Walker, 2007).

Disease Progression

Typically, Huntington's disease is divided into five stages of symptom progression with a prediagnostic stage representing life prior to diagnosis and onset of cardinal signs. Early signs of the disease that sometimes present in the prediagnostic stage are restlessness, difficulty sleeping, incoordination, anxiety, and/or irritability (Walker, 2007). However, these early signs have an insidious onset and can go unnoticed, unrecognized, or be misdiagnosed.

Eventually, with the onset of the distinctive motor signs, the diagnosis of Huntington's is made and the affected individual moves into the five-stage progression of the disease. During stages 1 and 2, the motor symptoms of the chorea are typically present, although affected individuals at times present with motor symptoms characterized more by rigidity and bradykinesia than chorea. This presentation can lead to a misdiagnosis of Parkinson's disease. After diagnosis, in stages 1 and 2, emotional problems such as sadness and personality changes occur as well as mild cognitive dysfunctions such as difficulties with executive functioning. During the early phases, those with Huntington's disease report concerns regarding physical and functional activities such as sleeping and swallowing, as well as concerns regarding cognitive difficulties such as maintaining concentration, memory problems, and difficulties with executive functioning (Ho & Hocaoglu, 2011). Generally, affected individuals in the first two stages of this disease are still quite functional and can carry on with employment.

In stages 3 and 4, or roughly during the fourth year after diagnosis (Phillips, Shannon, & Barker, 2008), chorea and hyperkinesias begin to interfere with speech production (Ho & Hocaoglu, 2011). The irregular, unpredictable movements of the face, mandible, vocal folds, tongue, palate, and muscles of respiration create the form of hyperkinetic dysarthria associated with Huntington's disease. At this point, affected individuals become more dependent on others and can no longer manage their households or complete ADLs without some level of assistance. Typically, those in stages 3 and 4 can still live at home with a great deal of assistance. Ambulation might remain, though affected individuals are at heightened risk of experiencing a fall (Pollard et al., 1999). Although individuals in these stages retain overall expressive abilities, typically training begins on an alternative or augmentative form of communication (AAC device) to prepare for the possible full loss of verbal and written expression resulting from motor deficits.

Over the course of the disease leading to the advanced stage, stage 5, cognitive deficits become less of a concern for those with Huntington's, and physical symptoms become more of a concern as they worsen (Ho & Hocaoglu, 2011). During stage 5, affected individuals are fully dependent on others. They are non-ambulatory and at high risk for aspiration, though receptive language is mostly intact as are sense of self and recognition of family. However, verbal expression can be inhibited by choreic movements and an AAC device can be used to meet basic communicative needs. Rigidity, bradykinesia, and incoordination become more problematic in the advanced stage and often are more functionally disabling than the chorea (Rosenblatt et al., 2003). Memory loss becomes more severe in the later stages of this disease. Degeneration of the basal ganglia becomes detectable with neuroimaging technology. Eventually, death occurs as a result of a fall, anorexia, or dysphagia causing aspiration pneumonia.

Neuropathology

The pathogenesis of Huntington's disease is the mutation of a protein-producing gene commonly referred to as the *HD* gene (Walker, 2007). Normally, the *HD* gene produces a protein known as Huntingtin, but this protein's role in the body is not yet clearly understood. However, a mutated version of the *HD* gene present in those with Huntington's disease produces an altered and abnormal form of the Huntingtin protein known as mutant Huntingtin. The effects on the body of mutant Huntingtin produce Huntington's disease.

Huntingtin protein is produced throughout the body, not just in the brain; however, there are high amounts in the brain. Mutant Huntingtin is also produced throughout the body but creates more conspicuous and greater degeneration among the various components of the basal ganglia, its connections and pathways, the hippocampus, substantia nigra, as well as the Purkinje cells associated with the cerebellum's attachment to the pons (Walker, 2007). These changes to extrapyramidal structures such as the basal ganglia are responsible for creating the motor deficits associated with this disease.

Mixed Dementias

Vascular Dementia

Vascular dementia is the second leading cause of dementia (Alzheimer's Association, 2011). This is a dementia created by usually small ischemic strokes within the cortex, subcortex, or both. Risk factors for vascular dementia mirror classic risk factors for stroke such as hypertension and inactivity and are related to the presence of atherosclerosis. Medical treatment for vascular dementia therefore focuses on minimizing the likelihood of further ischemic strokes. The diagnostic criteria for vascular dementia, as stated in the *DSM-IV*, are as follows:

- Multiple cognitive deficits must be present, including memory impairment and one or more of these: aphasia, apraxia, agnosia, disturbance in executive function.
- Also, these cognitive deficits must cause impairment in the ability to execute social and/or occupational skills.
- Neurologic signs of stroke such as hyperactive reflexes and weakness must be present as well as documented evidence of infarctions on laboratory tests (brain imaging).
- Finally, it is required that these deficits do not occur only during episodes of delirium.

Vascular dementia often has a more sudden onset than does Alzheimer's disease and can often be traced to a single ischemic stroke or episode where stroke-like symptoms were displayed by the affected individual. However, in older individuals vascular dementia and Alzheimer's disease often co-occur (Roman, 2004). Individuals who develop vascular dementia usually have a medical history that predisposes them to stroke. They often have histories positive for hypertension (high blood pressure), stroke, and heart disease. Vascular dementia can also play a role in releasing or revealing signs of Alzheimer's disease that were previously unknown or compensated for by the affected individual. For unknown reasons, Alzheimer's disease often accompanies vascular dementia (Dickson, 2001).

Neuropathology

Vascular dementia is the presence of cognitive changes as a result of damage to the brain by, usually, multiple small or even unnoticed (silent) ischemic strokes. The effects of each of these individual strokes are usually not in themselves devastating to the functioning of the individual. However, as more occur over time, the detrimental effects on the ability of the brain to function build incrementally, creating possible memory loss, confusion, and dementia.

Multi-infarct dementia is the most widely recognized form of vascular dementia and is caused by many small infarcts (i.e., areas of tissue death caused by a lack of blood flow) usually to various areas of the brain. **Cortical multi-infarct dementia** is the result of small recurrent ischemic strokes to the cortex. When multi-infarct dementia occurs in the subcortex, it is known as lacunar state. **Lacunar state**, or lacunar syndrome, is the result of multiple subcortical thrombotic ischemic strokes occurring in small and deep blood vessels that supply blood flow to the brain stem, basal ganglia, and other subcortical structures. These small ischemic strokes cause tissue necrosis, which results in many small yet discrete cavities in the tissue of affected structures that, because of their subcortical nature, create motor signs such as dysarthria, dysphagia, and extrapyramidal

> **Multi-infarct dementia** A form of vascular dementia caused by many small infarcts usually to various areas of the brain.
>
> **Cortical multi-infarct dementia** A form of vascular dementia that is caused by small recurrent ischemic strokes within the cortex.
>
> **Lacunar state** A form of vascular dementia that is the result of multiple subcortical thrombotic ischemic strokes occurring in small and deep blood vessels that supply circulation to the brain stem, basal ganglia, and other subcortical structures.

signs including hyperactive reflexes, abnormal reflexes, hypertone, balance difficulties, or extremity weakness. Nonetheless, vascular dementia can present as a combination of cortical as well as subcortical damage and a combination of consequent signs and symptoms.

Disease Progression

Unlike Alzheimer's disease and other progressive dementing illnesses that have an insidious and often steady profile of degeneration, vascular dementia usually has an acute onset followed by a stepwise progress of degeneration. This stepwise degeneration is accounted for by subsequent strokes in which the affected individual's cognition might suddenly decrease and then level off until the next stroke occurs, at which time further degeneration is seen. Of course, the rate of degeneration and nature of the resulting deficits depend on the location and severity of the accumulating strokes. Typically, the memory

deficits associated with vascular dementia are not as severe as those associated with Alzheimer's disease, and individuals with vascular dementia present earlier with motor difficulties. Table 9-2 is a comparison of the clinical features of vascular dementia and Alzheimer's disease.

Lewy Body Disease

The defining neuropathologic change in the brains of those with Lewy body disease is the presence of abnormal spherical deposits of proteins in the cell bodies of neurons. These pathologic protein deposits are known as Lewy bodies (Figure 9-4), named for Friederich Lewy, who described their presence in 1912 (Del Tredici & Duda, 2011). Although the presence of Lewy bodies is a primary pathology of Lewy body disease, Lewy bodies have also been found in individuals affected with Alzheimer's and Down syndrome (Simard & van Reekum, 2001).

Table 9-2 Clinical Features that Differentiate Vascular Dementia from Alzheimer's Disease

Clinical Feature	Vascular Dementia	Alzheimer's Disease
Onset and progression	Abrupt onset; stepwise progression	Insidious onset; gradual progression
Neuroimaging findings	Evidence of multiple ischemic lesions, hemorrhagic events, and white matter lesions required for diagnosis, per *DSM-IV-TR guidelines*	Evidence of hypoperfusion of the medial temporal lobe areas, including the hippocampus, entorhinal and perirhinal cortices, and parahippocampal gyrus

No evidence of a cerebrovascular event, per *DSM-IV-TR guidelines* |
Focal neurologic signs	Present	Usually absent
Hachinski Ischemia Scores (HIS)*	Score of 7 or greater	Score of 4 or lower
Attention	Worse performance than Alzheimer's disease	Better performance than vascular dementia
Episodic memory impairment	Better performance on immediate and delayed verbal memory measures, compared to persons with Alzheimer's disease	Cardinal, early-appearing, severe deficit on delayed verbal memory measures
Gait alterations	Present early and are more common	May present later; not as common
Personality changes	More likely; tend to occur earlier in the course	Less likely than in vascular dementia; tend to present in the middle to late stages

Source: Reproduced from Papathanasiou, I (2013). Aphasia and Related Neurogenic Communication Disorders. Burlington, MA: Jones & Bartlett Learning.

*A tool used to determine the likelihood of a vascular component to dementia in order to differentiate Alzheimer's disease from vascular dementia.

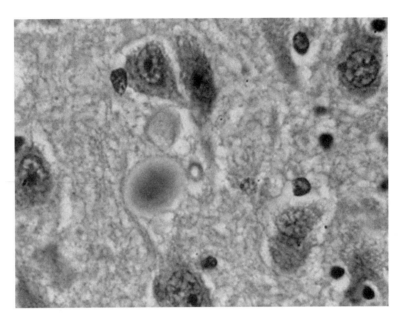

Figure 9-4 Lewy body (the large light sphere near the center of the image).

Source: Courtesy of Kondi Wong, Armed Forces Institute of Pathology.

There are two primary variants of Lewy body disease: Parkinson's disease and dementia with Lewy bodies; both are the result of the formation of Lewy bodies in the brain. However, there is disagreement over the categorization of Parkinson's disease as a form of Lewy body disease, and many consider it to be a standalone diagnosis. Clinically, this is certainly the case. Parkinson's disease has a very rich history of research and is a well-documented syndrome of deficits that are manifestly different from dementia with Lewy bodies, which has received far less attention and really just began to be recognized and labeled consistently in the 1960s.

Parkinson's Disease

In 1817, James Parkinson first identified Parkinson's disease. He described six cases of an incipient loss of motor movement, which he then called the shaking palsy but which is now known as Parkinson's disease (Parkinson, 2002 [reprinted]). Men are more likely to develop Parkinson's disease than women are, and it is estimated that 10 million people worldwide are living with Parkinson's disease.

This disease is primarily associated with motor abnormalities characterized by rigidity, tremor, and slowness of volitional movement. Nonetheless, cognitive deficits do present with this disease and can at times reach a degree of severity to be called dementia. Parkinson's disease is not to be confused with the more general term *Parkinsonism*, which implies Parkinson's disease-like symptoms but without the disease's etiology.

Neuropathology

With the formation of Lewy bodies in the pigmented cells of the substantia nigra in the midbrain, the neuropathologic process of Parkinson's disease begins with the loss of dopamine-producing cells within the substantia nigra. Once a large enough number of these cells disappear, a substantial loss of dopamine is created. With the lack of dopamine, certain areas of the brain are unable to function properly. The first area to malfunction as a result of the loss of dopamine is the basal ganglia. The basal ganglia plays a large role in regulating and refining motor movement, learning new sequences of motor movement, and maintaining postural reflexes. As such, the presenting symptoms of this disease are motoric in nature and involve the reduction of voluntary motor movements and the release of involuntary movements and postural abnormalities.

There is no known treatment to slow or stop this disease process. Symptom reduction and control in Parkinson's disease are usually accomplished, at least for a time, by administering the synthetic form of dopamine Levodopa, or L-Dopa. However, the beneficial effects of L-Dopa decrease over time and become less useful to the affected individual as the side effects of the drug increase. ▶ See the videos, *Parkinson's Disease Caregiver and Advocate* as well as the video, *Multiple Systems Atrophy Parkinsonism* for discussions of this disease.

Disease Progression

The initial symptoms of Parkinson's disease are motor abnormalities. Often, a tremor at rest begins in the thumb or forefinger, hand, or lips of the affected individual. Tremor usually appears unilaterally, and as the disease progresses the other side of the body begins to show signs of tremor as well. Early physicians made their own medications for patients by rolling soft materials into little pills using their thumb and forefinger. The initial, distinctive tremor in Parkinson's disease resembles this action and therefore is known as a *pill-rolling tremor*.

Along with the nonvolitional movements in certain body parts when at rest, Parkinson's disease also presents with a general slowness or bradykinesia. Volitional movements are reduced in speed, force, and range of motion. In the muscles of the face, this creates the iconic frozen, mask-like expression typical of those with Parkinson's disease. Though the lack of movement in the face makes the affected individual appear affectless and emotionally neutral, this is usually not truly representative of the affected individual's emotional state. Those with Parkinson's disease often report that their lack of facial expression creates communicative difficulties

because their loved ones cannot determine their emotional reactions to events or communications and assume them to be uncaring or insensitive simply because their emotions are no longer displayed on their face.

Difficulties with the initiation of volitional movement also appear in Parkinson's disease. These can manifest in the form of difficulty starting speech or starting to walk. Interestingly, when an affected individual has difficulty initiating the motor plans for walking, if an obstacle is placed in front of her, it often primes or cues the motor plans, making initiation of movement occur more readily. For instance, individuals with Parkinson's often stand, unable to initiate gait, but if a line of tape is put down on the floor and the affected individual is asked to step over the line, he might be able to do this readily and so begin the process of walking. This same phenomenon occurs when the affected individual is placed near a staircase. The automaticity of and natural context in which the movement is initiated makes the requisite movements more likely to be initiated. However, this is not always the case. ▶ See the video *Multiple Systems Atrophy Parkinsonism* to hear a woman with Parkinsonism discuss difficulties getting her body to walk through door frames.

Another motor sign in Parkinson's disease is known as festination (Latin for *to hurry*). Festination is a progressive speeding up of repetitive movements. This increase in speed usually occurs with a simultaneous reduction in range of movement of a repeated action, such as walking. Festination of gait is a Parkinsonian trait that occurs when affected individuals begin to walk but then increase the speed of their stride while decreasing the range of motion of their legs, thereby taking faster yet smaller steps. This creates the iconic shuffling walk of individuals affected with Parkinson's disease. At times, because of festination the affected individual cannot move his feet fast enough to keep up with his body, and a forward fall may become inevitable.

Festination is seen in speech acts as well as nonspeech acts. In speech, the speeding up of articulation can often be evoked using diadochokinetic rates. Individuals with Parkinson's disease initiate speech or diadochokinetic tasks at an already quick rate. Within a few repetitions, these verbalizations can grow so fast that the movements necessary for appropriate articulation begin to disappear because the repetitive movements of the mobile articulators become more reduced in force and range of motion. This speech disorder created by Parkinson's disease is known as hypokinetic dysarthria.

The small and often illegible handwriting of individuals with Parkinson's disease is known as micrographia. It should be noted that not only do difficulties with initiation of movement present, but also affected individuals can experience difficulties ceasing certain movements. In the case of festination of gait, difficulty ceasing movement presents a high risk of a fall because the individual cannot stop walking while their stride grows smaller and faster.

Motor symptoms present early in this disease along with sensory signs such as paresthesia. **Paresthesia** is a sensory abnormality usually characterized by the sensation of pins and needles, or tingling, or burning on the skin as well as general body aches. ▶ See the video, *Brain Stem Stroke* to hear an individual discuss his experiences with paresthesia. Individuals with Parkinson's disease usually die from medical complications caused by the motor deficits associated with the disease, such as aspiration pneumonia resulting from dysphagia.

> **Paresthesia**   A sensory abnormality usually characterized by sensation of pins and needles, or tingling, or burning on the skin as well as general body aches.

Dementia with Lewy Bodies

The deficit profile of dementia with Lewy bodies can be thought of as a combination of deficits from Parkinson's disease and Alzheimer's disease. Dementia with Lewy bodies presents with an overall decrease in volitional movement and difficulties initiating motor movement (as seen in Parkinson's disease) paired with cognitive deficits similar to those present in Alzheimer's disease. As such, dementia with Lewy bodies is often misdiagnosed as either Alzheimer's or Parkinson's disease. However, the presence of significant Parkinsonism and motor deficits early in the progression of dementia with Lewy bodies counterindicates a diagnosis of Alzheimer's disease. Meanwhile, the presence of significant cognitive deficits that fluctuate in severity counterindicates the diagnosis of Parkinson's disease.

The hallmark symptoms of dementia with Lewy bodies can be used to differentiate dementia with Lewy bodies from Alzheimer's and Parkinson's. These are the presence of significant sleep disturbances early in the disease with vivid and disquieting dreams as well as detailed hallucinations and delusions. Typically, those with Alzheimer's disease and Parkinson's disease do not present early in the disease process with such symptoms. Another differentiating characteristic is that those with dementia with Lewy bodies typically have severe and adverse reactions to the administration of L-Dopa, which is given to those with Parkinson's disease. A negative reaction to L-Dopa in the presence of Parkinsonism is an indicator of possible dementia with Lewy bodies.

Neuropathology

Whereas Alzheimer's disease is primarily the result of deterioration at the cortical level (creating mostly cognitive symptoms) and Parkinson's disease is the result of degeneration of the subcortex (creating mostly motor symptoms), dementia with Lewy bodies is the result of degeneration of both the cortex and the subcortex because of the formation and presence of Lewy bodies within these areas.

Disease Progression

Disease progression of individuals with dementia with Lewy bodies varies highly among affected

Table 9-3 Clinical Features that Differentiate Dementia with Lewy Bodies and Parkinson's Disease from Alzheimer's Disease

Clinical Feature	Dementia with Lewy Bodies and Parkinson's Disease	Alzheimer's Disease
Onset and progression	Insidious onset; relatively rapid progression	Insidious onset; gradual progression
Histopathology	Hallmark: Abnormal intracellular inclusion bodies called Lewy bodies, composed of alpha-synuclein protein Neuritic plaques might be present; neurofibrillary tangles rarely present	Hallmark: Neurofibrillary tangles and neuritic plaques, composed of beta-amyloid
Extrapyramidal signs and Parkinsonian features	Present (tremors, rigidity, bradykinesia)	Rare but possible
Visuospatial impairments	Worse than Alzheimer's disease	Better than dementia with Lewy bodies and Parkinson's disease
Executive function impairments	Worse than Alzheimer's disease	Better than dementia with Lewy bodies and Parkinson's disease
Visual hallucinations and fluctuations in consciousness	Present early and are more common	Infrequent

Source: Reproduced from Papathanasiou, I (2013). Aphasia and Related Neurogenic Communication Disorders. Burlington, MA: Jones & Bartlett Learning.

individuals and can reflect more of a cortical or subcortical symptomatology depending on which areas are most affected. Ultimately, the progression of this disease ends nearly the same as most of the other degenerative diseases discussed: Affected individuals are bedridden and severely affected by dementia and often die from medical complications associated with refusing to eat, being unable to eat, or other complications such as bedsores. Table 9-3 presents the clinical features that differentiate dementia with Lewy bodies and Parkinson's from Alzheimer's diseases.

Other Etiologies of Dementia

Aside from the neurodegenerative diseases discussed previously, there are other common etiologies of dementia. It is important to rule out any nonfatal etiologies of dementia before proceeding with the assumption of a more serious disease diagnosis.

Drug-induced dementia can occur in those who take prescription medications or abuse illegal substances. **Polypharmacy** is the term used to describe negative side effects (including unexpected drug interactions) of taking many prescription drugs at once. The elderly population is at particularly high risk for polypharmacy because of their increased use of medications for short-term health issues that then are not discontinued when the health issue resolves. Polypharmacy creates a heightened risk of dementia induced by pharmaceuticals. Because of this, it is imperative for medical professionals to examine all medications being taken by an affected individual to rule out polypharmacy as the cause of any cognitive issues or dementia.

> **Polypharmacy** The unexpected and unknown side effects of taking many prescription drugs at once.

Depression also plays a role, though poorly understood, in the manifestation of dementia. It is estimated that a full half to a third of those with dementia also have depression (Lyketsos, 2010). In the past, the term **pseudodementia** was used to indicate the cognitive changes and deficits brought on by depression, though the term has fallen out of use.

Pseudodementia An outdated term once used to indicate cognitive changes and deficits brought on by depression.

Partly this is because the relationship between depression and dementia is far more complex (or at least confusing) than previously believed. It was once believed that the presence of late-life depression predisposed one to a greater risk of developing dementia in older age (Li et al., 2011). This relationship was confirmed because many of those who had depression later in life went on to develop Alzheimer's disease. However, recent studies suggest that depression is simply an early manifestation of the disease process leading to dementia (Brommelhoff, Johansson, McArdle, Fratiglioni, & Pedersen, 2009; Li et al., 2011). Nonetheless, the boundaries between depression and dementia are murky at best. In reaction, Jorm (2000) proposes these six possible scenarios to account for the relationship between depression and dementia:

1. The treatment used to reduce depression increases risk for dementia (specifically electroshock therapy).
2. The risk factors for depression and dementia are the same.
3. Depression is an early sign of dementia.
4. Depression is a reaction to the early cognitive changes experienced by those with dementia.
5. The presence of depression reveals an already present dementia syndrome that the person was able to compensate for and hide prior to developing depression.
6. The presence of depression actually increases the risk of developing dementia.

Of course, reality does not have to reflect any single one of Jorm's hypotheses. More than one, or possibly many, of these hypotheses could be true given different circumstances and different individual cases.

Role of the Speech-Language Pathologist in Treating Those with Dementia

During the early stages of dementia, the role of the speech-language pathologist is to recognize, appropriately diagnose, and provide therapy for cognitive, communication, or swallowing deficits occurring as a result of dementia or dementia-producing illnesses. Often, early in the dementia process speech-language pathologists can teach behavioral or dietary modifications to manage or minimize swallowing difficulties. The therapist can also teach the patient to adapt to mild declines in language, speech, and cognition using compensatory strategies.

The speech-language pathologist regularly reevaluates the patient's mastication and swallow abilities as cognitive and motor deficits progress. As the negative effects of the disease grow to affect the patient's ability to eat and drink, the speech-language pathologist continues to alter the patient's position during eating, changes consistency of the patient's diet to facilitate safe swallowing, and adds further precautions during mealtimes to minimize aspiration risk. As the disease progresses, the patient will reach a point when, despite all modifications and precautions, safely taking food and/or fluids by mouth becomes impossible and the individual is forced to choose between the high likelihood of developing aspiration pneumonia or having a feeding tube placed to bypass the swallow mechanism entirely and provide nutrition and hydration straight to the stomach or gastrointestinal tract to minimize the risk of aspiration pneumonia.

More often than not, interventions by the speech-language pathologist for cognitive, speech, and language deficits focus on compensatory measures that allow the patient to function for as long as possible despite the deficits. An example of a compensatory intervention for memory deficits is a memory folder tied to the patient's wheelchair that is filled with the patient's personal and relevant information; the individual can look at or read the information in the folder if confused and in need of reorientation.

The presence of a degenerative and fatal illness, while making restoration of lost abilities impossible, does not rule out the possibility of short-term gains that can increase quality of life of the affected individuals. Although restoring actual cognitive abilities for the long term is usually impossible in these diseases, federal legislation (Omnibus Budget Reconciliation Act of 1987; Bayles & Tomoeda, 2007) requires that residents of nursing homes are evaluated regularly and that plans are developed to keep them functioning at the highest possible level. So, although a speech-language pathologist might not be able to restore lost cognitive abilities, the speech-language pathologist can determine that the life of a resident with dementia can be improved by maximizing intact but unused cognitive skills, and then he or she is justified in performing therapy toward that end and these services are reimbursable by law. If there is no potential for a nursing home resident to improve, the speech-language pathologist can create a functional maintenance plan that outlines the arrangements necessary to keep the patient functioning at a certain level.

Cognitive-Communication Assessment of Those with Dementia

Purpose of Assessment

There are many reasons to assess individuals for the cognitive and communication changes associated with dementia. The purpose of assessment usually varies according to the particular situation of the affected individual. Around the onset of dementia, the purpose of assessment is to document changes toward deficit in language and cognition that are beyond those associated with normal aging. In other words, the purpose is to establish that there is a problem. Later in the disease process, when it is obvious

that there are problems, the purpose of assessment is to establish the strengths, deficits, and severity of deficits affecting the individual and to help with accurate diagnosis of the primary etiology (the disease causing the deficits). Assessment also serves to identify deficits for which to set goals and to determine the best methods for achieving those goals. Also during assessment, counseling of the family and caregivers is necessary.

Assessment of Dementias

Assessment of an individual with dementia begins with a thorough case history of the person. This involves an in-depth review of any available medical records or medical charts as well as an interview with the individual and the family or caregiver. Information gathered in the chart review and interview portion of the assessment should agree and reinforce one another. The speech-language pathologist must follow-up on any discrepancies and make appropriate referrals. Important information that needs to be gathered in an individual's history includes the following items:

- A complete list of medications currently being used
- A description by the affected individual of problems he or she is having and how it is affecting the individual's life
- A description by the family of the problems they see the affected individual is having
- A social, educational, and medical history of the patient, especially including an exploration of risk factors such as family history of dementia, personal history of depression, and personal history of traumatic brain injury

In addition to taking a detailed case history, therapists can administer evaluative tools to establish the presence and severity of cognitive and language deficits. Rating scales are used as screening tools by nurses and medical personnel to get a quick, mostly informal idea of the possible presence and severity of dementia. A rating scale enables the clinician to observe the reactions of the individual to a small number of stimuli and gauge the individual's level of function on certain abilities. Rating scales can be used to assess orientation to time, place, and person, as well as attention, short-term memory, long-term memory, motor abilities, and different modalities of language. However, they are not sensitive to mild or more subtle deficits and instead are better suited to moderate to severe cases of dementia. Rating scales commonly administered to those with dementia include the following:

- *Mini-Mental State Examination (MME; Folstein, Folstein, & McHugh, 1975):* Also known as the Folstein test. Takes approximately 10 minutes to administer. This is the most commonly used screen and is used with a variety of disorders, not just dementia. No training is required to administer.
- *Alzheimer's Disease Assessment Scale (ADAS; Rosen, Mohs, & Davis, 1984):* Takes approximately 45 minutes to administer. This scale is designed to evaluate the cognitive and noncognitive manifestations of Alzheimer's disease.
- *Global Deterioration Scale (GDS; Reisberg, Ferris, de Leon, & Crook, 1982):* Takes approximately 2 minutes to administer. Used to rate level of dementia with a seven-stage scale and to track deterioration over time.
- *Dependence Scale (Stern et al., 1994):* Takes approximately 5 minutes to administer. This rating scale is designed to assess the level of dependence of the individual with dementia. It is used generally to assess the need for institutionalization.
- *Geriatric Depression Scale (GDS; Yesavage et al., 1983):* Takes approximately 10 minutes to administer. Used to assess the presence of depression in older adults. The presence of dementia can confound results, so the possibility and presence of dementia needs to be assessed

separately so that the speech-language pathologist can differentiate whether the results are from dementia or depression.

However, screening tools are of limited usefulness and a comprehensive evaluation of cognition and communication abilities is usually warranted in a therapy setting. Few comprehensive tests include individuals with dementia in their normative sample. Therefore, few comprehensive tests can give detailed information about level of deficits and the relation of those deficits to the deficits of others with dementia. For instance, standardized tests such as the Wechsler Adult Intelligence Scale—Revised (WAIS–R; Wechsler, 1981) can be used to detect deterioration in cognitive status away from normal and can be used by the speech-language pathologist to detect deficits and set goals, but the WAIS–R cannot further analyze results to give additional information about type or severity of dementia.

One example of a comprehensive and standardized test for dementia is the Arizona Battery for Communication Disorders of Dementia (ABCD; Bayles & Tomoeda, 1993). In addition to having unimpaired individuals in the normative sample, individuals with a variety of different dementias at varying levels of severity were also included. The ABCD assesses expressive and receptive language abilities, verbal memory, visuospatial skills, and mental status. Results from the ABCD indicate severity level of dementia, possible dementia type, and deficit to be targeted in therapy.

Medical Management of Cognitive Deficits in Dementia

In the progressive diseases detailed in this chapter, no known medical treatments can halt or reverse the cognitive and language deficits associated with dementia. Medical treatment for these deficits involves allowing the affected individual's brain to maximize the abilities left intact.

Two medications are now almost universally prescribed to individuals with Alzheimer's disease: donepezil (Aricept) and memantine (Namenda). Although there are no indications that either of these medications slow or halt the progression of Alzheimer's disease, donepezil and memantine are used for palliative care, meaning they are administered to reduce the symptoms of the disease. These medications improve cognitive function in affected individuals, although increases are usually very modest improvements and disappear as the medication wears off. Donepezil and memantine can also reduce the behavioral and psychological symptoms associated with Alzheimer's (Lockhart, Orme, & Mitchell, 2011). Typically, donepezil has been shown to best improve cognition in the early and moderate stages of Alzheimer's disease while memantine has been found to be more efficacious in improving cognition in the moderate and late stages of Alzheimer's (Schneider, Dagerman, Higgins, & McShane, 2011). Recent research has begun to examine the effects of using these drugs in combination to treat the symptoms of Alzheimer's disease and has found positive results (Patel & Grossberg, 2011).

Management of Cognitive-Communication Deficits in Dementia

As previously mentioned, therapy for cognitive-communication disorders in dementia might not restore lost abilities, but the modern focus is on improving quality of life and ensuring that a person with dementia is operating at the highest possible level, given the deficits. Bayles and Tomoeda (2007) provide guidelines to assist in designing a plan of care for individuals with dementia to ensure they reach a maximum level of functioning.

1. First, therapy should focus on strengthening abilities and knowledge bases that are capable of improving. For example, if a resident at a nursing home keeps getting lost on the way to the bathroom, does she have the cognitive ability to ask for directions? If so, then strengthening and training her to ask for directions can reduce her difficulties finding the bathroom and significantly increase her quality of life.

2. Next, therapy should reduce demands on impaired cognitive abilities while increasing use of intact cognitive abilities. Continuing the last example, if the nursing home resident who cannot find the bathroom lacks the cognitive skills to ask for directions, can the therapist employ another one of her intact abilities to enable her to compensate? For instance, putting up signs leading from her bed all the way to the bathroom can capitalize on the patient's ability to attend to visual stimuli and operate on working memory long enough to get from one sign to the next and eventually to the bathroom to compensate for her lack of ability to request directions.

3. Last, therapy should provide stimuli that evoke positive memories and positive emotion, not negative. The presence of negative emotions such as withdrawal and depression is common in those with dementia and negatively affects their quality of life and the quality of life of their caregivers. Speech-language pathologists should take great care to avoid evoking negative emotions during therapy sessions.

Bayles and Tomoeda (2007) define two primary categories of interventions for dementia as direct and indirect therapies. Direct therapy strategies are those in which the speech-language pathologist provides individual or group therapy sessions to target deficits. Indirect therapy strategies are strategies that focus on modifying or manipulating the physical or communicative environment of the affected individual to best support communication and activities of daily living.

Direct Therapies

Reminiscence Therapy

Reminiscence therapy is a semicued conversation regarding past events or the affected individual's past experiences and activities that is meant to increase orientation and to trigger recall of pleasant long-term or episodic memories. Individuals with Alzheimer's disease usually have mostly intact long-term memory through a good portion of the disease's progression. Reminiscence therapy allows the speech-language pathologist to capitalize on intact long-term memory ability to increase orientation and to facilitate functional communication. Usually, the speech-language pathologist uses tangible prompts such as objects, videos, music, or scents to cue the conversation. Family members can bring in objects that hold some deep and personal meaning such as old photographs or items from a previous workplace or career to be used in therapy. Reminiscence therapy sessions are held one on one or in groups. Utilizing this form of therapy in group settings allows for a greater level of interaction and facilitation of social skills (Akanuma et al., 2011).

Errorless Learning Therapy

Errorless learning therapy capitalizes on intact procedural memory for rehabilitation of anomia and memory deficits. The primary basis for errorless learning therapy is that difficulty level of the therapy task is set well within the ability level of the patient. This is done to maximize patient success and minimize the possibility of patient failure. The rationale is to avoid the production of errors by the patient entirely. It is believed that when patients produce errorful responses to therapy stimuli, they are in effect practicing the production of errors, which increases the odds of future failures. Of course, minimizing the number of errors produced by a patient in therapy is a primary responsibility of speech-language pathologists even in traditional therapy sessions.

Clinical Note

Negative Emotions in Reminiscence Therapy

It should be emphasized that in reminiscence therapy the speech-language pathologist must focus on stimulating positive memories and evoking positive emotions. Emphasizing or discussing negative experiences and evoking negative emotions are not likely to pay off in a positive way. In fact, they are likely to guide the affected individual to a possible crisis and ruin any possibility of a productive therapy session.

I saw a relevant example of this a while back. A young, enthusiastic student of speech-language pathology entered the therapy room with her patient. There was much positive discussion about this and that from the patient's past, and everything was jovial and positive. Then, quite innocently and offhandedly, the student inquired about the cap the client was wearing because he usually wore a different cap to therapy. This patient had spent his life working as a Methodist minister. Upon removing his hat, the patient saw that he was wearing a hat with the name and number of a fire station. Unknown to the student, this was the hat that the men of a fire station in New York City had given him in token of appreciation of his efforts and work at Ground Zero in New York City after the World Trade Center was destroyed. The recall of the horrible tragedy, human suffering, and loss experienced by all those at Ground Zero on September 11, 2001, mistakenly cued by the student deeply upset the patient. We were unable to get his mind off it for the rest of the therapy session. Indeed, the caregiver reported that the patient had difficulties getting past his memories of 9/11 for the rest of the day.

Researchers who have examined errorless learning approaches conclude that errorless learning therapies for anomia and memory deficits are effective in remediation of these deficits to some degree (Fillingham, Sage, Lambon Ralph, 2006; McKissock & Ward, 2007; Mulholland, Donoghue, Meenagh, & Rushe, 2008; Ruis & Kessels, 2005). Results from Kessels and

Hensken (2009) indicate that procedural learning of tasks was better in early- and midstage Alzheimer's disease using errorless strategies than with traditional errorful learning strategies. However, in severe dementia, any gains produced by errorless learning are limited and short-lived (Ruis & Kessels, 2005).

Spaced Retrieval Training

Spaced retrieval training (SRT) is a therapy procedure in which speech-language pathologists present new or previously known information to those with memory deficits and then prompt them to recall that information over increasingly greater intervals of time. The intervals are initially very short but are slowly increased by the speech-language pathologist over time while the amount of information presented to the affected individual is also increased. Spaced retrieval training should work in an errorless fashion. The speech-language pathologist should set the difficulty well within the ability level of the patient, cue many repetitions (massed practice), and the patient should rarely make an error. In fact, Balota, Duchek, Sergent-Marshall, and Roediger (2006) compared the use of expanding intervals with equal intervals in SRT and found no difference in the gains between conditions. These results suggest that it might not be the expanding interval between cued recalls but merely the errorless learning component that is the active component in SRT.

Nonetheless, in early Alzheimer's disease, SRT has been used successfully to retrain functional information such as face–name associations with friends and family (Abrahams & Camp, 1993) and techniques for a safe swallow and transfers (Mahendra & Hopper, 2013). Spaced retrieval training is particularly well fit for targeting the establishment of very important and functional knowledge such as names of family and friends, important locations such as bathroom and cafeteria, and emergency procedures such as how to call for a nurse or get help.

Bayles and Tomoeda (2007) highlight that this therapy technique can be nested among other techniques in a therapy session, meaning that other strategies and activities can be taking place while the speech-language pathologist periodically cues the patient to produce the information targeted using SRT. Results from Hopper, Drefs, Bayles, Tomoeda, and Dinu (2010) support this assertion and indicate that the intervals can be filled with tasks unrelated to the SRT task without compromising the success of SRT.

Memory Prostheses

The use of external memory aids to augment the memory capacity of those with memory deficits is a common and effective intervention for chronic memory deficits. When an individual with memory deficits carries and actively uses the memory aid the term *memory prosthesis* is often applied. Examples of memory prostheses are memory books, wallets, calendars or appointment books, and more recently smartphones and personal digital assistants (PDAs).

Memory prostheses usually contain personal and biographic information in written and/or pictorial form. A memory book might contain a life history timeline complete with pictures of friends and family members, information for orienting the affected person to his or her surroundings (location, time, etc.), and perhaps even an explanation concerning why the person is in therapy or a hospital or nursing home. This strategy is widely applied to individuals with memory loss from many etiologies from traumatic brain injury to dementia.

Bourgeois (1990) found that communicative effectiveness in her participants with Alzheimer's disease was increased and that they were able to use their memory prostheses effectively with caregivers and even when communicating with another individual with dementia (Bourgeois, 1993). Of course, an inherent difficulty is that those with memory deficits might not remember that they have a memory book and must be cued to look at it. Also, the memory book must be attached to the patient in some way, usually by tying or chaining the memory book (usually a three-ring binder) to the patient's wheelchair, so that it is not lost or forgotten. If the patient has no wheelchair, than a more compact version, a memory wallet, can be devised to fit into a pocket.

Montessori Approach

One of the latest additions to the list of approaches to increase function in individuals with dementia is the utilization of Montessori methods. Montessori methods are used to increase the ability of those with dementia to participate in their daily routines while improving mood and increasing social skills (Orsulic-Jeras, Judge, & Camp, 2000). In the late 1800s, Maria Montessori began to develop her theory of early childhood education that focuses on encouraging a child's independence and self-discovery, rather than direct instruction. The most important aspects of Montessori's principles summarized by Mahendra (2001) are as follows:

1. Breaking down complex tasks into individual parts and arranging these individual tasks hierarchically from simple to difficult, and from concrete to abstract
2. Providing extensive cues to guide the individual and facilitate success
3. Providing feedback about the accuracy and appropriateness of performance to minimize frustration and failure
4. Utilizing materials that yield cognitive and sensory stimulation

Individuals at all levels of dementia can participate in Montessori-based activities. Orsulic-Jeras, Judge, and Camp (2000) found that the use of Montessori-based activities elicited more active levels of engagement and more pleasure than the regularly scheduled non-Montessori activities used in the nursing home. Camp and Skrajner (2004) found that individuals with milder levels of dementia can be taught to

operate as group leaders of Montessori-based activities. Although more research is needed to focus on the effects of using Montessori methods to target communication and cognitive skills, the general use of Montessori methods in nursing homes to increase engagement and pleasure and decrease frustration and aggression is well supported.

Indirect Therapies

Life History Videos

Custom-made personal videos, or life history videos, are videos composed by the family of the individual with dementia and/or the speech-language pathologist. The purpose of the video is to provide an audiovisual presentation of relevant personal facts such as relationships and past events to increase orientation and decrease confusion and behavioral disturbances of the individual with dementia. Yasuda, Kuwabara, Kuwahara, Abe, and Tetsutani (2009) used a slideshow of personal photos with narration and music and found that their participants were more likely to attend to a personalized video than to any regularly programmed television show. Hatakeyama and colleagues (2010) constructed personalized life history videos for individuals from home movies and recordings, photos of children and grandchildren, and recordings of their favorite singers. The researchers found that after viewing these life history videos, participants with dementia showed significant improvements on measures of cognition.

Environmental Manipulations

Altering the environment of the individual with dementia to keep the person calm, safe, and oriented is a very important strategy that is used in long-term care facilities as well as in the homes of those with dementia.

First and foremost, the environment should be altered to keep the individual with dementia safe. If the individual lives at home or with family, important environmental manipulations include (Bayles and Tomoeda, 2007):

1. Remove all firearms and weapons from the house.
2. Minimize the number of mirrors in the house (which some individuals with dementia find to be agitating).
3. Lock up poisonous substances.
4. Use nightlights.
5. Place decals on glass doors to keep the individual with dementia from walking into or through the glass.
6. Utilize nonslip mats in the bathrooms.
7. Post signs on doors identifying which room is which (e.g., bathroom, bedroom).
8. Keep the keys to the car secured to prevent the individual from driving (if it is deemed dangerous for him or her to do so).
9. Have an identification bracelet made with the individual's name and address.

Indirect strategies for manipulating the environment of those with dementia are the use of external memory aids. Posting relevant information where an individual with dementia can see and access the information helps to keep the affected individual oriented and calm. This can include calendars that highlight the date, digital clocks that give the time of day, and photos of family and loved ones. Labeling cupboards, cabinets, and drawers in the kitchen and bathroom and other important locations in the house can also keep an individual with dementia functioning at higher levels for longer periods of time. Playing music that is familiar and preferred by the affected individual also helps maintain orientation and reduce agitation.

Also important is manipulating the communicative environment to facilitate appropriate communication among the individual with dementia and others. This usually begins with limiting distractions in the room before engaging the individual in conversation. For instance, this might involve turning off the television or radio, closing the door or window to limit noise, and closing the blinds to limit visual distractions. Other important changes to facilitate communication are limiting the number of individuals involved in a conversation, sitting close enough to hear the speech of a person with dementia, and speaking loudly enough for the affected individual to hear.

Sometimes caregivers as well as some speech-language pathologists automatically change the way they speak when talking to someone with dementia in an attempt to increase the affected individual's comprehension or attention to speech. This is called code switching, the altering of the way one speaks depending on to whom one is speaking. Code switching is an important skill for the speech-language pathologist to develop and it is a learned skill. But in some long-term care facilities, health professionals code switch very inappropriately and ineffectively when addressing individuals with dementia by speaking to them as they would address a small child. This is to be strongly avoided and usually is highly offensive to the individual's caregivers and the affected individual. Appropriate code-switching behavior should be subtle. When code switching to speak to someone with dementia to increase comprehension and attention it is important to do the following:

1. Speak slower (though not abnormally so).
2. Use shorter sentences.
3. Augment what you are saying with appropriate gestures and facial expressions and possibly write out any words not readily understood.
4. Avoid abstract topics and focus on more concrete topics.
5. Use frequently used words and avoid less frequently used words or jargon.
6. Repeat important points often and rephrase important information if not understood.
7. Give the individual with dementia plenty of time to process what is said.
8. Give the individual with dementia plenty of time to respond to what has been said.
9. Avoid teasing and sarcasm, which often leads to confusion (Bayles & Tomoeda, 2007).

Caregivers and health professionals often require training or counseling on ways to change the communicative environment to best facilitate communication with those with dementia. They might also need coaching on appropriate code-switching behaviors to facilitate communication.

Main Points

- Dementia is an acquired global loss of brain function with a slow, insidious onset that is caused by a variety of diseases. Dementia is a syndrome created by disease, not a disease itself.
  - The *DSM-IV* describes dementia as memory loss plus deficits in at least one other of the following areas: verbal expression or auditory and written receptive language skills, recognition and identification of objects, ability to execute motor activities, abstract thinking, judgment, and execution of complex tasks. Also, deficits must affect the individual's ADLs.
- Delirium is a sudden disturbance in consciousness or a change in cognitive ability that fluctuates throughout the course of a day with an onset usually resulting from a general medical condition.
- Mild cognitive impairment is changes that are significant enough not to be within the spectrum of changes associated with normal aging, though not severe enough to significantly affect the daily lives of affected individuals. Symptoms of mild cognitive impairment include decreased ability to concentrate, decreased word finding abilities, decreased short-term memory, and difficulty following detail-heavy conversations or writings.
- Speech-language pathologists must assess and treat cognitive and communicative deficits that are the result of dementia. Difficulties in communication often occur when cognitive functions are disrupted.
- Alzheimer's disease is a cortical dementia that is the most common cause of dementia. Alzheimer's disease is a progressive and fatal disease with no known treatments to stop or slow its progression.
- The neuropathology of Alzheimer's disease includes neurofibrillary tangles, amyloid plaques, and granulovacuolar degeneration.
- Alzheimer's disease is divided into early, mid, and late stages.
  - Early-stage indications of the disease are short-term memory loss, word finding difficulties, difficulties comprehending verbal language, and personality changes.
  - Deficits in the midstage of the disease begin to affect ADLs. The midstage is characterized by significant memory loss, attention deficits, more dramatic personality changes, visuospatial and visuoconstructive deficits, and expressive language deficits.
  - The late stage is when individuals lose motor function and become nonambulatory, bedridden, incontinent, and unresponsive. Memory, cognition, and expressive language deficits are severe to profound and can lead to institutionalization, muteness, and dysphagia.
- Frontotemporal dementia is the degeneration of the frontal and temporal lobes. This category of dementia includes Pick's disease, the primary progressive aphasias, and semantic dementia.
- Pick's disease is a dementia resulting from progressive degeneration of the frontal and

temporal lobes. It is characterized by changes in personality, antisocial and inappropriate behavior, and memory loss.

- The neuropathology of Pick's disease includes Pick bodies and ballooned neurons.
- Pick's disease is a progressive terminal illness that is characterized by early behavioral, emotional, and personality changes in the absence of significant language deficits.

- Huntington's disease is a subcortical dementia that is a progressive terminal illness characterized by distinctive, involuntary, erratic body movements. Huntington's disease can also cause changes in personality, cognition, language, and emotions.

  - The neuropathology of Huntington's disease is the production of mutant Huntingtin by the *HD* gene. Mutant Huntingtin creates degeneration of the basal ganglia, hippocampus, substantia nigra, and Purkinje cells of the pons.
  - Huntington's disease is divided into five stages:

    Stages 1 and 2 are characterized by the motor symptoms of chorea, emotional problems, difficulty concentrating, memory problems, difficulties with executive functioning, as well as concerns regarding sleeping and swallowing.

    Stages 2, 3, and 4 are characterized by chorea and hyperkinesias that begin to interfere with speech production. Training the individual on an AAC device during these stages helps prepare the individual for the full loss of verbal and written expression caused by motor deficits.

    Stage 5 is when individuals are nonambulatory, dependent on others, at high risk for aspiration, and often use AAC devices to communicate.

- Vascular dementia is caused by small ischemic strokes within the cortex, subcortex, or both.

The diagnostic criteria required for vascular dementia, as stated in the *DSM-IV*, is that multiple cognitive deficits must be present, including memory impairment and one or more of these: aphasia, apraxia of speech, agnosia, and disturbance in executive function. These cognitive deficits must cause impairment in the ability to execute social and/or occupational skills. Neurologic signs of stroke such as hyperactive reflexes and weakness must be present as well as documented evidence of infarctions on laboratory tests (brain imaging). It is finally required that these deficits do not occur only during episodes of delirium. Vascular dementia has acute onset followed by a stepwise progression of degeneration.

- The defining neuropathologic change in the brains of those individuals with Lewy body disease is the presence of abnormal spherical deposits of proteins in the cell bodies of neurons that are referred to as Lewy bodies. Lewy body disease is a category of diseases with variants including Parkinson's disease and dementia with Lewy bodies.

- Parkinson's disease is characterized by motor abnormalities such as rigidity, tremor, and slowness of volitional movement as well as cognitive deficits. There is no treatment known to slow or stop this disease process.

  - The neuropathology of Parkinson's disease is the loss of dopamine-producing cells within the substantia nigra; certain areas of the brain, including the basal ganglia, need dopamine to function.

- Dementia with Lewy bodies presents with the overall decrease of volitional movement and difficulties initiating motor movement seen in Parkinson's disease paired with the cognitive deficits present in Alzheimer's disease. Hallmark characteristics that differentiate dementia with Lewy bodies from Alzheimer's disease and Parkinson's disease are the presence of significant sleep disturbances with vivid dreams, hallucinations, as well as negative reactions to L-Dopa.

- The neuropathology of this disease is deterioration resulting from the proliferation of Lewy bodies within the cortex and subcortex.

- Other etiologies of dementia include polypharmacy and depression.

- The speech-language pathologist should be able to recognize, diagnose, and provide treatment for cognitive, communicative, and swallowing deficits as a result of dementia or dementia-producing illnesses.

- The purpose of assessing communication and cognition deficits as a result of dementia is to document that there are changes, establish strengths, delineate deficits, set goals and therapy strategies, as well as counsel the family and caregivers.

- Assessment of dementia often includes the following:

  - A detailed case history, review of medical history and interviews with the family and patient.

  - Rating scales such as the Mini-Mental State Examination, which are used to assess an individual's level of function on certain abilities through observation. Other rating scales include the Alzheimer's Disease Assessment Scale, Global Deterioration Scale, the Dependence Scale, and the Geriatric Depression Scale.

    - Comprehensive, formal tests, such as the Arizona Battery for Communication Disorders of Dementia, which can be given to warrant therapy.

- Medical management of cognitive deficits in dementia is used to maximize the abilities that an individual has left. Two commonly used medications include donepezil (Aricept) and memantine (Namenda).

- Therapy for cognitive-communication disorders in progressive dementia is usually meant to improve quality of life and ensure that the individual is operating at his or her highest possible level given the deficits.

- Therapy should focus on strengthening abilities and knowledge bases that are capable of improving, reducing demands on impaired cognitive abilities while increasing use of intact cognitive abilities, and providing stimuli that evoke positive memories and emotion.

- Direct therapy strategies are individual or group therapy sessions that target deficits.

  - Reminiscence therapy is a semicued conversation regarding past events or the affected individual's past experiences and activities that work to increase orientation and trigger recall of pleasant long-term or episodic memory.

  - Errorless learning therapy is when the difficulty level of a task is set well within the ability of the patient to maximize patient success and minimize patient failure.

  - Spaced retrieval training is the presentation of new or previously known information to those with memory deficits that they must recall over increasingly greater intervals of time.

  - Memory prostheses are external memory aids to augment the memory capacity of those with memory deficits such as memory books, wallets, calendars, smart phones, and personal digital assistants.

  - The Montessori approach includes the breaking down of complex tasks into individual parts and arranging these individual component tasks for practice into hierarchical order of difficulty.

- Indirect therapy strategies are strategies that focus on modifying or manipulating the physical or communicative environment.

  - Life history videos are custom-made personal videos that are composed by the speech-language pathologist or the family of the individual with dementia to provide an audiovisual presentation of relevant personal facts such as relationships and past events to increase orientation and decrease confusion.

- Environmental manipulations are meant to keep the individual with dementia safe, calm, and oriented.

Review Questions

1. Define dementia.
2. How do delirium and mild cognitive impairment differ?
3. Why must speech-language pathologists treat both communication and cognition deficits that are the result of dementia?
4. Describe the three stages of Alzheimer's disease.
5. List deficits associated with Pick's disease.
6. Describe the progression of Huntington's disease.
7. Describe the diagnostic criteria for vascular dementia.
8. How does the neuropathology associated with lacunar state differ from the neuropathology associated with cortical multi-infarct dementia?
9. How does dementia onset differ between Alzheimer's disease and vascular dementia?
10. Describe the role of the substantia nigra in relation to Parkinson's disease.
11. How is dementia with Lewy bodies similar to both Parkinson's disease and Alzheimer's disease?
12. What is polypharmacy and why is the aging population at risk for polypharmacy?
13. What is the speech-language pathologist's role with individuals with dementia?
14. Why is assessment important in dementia?
15. What are two medications popularly used to reduce symptoms of dementia ?
16. How are direct and indirect therapy strategies different?
17. How might reminiscence therapy be used with an individual with dementia?
18. How might the Montessori approach be used with an individual with dementia?
19. Why might life history videos be useful with individuals with dementia?
20. Why are environmental manipulations important for individuals with dementia?

References

1. Abrahams, J., & Camp, C. (1993). Maintenance and generalization of object naming training in anomia associated with degenerative dementia. *Clinical Gerontology, 12*, 57–72.
2. Akanuma, K., Meguro, K., Meguro, M., Sasaki, E., Chiba, K., Ishii, H., & Tanaka, N. (2011). Improved social interaction and increased anterior cingulate metabolism after group reminiscence with reality orientation approach for vascular dementia. *Psychiatry Research, 192*(3), 183–187.
3. Alzheimer's Association. (2011). *2011 Alzheimer's disease facts and figures*. Chicago, IL: Author.
4. American Psychiatric Association. (2000). *Diagnostic and statistical manual of mental disorders* (4th ed.). Washington, DC: Author.
5. American Speech-Language-Hearing Association. (2005). *The roles of speech-language pathologists working with individuals with dementia-based communication disorders: Position statement*. Rockville, MD: Author.

6. Balota, D., Duchek, J., Sergent-Marshall, S., & Roediger, H. (2006). Does expanded retrieval produce benefits over equal-interval spacing? Explorations of spacing effects in healthy aging and early-stage Alzheimer's disease. *Psychology and Aging, 21*(1), 19–31.

7. Bates, G., Harper, P., & Jones, L. (2002). *Huntington's disease*. Oxford, England: Oxford University Press.

8. Bayles, K., & Tomoeda, C. (1993). *The Arizona Battery for Communication Disorders of Dementia*. Austin, TX: Pro-Ed.

9. Bayles, K., & Tomoeda, C. (2007). *Cognitive-communication disorders of dementia*. San Diego, CA: Plural.

10. Bourgeois, M. (1990). Enhancing conversation skills in patients with Alzheimer's disease using a prosthetic memory aid. *Journal of Applied Behavior Analysis, 23*(1), 29–42.

11. Bourgeois, M. (1993). Effects of memory aids on the dyadic conversations of individuals with dementia. *Journal of Applied Behavior Analysis, 26*(1), 77–87.

12. Brommelhoff, J., Johansson, B., McArdle, J., Fratiglioni, L., & Pedersen, N. (2009). Depression as a risk factor or prodromal feature for dementia? Findings in a population-based sample of Swedish twins. *Psychology of Aging, 24*(2), 373–384.

13. Camp, C., & Skrajner, M. (2004). Resident-assisted Montessori programming (RAMP): Training persons with dementia to serve as group activity leaders. *The Gerontologist, 44*(3), 426–431.

14. Collie, A., & Maruff, P. (2000). The neuropsychology of preclinical Alzheimer's disease and mild cognitive impairment. *Neuroscience and Behavioral Reviews, 24*, 365–374.

15. Craik, F. (2000). Age-related changes in human memory. In D. Park & N. Schwarz (Eds.), *Cognitive aging: A primer* (pp. 75–92). Philadelphia, PA: Psychology Press.

16. Cummings, J. (1984). Dementia: Definition, classification, and differential diagnosis. *Psychiatric Annals, 14*(2), 85–89.

17. Del Tredici, K., & Duda, J. (2011). Peripheral Lewy body pathology in Parkinson's disease and incidental Lewy body disease: Four cases. *Journal of the Neurological Sciences, 310*, 100–106.

18. Dickson, D. (2001). Neuropathologies of Alzheimer's disease and other dementias. *Clinics in Geriatric Medicine, 17*(2), 209–228.

19. Ferri, C., Prince, M., Brayne, C., Brodaty, H., Fratiglioni, L., Ganguli, M., . . . Scazufca, M. (2005). Global prevalence of dementia: A Delphi consensus study. *Lancet, 366*(9503), 2112–2117.

20. Fillingham, J., Sage, K., & Lambon Ralph, M. (2006). The treatment of anomia using errorless learning. *Neuropsychological Rehabilitation, 16*(2), 129–154.

21. Folstein, M., Folstein, S., & McHugh, P. (1975). "Mini-Mental State": A practical method for grading the cognitive state of patients for the clinician. *Journal of Psychiatric Research, 12*(3), 189–198.

22. Green, R., Cupples, L., Go, R., Benke, K., Edeki, T., Griffith, P., . . . Farrer, L. (2002). Risk of dementia among white and African-American relatives of patients with Alzheimer's disease. *Journal of the American Medical Association, 287*(3), 329–336.

23. Grober, E., Lipton, R., Hall, C., & Crystal, H. (2000). Memory impairment on free and cued selective reminding predicts dementia. *Neurology, 54*, 827–834.

24. Hatakeyama, R., Fukushima, K., Fukuoka, Y., Satoh, A., Kudoh, H., Fujii, M., & Sasaki, H. (2010). Personal home-made digital video disk for patients with behavioral psychological symptoms of dementia. *Geriatrics and Gerontology, 10*, 272–274.

25. Ho, A., & Hocaoglu, M. (2011). Impact of Huntington's across the entire disease spectrum: The phases and stages of disease from the patient perspective. *Clinical Genetics, 80*, 235–239.

26. Hopper, T., Drefs, S., Bayles, K., Tomoeda, C., & Dinu, I. (2010). The effects of modified spaced-retrieval training on learning and retention of face–name associations by individuals with dementia. *Neuropsychological Rehabilitation, 20*(1), 81–102.

27. Jorm, A. (2000). Is depression a risk factor for dementia or cognitive decline? A review. *Gerontology, 48*, 219–277.

28. Kessels, R., & Hensken, L. (2009). Effects of errorless skill learning in people with mild-to-moderate or severe dementia: A randomized controlled pilot study. *NeuroRehabilitation, 25*, 307–312.

29. Klunk, W., Engler, H., Nordberg, A., Wang, Y., Blomqvist, G., Holt, D., . . . Langstrom, B. (2004). Imaging brain amyloid in Alzheimer's disease with Pittsburgh Compound-B. *Annals of Neurology, 55*, 306–319.

30. Klunk, W., Mathis, C., Price, J., Lopresti, B. Dekosky, S. (2006). Two-year follow-up of amyloid deposition in patients with Alzheimer's disease. *Brain, 129*(11), 2805–2807.

31. Kramer, A., Humphrey, D., Larish, J., Logan, G., & Strayer, D. (1994). Aging and inhibition: Beyond a unitary view of inhibitory processing attention. *Psychology and Aging, 9*, 491–512.

32. Li, G., Wang, L., Shofer, J., Thompson, M., Peskind, E., McCormick, W., . . . Larson, E. (2011). Temporal

relationship between depression and dementia. *Archives of General Psychiatry, 68*(9), 970–977.

33. Lockhart, I., Orme, M., & Mitchell, S. (2011). The efficacy of licensed-indication use of donepezil and memantine monotherapies for treating behavioral and psychological symptoms of dementia in patients with Alzheimer's disease: Systemic review and meta-analysis. *Dementia and Geriatric Cognitive Disorders, 1*, 212–227.

34. Lyketsos, C. (2010). The interface between depression and dementia: Where are we with this important frontier? *American Journal of Geriatric Psychiatry, 18*(2), 95–97.

35. Mahendra, N. (2001). Direct interventions for improving the performance of individuals with Alzheimer's disease. *Seminars in Speech and Language, 22*(1), 291–304.

36. Mahendra, N., & Hopper, T. (2013). Dementia and related cognitive disorders. In I. Papathanasiou, P. Coppens, & C. Potagas (Eds.), *Aphasia and related neurogenic disorders*. Burlington, MA: Jones & Bartlett Learning.

37. Mathers, C., & Leonardi, M. (2000). Global burden of dementia in the year 2000: Summary of methods and data sources. In *Global Burden of Disease 2000*. Geneva, Switzerland: World Health Organization.

38. McKissock, S., & Ward, J. (2007). Do errors matter? Errorless and errorful learning in anomic picture naming. *Neuropsychological Rehabilitation, 17*(3), 355–373.

39. Mulholland, C., Donoghue, D., Meenagh, C., & Rushe, T. (2008). Errorless learning and memory performance in schizophrenia. *Psychiatry Research, 159*, 180–188.

40. Orsulic-Jeras, S., Judge, K., & Camp, C. (2000). Montessori-based activities for long-term care residents with advanced dementia: Effects on engagement and affect. *The Gerontologist, 40*(1), 107–111.

41. Parkinson, J. (2002). An essay on the shaking palsy. *Journal of Neuropsychiatry and Clinical Neuroscience (Neuropsychiatry Classics), 14*(2).

42. Patel, L., & Grossberg, G. (2011). Combination therapy for Alzheimer's disease. *Drugs and Aging, 28*(7), 539–546.

43. Phillips, W., Shannon, K., & Barker, R. (2008). The current clinical management of Huntington's disease. *Movement Disorders, 23*, 1491–1504.

44. Plude, D., & Doussard-Roosevelt, J. (1989). Aging, selective attention, and feature integration. *Psychology and Aging, 4*, 98–105.

45. Pollard, J., Best, R., Imbrigilo, S., Klasner, E., Rubin, A., Sanders, G., & Simpson, W. (1999). *A caregivers handbook for advanced-stage Huntington's disease*. New York, NY: Huntington's Disease Society of America.

46. Reisberg, B., Ferris, S., de Leon, M., & Crook, T. (1982). The global deterioration scale for assessment of primary degenerative dementia. *American Journal of Psychiatry, 139*(9), 1136–1139.

47. Rickards, H., De Douza, J., van Walsem, M., van Duijn, E., Simpson, S., Squitieri, F., & Landwehmeyer, B. (2011). Factor analysis of behavioral symptoms in Huntington's disease. *Journal of Neurology and Neurosurgical Psychiatry, 82*, 411–412.

48. Roman, G. (2004). Facts, myths, and controversies in vascular dementia. *Journal of Neurological Sciences, 226*, 49–52.

49. Rosen, W., Mohs, R., & Davis, K. (1984). A new rating scale for Alzheimer's disease. *American Journal of Psychiatry, 141*(11), 1356–1364.

50. Rosenblatt, A., Abbott, M., Gourley, L., Troncoso, J., Margolis, R., Brandt, J., Ross. C. (2003). Predictors of neuropathological severity in 100 patients with Huntington's disease. *Annals of Neurology, 54*, 488–493.

51. Ross, C., Tabrizi, S. (2011). Huntington's disease: From molecular pathogenesis to clinical treatment. *The Lancet Neurology, 10*, 123–130.

52. Ruis, C., & Kessels, R. (2005). Effects of errorless and errorful face–name associative learning in moderate to severe dementia. *Aging Clinical and Experimental Research, 17*(6), 514–517.

53. Schneider, L., Dagerman, K., Higgins, J., & McShane, R. (2011). Lack of evidence for the efficacy of memantine in mild Alzheimer disease. *Archives of Neurology, 68*(8), 991–998.

54. Simard, M., & van Reekum, R. (2001). Dementia with Lewy bodies in Down syndrome. *International Journal of Geriatric Psychiatry, 16*, 311–320.

55. Stern, Y., Albert, S., Sano, M., Richards, M., Miller, L., Folstein, M. . . . Lafleche G. (1994). Assessing patient dependence in Alzheimer's disease. *Journal of Gerontology, 49*, 216–222.

56. Verghese, J., Buschke, H., Viola, L., Katz, M., & Hall, C. (2002). Validity of divided attention tasks in predicting falls in older individuals: A preliminary study. *Journal of the American Geriatric Society, 50*, 1752–1756.

57. Walker, F. (2007). Huntington's disease. *The Lancet, 363*, 218–228.

58. Wechsler, D. (1981). *Wechsler Adult Intelligence Scale—Revised*. San Antonio, TX: Psychological Corporation.

59. Xu, J., Kochanek, K., Sherry, L., Murphy, B., & Tejada-Vera, B. (2010). Deaths: Final data for 2007. In *National*

Vital Statistics Reports. Hyattsville, MD: National Center for Health Statistics.

60. Yasuda, K., Kuwabara, K., Kuwahara, N., Abe, S., & Tetsutani, N. (2009). Effectiveness of personalized reminiscence photo videos for individuals with dementia. *Neuropsychological Rehabilitation, 19*(4), 603–619.

61. Yesavage, J., Brink, T., Rose, T., Lum, O., Huang, V., Adey, M., & Leirer, V. (1983). Development and validation of a geriatric depression screening scale: A preliminary report. *Journal of Psychiatric Research, 17*, 37–49.

Chapter 10

Counseling

Cari M. Tellis, Nicholas A. Barone, and Orlando R. Barone

 Where this icon appears, visit http://go.jblearning.com/ManascoCWS to view the corresponding video.

Communication and swallowing disorders affect individuals across the life span. These disorders affect infants born with cleft palates who have difficultly feeding. Toddlers experience the effects of communication disorders when apraxia of speech prevents them from expressing their wants and needs. Adolescents who stutter might become apprehensive about speaking in public. A voice disorder can prevent a middle-aged individual from performing routine job-related activities. Dementia can cause elderly persons to forget the faces and names of loved ones. Not only do these disorders affect the patients who have them, but they also affect members of that patient's support network (friends and family).

Throughout the therapeutic process, speech-language pathologists provide information, assistance, and guidance to individuals experiencing communication and related disorders. Remediation of the disorder or reduction of its impact on patients' quality of life is the main goal of therapy. In pursuit of that objective, patients and their family and friends display a range of strong feelings and emotions, attitudes and reactions, thoughts and behaviors. Traditional therapy goals might not adequately address these concerns. For that reason, speech-language pathologists should be knowledgeable about the role counseling plays in the therapeutic process.

Counseling and Therapy

To **counsel** is to provide information, assistance, and guidance. Within every therapy activity, then, there is an element of counseling. Speech-language pathologists engage in counseling without realizing that they are doing so. Differentiating therapy and counseling is necessary only in clinicians' minds when distinguishing between how to target a patient's communication disorder and how to determine the ways the patient's communication disorder affects his or her life.

This chapter focuses on why counseling is important to speech-language pathology, especially in the treatment of individuals with neurogenic communication disorders. Also discussed are concerns that arise during therapy that can require counseling, individuals who are counseled during therapy, and counseling strategies to deal with specific issues.

Counsel To provide information, guidance, and assistance.

The Role of the Speech-Language Pathologist in Counseling

Speech-language pathologists provide a pathway to communication for individuals with neurogenic communication disorders. They are often the first rehabilitation professionals that patients see in the hospital after onset of their brain injury or diagnosis. Speech-language pathologists work with patients from the initial onset of their disorder through its entire progression. They cheer when communication is regained and persevere when communication is lost. Speech-language pathologists encounter many patient issues throughout the therapy process; it is the speech-language pathologist's job to define and deal with these issues as they arise.

Many clinicians believe that counseling is essential in the delivery of speech-language pathology services (Shipley & Roseberry-McKibbin, 2006). The main purpose of counseling patients and caregivers is to reduce the impact that negative reactions have on the therapeutic process and to promote positive progress in therapy. Not all emotions and reactions, however, are within a speech-language pathologist's scope of practice.

Speech-language pathologists' counseling should focus only on the emotions, thoughts, and behaviors patients or caregivers have that are directly related to communication disorders. If patients are depressed because they cannot remember names of common objects, understand the speech of their grandchildren, or produce intelligible speech to communicate with their spouse, speech-language pathologists can discuss with the patient how those negative emotions affect their progress in therapy. If patients are depressed because of events unrelated to their communication disorder (e.g., they have gone through a recent family or personal tragedy), speech-language pathologists should always consider referring the patient to a psychologist or psychiatrist to help the

patient deal with those negative emotions. Diagnosed or undiagnosed mental health issues are not within the speech-language pathologist's scope of practice.

Patients affected by neurogenic communication disorders are susceptible to many different forms of psychological reactions resulting from the sudden or progressive onset of communication deficits. These reactions play a key role in how patients progress or do not progress in therapy.

Speech-language pathologists cannot merely treat the communication symptoms of patients with a neurogenic communication disorder and ignore the psychological effects involved in coping with the loss of those communicative abilities, especially if these effects are inhibiting rehabilitation. Speech-language pathologists should have an understanding of the different types of emotional reactions that patients or caregivers might have following the onset of a neurogenic communication disorder and understand how to counter them to create more productive treatment outcomes.

Emotional Reactions: Cause and Effect

Certainly after a brain injury of any kind, patients experience some degree of loss of function as well as the accompanying emotional reactions associated with impairments of communication, swallowing, and the impacts these deficits have on activities of daily living (ADLs). Many debate, however, the extent to which the brain injury itself is the direct organic cause of these emotional reactions or whether the emotions are a psychological effect of the loss from the injury (Binder, Robling, & Larrabee, 1997; King, 1996; Lishman, 1988; Tanner, 2003).

The speech-language pathologist must consider the location of the brain injury and any known psychoemotional signs associated with damage to that area. For example, individuals with right hemisphere brain damage are often jovial, euphoric, or lack appropriate expression of emotion while individuals with left hemisphere injuries often experience anxiety or depression (Tanner, 2010). Individuals with injury to the frontal lobe and limbic system might exhibit disinterest, apathy, mania, irritability, and emotional lability (Absher & Cummings, 1995; Malia, Powell, & Torode, 1995; Mattson & Levin, 1990; Stuss & Benson, 1984, 1986; Stuss, Gow, & Hetherington, 1992). Focal brain lesions, however, are not the only organic cause for an emotional response. Individuals with mild traumatic brain injury (concussion) exhibit higher levels of depression than normal controls (Mathias & Coats, 1999).

Separating out the effects of the primary injury or disease from the psychological reaction to the disorder is difficult. Some researchers believe that the emotional response to the deficit and the emotional lability caused by the deficit are not easy to distinguish. These researchers believe that the emotional reactions are a result of the primary injury or disease as well as the psychological reaction to the loss of function (communication or otherwise) (Binder et al., 1997; King, 1996; Lishman, 1988). Organic causes for emotional response following injury or disease to the brain can be a decrease in serotonin and/or dopamine levels (Tanner, 2010). Preexisting psychological conditions could also contribute to patients' psychological response to the injury. The presence of preexisting psychological disorders should be determined prior to the evaluation by speech-language pathologists.

Negative emotional reactions can significantly affect progress in therapy for patients with disease or trauma to the brain. Speech-language pathologists should work closely with psychologists or psychiatrists to determine if medical management for some of these psychological issues is warranted. Masand and Chaudhary (1994) describe a patient with aphasia who exhibited signs of depression following his stroke. This patient was very resistant to therapy and was unwilling to participate in any of the activities the speech-language pathologist planned for him. However, once the patient began taking an antidepressant, his willingness to participate in therapy increased and he made significant progress toward his goals. When the antidepressant was removed, however, he quickly regressed and stopped making gains in therapy. The job of speech-language pathologists in these cases is to recognize the emotion, consider its cause, and refer to a professional trained in the medical management of these psychological issues.

Author's Note

Power of Emotion

One weekend I covered for a speech-language pathologist at a rehabilitation hospital. The first patient I saw that morning was a 66-year-old professor who sustained a bilateral brain stem stroke following surgery on his leg 3 weeks prior. He had been receiving speech-language pathology services for 2 weeks. The patient presented with a severe delay in speech initiation (30+ seconds). He lacked the ability to initiate speech even when in pain and was unmotivated in therapy. He had a severe bilateral paresis from the neck down. The physical and occupational therapists said his progress was slow because of his lack of motivation. The speech-language pathologist's note stated that his wife was very involved and was present at nearly every speech therapy session. The speech-language pathologist attributed all communication deficits to the injury he incurred from the stroke.

When I entered his room I could clearly observe that his speech was severely delayed. The nurse in the room asked him a couple of questions, "How are you feeling?" and "How has your day been so far?" His answers were short and concise, "Fine." She introduced me, and I spoke to him briefly about him growing up in the same area where my family had resided. As we spoke, I noticed his delay became nearly nonexistent.

(Continues)

After we conversed for a minute or two, the nurse left the room and said goodbye. He nodded at her. He followed this gesture with a question directed at me, which he initiated without any prompts. He fluently asked, "Do you have any questions for me?" Surprised, but quick to jump at the opportunity, I responded with, "Do you find that it is hard to get the words out sometimes?" After a moment of apparent reflection (not a disordered delay), he replied, "Sometimes it is hard to get the words out when you are so sad all the time."

Later in my visit, while his wife waited outside in the hall, I discussed with the gentleman how hard it must be to be thrust suddenly from a position of strength and importance, taking care of and providing for his wife, to being completely dependent on others for everything. With a mild speech delay, he recounted how he had once dug a pond in his backyard. With his hands, he had moved several yards of dirt to landscape a large garden pond for his wife. He then pointed out that every day in physical therapy they had him digging with his hand in small buckets of dirt. How far he had fallen. He had physical therapy directly before speech therapy every day, and he was angry, upset, and ashamed by the reminders of the degree of his loss even before speech therapy began. He then said that he had to control his emotions in front of his wife and the other speech-language pathologist because it was "unmanly to cry in front of a woman." He had no problem expressing his emotions to another man, but as his wife came back in the room, the tears stopped and the severely delayed speech returned.

Given the negative emotional reactions detailed in this anecdote, how can this man's deficits in communication be perceived? Were the behaviors he exhibited caused solely by the stroke, or was he exhibiting negative emotional reactions to the loss he incurred? Was he crying because of an emotional lability caused by the injury to his brain, or was there another reason he was having such a strong emotional response?

There are many possible answers to these questions. Regardless of the exact cause of his emotional response there was an error made in the diagnosis of a severe speech delay. The man's loss of physical abilities along with his need to be strong and stoic when in the presence of women created a scenario where a mild speech delay presented itself and then was diagnosed as severe. His lack of initiation of speech occurred because he was ashamed to admit he was struggling with his loss of physical ability.

Taking into account the patient's emotional state and using counseling strategies such as asking open-ended questions, probing, and using listening skills, the speech-language pathologist treating this man might have made a more accurate assessment of the patient's speech delay. Therapy could have taken a different route. By finding out more about the patient, the speech-language pathologist could have developed better rapport and credibility, and thus had more success in therapy.

Communicating with the physical therapist about using alternatives to digging in dirt, the speech-language pathologist could have spared the patient the pain and embarrassment he felt during the speech therapy sessions. Talking about how his loss, sadness, guilt, and shame negatively affected his speech and hindered his progress might have given him more ownership of his goals and provided a purpose to therapy. Considering the extent of his depression, the speech-language pathologist could have referred the patient to a social worker, psychologist, or psychiatrist for further counseling or possible medical management. When a patient lacks motivation, the speech-language pathologist needs to consider the cause and then address the issues systematically.

Stages of Grief

Kübler-Ross (1969) suggests five stages in the grieving process: denial, anger, bargaining, depression, and acceptance. Struggling through the stages of grief is completely natural and healthy for people experiencing a loss (Tanner, 2003). Problems begin when people become bogged down in the emotions of one stage or another and cannot find their way out. When this happens, any of the first four stages of grief can be categorized as negative reactions, with the fifth stage being the ultimate aim of anyone experiencing loss. Though there are clearly defined stages of grief, it is important to remember that patients and caregivers might not proceed through the stages in a linear process, they might not experience all stages, and they might revert to a previous stage once they have moved forward. People experiencing the stages of grief can also jump around from stage to stage or exhibit characteristics of more than a single stage at one time (Kübler-Ross, 1969; Shipley & Roseberry-McKibbin, 2006).

Denial

Stage one is denial. When patients experience a brain injury or are diagnosed with a progressive neurogenic communication disorder, denial can be their initial reaction. While in this stage, patients really believe there is nothing wrong and that there will never be anything wrong with their speech, language, cognition, or a related area. Denial is usually counterproductive to the therapeutic process but can sometimes be useful as patients work through the shock associated with the initial trauma or diagnosis.

When patients are in denial they readily confabulate or fabricate explanations for any change in their speech or communication. They might blame others for their issues and might even dismiss compelling evidence speech-language pathologists offer to support the reality of the problems they are experiencing. Speech-language pathologists need to be patient with individuals in this stage. Patients need time to fully digest the information if they are hearing bad news for the first time. The speech-language pathologist needs to be clear and straightforward with the information provided, including results of testing, recommendations, and referrals. Using objective data patients cannot dispute such as charts or standardized results can make it easier for patients to see the reality of their problem. The speech-language pathologist can provide handouts with information about the disorder to patients and their families. The patients and families need time to ask questions. Patients can remain in denial for a long time, but when they are ready to move on, they most likely enter stage two, anger.

Anger

Stage two is anger. In this stage, patients ask, "Why me?" They are furious that this terrible thing is happening to them. Counseling patients when they are angry is often difficult. They might feel a lack of ownership because they feel out of control. This anger can lead to frustration in therapy. Sometimes they project their anger as resentment toward the "lucky ones" who are not dealing with their disorder. Speech-language pathologists can also be a target of their anger. It is important for therapists to remain calm and not be defensive in these situations. Often becoming defensive makes patients become more angry and frustrated.

It is important for the speech-language pathologist to validate patients' feelings. Statements like, "I can see that this is very hard for you" or "You appear really angry right now" give patients an opportunity to talk about their anger and frustration. Focus should be on the patients' objectives and goals. Patients might be more likely to move through the anger stage if they begin to see improvement and feel they are making progress toward their goals. Many patients, however, revisit this stage when they advance to more difficult therapeutic goals or face new obstacles related to their disorder.

Bargaining

Stage three is bargaining. In this stage patients are looking for hope. They often look to a higher being to make a deal. In return for making their problem go away, patients promise to change something in their lives for the better or give up something they value. When counseling patients in this stage it is useful to remind patients that bargaining is a stage within the grieving process. Although it is natural for patients to want to bargain, speech-language pathologists need to stress that though the patient can find comfort in their belief in a higher being, there are no real bargains to be made. Therapists must not confuse bargaining with hopefulness. Patients in the bargaining stage are often expressing a sign of desperation. If the patients perceive that the bargain has not panned out, patients can find themselves in stage four.

Depression

Stage four is depression. Patients within this stage have lost their sense of purpose. They can appear apathetic, unmotivated, or discouraged. Discouragement actually means *a loss of heart*. These patients often display true sadness, a lack of hope, the feeling that therapy is worthless and that there is no use in trying. The job of speech-language pathologists at this point is to help the patient find their hopefulness; encourage them. Highlight the progress they have made so far. Keep the patient focused on what they know they can do, and keep them connected to their support system. Speech-language pathologists must be careful not to use slogans like, "Don't worry, be happy" or tell patients that their progress in therapy is all up to them. Neither of these tactics helps to empower patients. They might end up feeling more alone.

Patients in the depression stage can also become clinically depressed. If their sadness extends to their everyday living, and they stop eating, communicating, or getting out of bed, then the therapist must consider a referral to a licensed psychologist or psychiatrist. Whether the depression is organic to the brain injury or diagnosed as clinical depression, the attention of a medical professional is warranted.

Depression, regardless of whether it is clinical or not, is a difficult stage to work through. Be mindful that it is a stage in the grieving process and one that must run its course for patients to muster the strength to move forward.

Acceptance

Stage five is acceptance. This is the stage speech-language pathologists want their patients to reach in therapy. As patients move from one stage to another, they leave behind negative states to move in a positive direction toward acceptance. Their movement is a sign of progress because none of the first four stages are ideal stages to stay in for the long term. As they begin to accept their deficits and disorder, they begin to realize how they will need to integrate their communication issues into their lives to move forward. Acceptance should not be seen as complacency or simply succumbing to the disorder or loss. Acceptance signals the patients' willingness to participate in realistic therapy. There are limitations, but those are a matter of degree; no one has unlimited potential. Speech-language pathologists must work to set

Author's Note

Stages of Grief in the Real World

I have seen many individuals who have sustained traumatic brain injuries progress through the stages of grief in a typical manner. Once they are discharged from inpatient rehabilitation services, many of them begin to deny that there is a problem. Some attempt to return to work or resume their normal activities of daily living. Denial is apparent: "These are just the lingering effects of being in the hospital," they say. Once the deficits become obvious either through patients' own realization or the constant observations made by friends and families, patients typically contact their doctor, angry at the injustice of it all. "It's not fair" or "I should be able to do the things I want to do" are some of the ways they express their anger. Before coming back for therapy, patients start to bargain, "Please, God, if you get me through this, I'll live a better life." Upon the full realization that there are real communication issues, patients become unmotivated and depressed, "Why should I even try?" Once they arrive at acceptance, they often take responsibility for their own well-being and really begin the progress toward recovery. "I'm ready."

appropriate goals and make a plan to achieve those goals, while keeping in mind the patients' quality of life.

Negative Attitudes and Emotions

The onset of negative attitudes and emotions can occur at any time post acquisition of a neurogenic communication disorder (Hackett, Yapa, Parag, & Anderson, 2005). Patients experience a myriad of emotions throughout the five stages of grief. Some emotions are seen more in one stage than another (e.g., apathy in the stage of depression). Speech-language pathologists need to be cognizant of changes in the mood, attitude, motivation, and affect of patients and must deal with them when they are first noticed.

Negative reactions can also manifest later in recovery as trauma to the brain begins to heal and feelings of euphoria give way to the reality of patients' situation. The opposite can also occur as the brain heals; emotional lability can decline and emotional balance might be restored. This balance can reduce the occurrence of negative reactions that were present at the onset of treatment.

Speech-language pathologists must remember that clients are not the only individuals who can experience negative reactions to disease or diagnosis of a neurogenic communication disorder. Caregivers, family members, and friends of the patients have their own reactions. Speech-language pathologists should be prepared to counsel both patients and caregivers throughout the treatment process. Counseling strategies and techniques used to deal with members of the patients' support system are discussed later in this chapter.

Some of the more common negative emotional reactions and attitudes patients and their support system face are discussed in the following subsections.

Depression

Depression can be observed in people with any etiology that results in neurogenic communication disorders. **Depression** is a disorder characterized by an abnormally low mood that affects individuals' daily lives. Sometimes depression can be organic in nature, meaning that the depression is the result of a chemical imbalance in the brain caused directly by the injury sustained to the brain (Craig & Cummings, 1995; Tanner, 2003). Mathias and Coats (1999) found that patients and their caregivers reported an increased level of depression following the onset of a traumatic brain injury (TBI). Results of research on individuals who have had a stroke indicate that nearly 33% of these individuals showed symptoms of depression (Hackett et al., 2005). The co-occurrence of depression and dementia has been reported to be as high as 87% (Merriam, Aronson, Gaston, Wey, & Katz, 1988), but a more likely estimate is between 26% and 34% (Ballard, Bannister, Solis, Oyebode, & Wilcock, 1996; Panza et al., 2010). Successfully treating depression in individuals with dementia can lead to better cognition but not a full recovery from depression because it will typically continue to develop later in the progression of the dementia (Korczyn & Halperin, 2009). As mentioned previously, individuals showing signs of depression should be referred to the appropriate mental health professionals.

> **Depression** A disorder characterized by abnormally low mood that affects individuals' daily lives.

The ability to recognize the symptoms of clinical depression is imperative to speech-language therapy because appropriate medical treatment can increase the likelihood that patients will achieve their therapeutic goals. Following is a list of signs and symptoms of depression (National Institute of Mental Health [NIMH], 2011):

- Anxiety/agitation
- Irritability or uncharacteristic anger
- Crying for no apparent reason

- Persistent feelings of sadness, hopelessness, pessimism, guilt, helplessness, worthlessness
- Lack of interest in things that once brought pleasure, including hobbies and sex
- Abnormal levels of fatigue
- Sleep changes: Difficulty sleeping or sleeping too much
- Appetite changes: Eating too little or eating too much
- Changes in weight
- Thoughts of dying, death, or suicide
- Restlessness
- Difficulties with concentration, memory, and decision making

Demotivation

Motivation is the achievement of a balanced state among a patient's sense of purpose, perception of growth or improvement, and ownership of goals, therapy, and the therapy process (Barone, 1986; Tellis & Barone, in press). **Demotivation** is the lack of this balanced state and a lack of ownership of goals and the therapy process. The patient must feel connected to the goals by purpose, growth, and ownership. Counseling strategies are employed in therapy to maintain or create this balance. If even one connection is faulty or missing, patients can become demotivated, and therapy progress suffers.

Apathetic patients lack emotion or feeling. They might simply tune out during therapy sessions, shrug their shoulders, or procrastinate on assignments. These patients are experiencing a disconnection in purpose. Patients who are bored can appear apathetic, but these patients lack a balance in their growth connection. Therapy

Motivation The achievement of a balanced state among an individual's sense of purpose, perception of growth or improvement, and ownership of his or her goals, therapy, and the therapy process.

Demotivation The lack of a balance between ownership of goals and the therapy process.

tasks might be too hard or too easy. The job of speech-language pathologists is to figure out the right balance among tasks that are challenging, but not too challenging; achievable, yet not too simple. Frustrated patients are disconnected from the ownership connection; they feel the control has been taken from them. For these patients, speech-language pathologists must find a way to restore choices, remove what patients feel is forcing them to therapy, and help them feel that the therapy goals and the therapy process are theirs. Addressing demotivation by finding creative ways to balance the connections among purpose, growth, and ownership should be one of the first priorities of speech-language pathologists.

Anxiety

When frustration becomes extreme and patients feel an intense ownership disconnection, they can become anxious. Anxiety should be distinguished from fear. Whereas fear is an appropriate response to something that is threatening, **anxiety** is a generalized mood that might or might not have a known cause. Anxiety can lead to a catastrophic negative reaction in individuals with neurogenic communication disorders, for example, irritability, crying, anger, striking out, withdrawal, fainting, and/or depression (Tanner, 2003). Speech-language pathologists must attempt to restore ownership within these patients. If the cause of the anxiety is unknown and begins to permeate the patients' lives, then speech-language pathologists should recommend a referral to a psychologist or psychiatrist for further treatment.

Anxiety A generalized mood with primary emotional components of apprehensiveness and unease.

Avoidance The act of refusing engagement in a task that is deemed undesirable.

Avoidance or Escape Behaviors

Avoidance and escape behaviors are negative reactions people use to remove themselves from an unpleasant, stressful, or feared situation or task (Carlat, 1999; Carson, Butcher, & Coleman, 1988; Tanner, 2003). Avoidance is the act of refusing engagement in a task that is deemed undesirable by the patient. Resistance can be one of the initial signs of avoidance. Patients who are resistant are usually overwhelmed, obsessed, or frustrated. At first, obsession might appear to be a positive reaction. Once patients do nothing but therapy, however, they become too narrowly focused and growth becomes restricted. Patients can become overwhelmed when a task is too challenging. This can lead to a lack of control and ownership, resulting in frustration and then avoidance. When patients physically try to remove themselves from the situation or task, they are not only avoiding but are trying to escape. Speech-language pathologists should step back and make tasks or exercises more achievable. Assess why patients are resisting therapy and discuss any fears they might be having.

Displacement and Projection

Displacement and projection is when patients transfer their own feelings of anxiety, fear, loss, or stress onto another person for the sake of reducing those feelings within themselves (Stuart, 2001a). If the therapist notices that patients are exhibiting an emotional response that does not seem justified by interactions with the speech-language pathologist or with therapy tasks, he or she should consider that patients might be displacing an emotional response onto the clinician. This displaced response might be intended for a physician, nurse, family member, or friend with whom the patients are actually upset with but fail to confront. Displacement and projection are frequently directed toward speech-language pathologists when patients are experiencing pain or discomfort, undergoing an uncomfortable

Displacement and projection When patients transfer their own feelings of anxiety, fear, loss, or stress onto another person for the sake of reducing those feelings within themselves.

medical treatment or painful procedure, learning a new therapy technique, or encountering a difficult emotional situation (Tanner, 2003).

Speech-language pathologists should remain calm and not become defensive. Remember, if patients are projecting or displacing their emotions onto the speech-language pathologist, the reaction is really not meant for the clinician. They should encourage patients to talk about their emotions and then validate patients' feelings with empathetic responses such as, "I can see that you are very frustrated right now" or "You seem more upset today than you were yesterday." Provide time for patients to respond. They might be having difficulty expressing or communicating their feelings, and speech-language pathologists can work those goals into therapy.

Disassociation

Disassociation is when patients or caregivers unconsciously remove themselves emotionally from painful, stressful, or upsetting situations to alleviate emotional stress (Carlat, 1999; Stuart, 2001b; Tanner, 2003). This phenomenon is often seen in people who have aphasia (Tanner, 2003). An extreme form of disassociation is fainting. This catastrophic negative reaction results in a loss of consciousness, which can increase safety concerns and decrease motivation.

Disassociation When patients or caregivers unconsciously remove themselves emotionally from painful, stressful, or upsetting situations to alleviate emotional stress.

Speech-language pathologists should stay attuned to patients' and caregivers' reactions during interactions with them. If they seem to be newly distant toward the speech-language pathologist or inexplicably unbothered by their current situation, then the speech-language pathologist might have reason to believe they are dissociating themselves from their loss. Again, speech-language pathologists should encourage them to discuss or express their feelings in the way that they can. Sometimes just keeping the patient company, playing a game, or engaging in conversation apart from therapy helps patients to feel comforted and less alone.

Passive Aggression

Passive aggression is an indirect negative reaction expressed toward others that is masked by timidity and passivity (Burgess & Clements, 1998; Kolb, 1977). Patients exhibiting passive aggression might indicate that they are fine with therapy but then refuse to participate in therapy activities or make excuses for why they cannot participate. Passive aggression can present as hostility toward speech-language pathologists or therapy. Hostility is indirectly expressed toward others through frustrating behaviors such as procrastination, delaying, or a lack of interest and motivation (Tanner, 2003). These behaviors can seemingly manifest for unknown reasons. Passive aggression is often confused with memory deficits, delayed responses, erratic behavior, and apathy. Any person with a severe neurogenic communication disorder can exhibit passive-aggressive behavior (Tanner, 2003). The best recourse for passive aggression is to provide an open, nonthreatening environment for patients to discuss their feelings and emotions.

Passive aggression An indirect negative reaction expressed toward others that is masked by timidity and passivity.

Repression Occurs when an individual suppresses acknowledgment of the negative experiences that are the result of his or her deficits.

Repression

Repression is similar to denial in that patients consciously suppress the negative experiences that are the result of their deficits (Stuart, 2001a; Tanner, 2003). When patients repress their emotions, they often become more dependent on others to help them. By becoming more reliant on others and engaging in dependent relationships with therapists, nurses,

or doctors, patients can find comfort in the reduction of stressful or anxious situations. This negative reaction is particularly prevalent in the early stages of recovery. If enabled, people exhibiting regression show a lack of motivation to progress in therapy for fear that the object of their dependency will no longer be available to them (Tanner, 2003).

To counsel effectively in all these situations, speech-language pathologists need to build rapport and develop relationships with patients. They should, however, be sure to keep professional boundaries. Patients need to know that although speech-language pathologists are there for them, the patients themselves are in control of their therapy and have ownership of the process. Speech-language pathologists should always provide opportunities for patients to achieve small successes. When patients experience success independent of speech-language pathologists, they are likely to believe in themselves and their abilities and be less likely to rely on others.

Adoption of Learned Helplessness and the Sick Role

When patients feel they need to rely or depend on others for their care, they might begin to show signs of learned helplessness—a feeling of being comfortable with the uncomfortable. **Learned helplessness** is a condition in which a person behaves in a helpless manner even though he or she has opportunities to improve their situation. Patients who feel a lack of ownership and control might resort to owning the sick role or helpless role because it is the only part of their life they feel they have control over. This negative reaction is detrimental to the therapy process because learned helplessness stems from a lack of hope, the feeling that patients cannot escape their

Learned helplessness A condition in which a person behaves in a helpless manner even though he or she has opportunities to improve the situation.

current situation. No matter how bad it is, they begin to accept it, and give up trying to change.

Caregivers can enable patients' learned helplessness. Loved ones or family members might have had no prior experience at being caregivers. However, as a result of patients' disease or diagnosis, they have been thrown into the caregiver role. In the midst of so many new changes they cannot control, loved ones or family members begin to identify with the caregiver role and feel they have control over that responsibility. Although this is a natural response to the loss, counseling caregivers about this response is important. Speech-language pathologists should involve caregivers in the patients' therapy and provide them with responsibilities and assignments that encourage patients' independence. They should counsel caregivers about how important it is to keep patients motivated, remembering the balance between purpose, growth, and ownership. Patients and caregivers who feel that they have individual roles in a team approach to therapy can work together better to empower patients' improvement and recovery.

Loss

Loss is one of the most consistent reactions that people with neurogenic communication disorders experience (Tanner, 2003). People with neurogenic communication disorders and their caregivers and family can feel loss on many levels (Tanner, 1999). These include the loss of communicative abilities, separation from loved ones, loss of independence because of physical limitations, and loss of the life that they had previously known (Tanner, 2003). Many times the loss occurs suddenly, without notice or without time to prepare, but losses can also be drawn out, made deeper and more painful as an illness progressively degrades a person's ability to communicate over months or years.

Tanner (1980) categorizes loss as real or tangible, such as the loss of a loved one or ability, or symbolic,

which might be the loss of a person's self-concept such as a position of prominence in the family. There are three dimensions of real and symbolic loss (Tanner, 2003; Tanner & Gerstenberger, 1988). Loss of self is the sense that patients have lost their own identity, how they define themselves related to their loss of ability and/or function. Loss of person is the psychological separation from a loved one a person can experience after the acquisition of a neurogenic communication disorder. Loss of object is loss caused by the resulting disability following the acquisition of a neurogenic communication disorder. Objects patients might feel they have lost are a real sense of home or workplace.

Loss can be the result of organic changes to the brain caused by injury or disease, or it can be an expression of the emotional reactions of patients or caregivers. Regardless of the cause of the loss, speech-language pathologists should always acknowledge a grievous loss by listening to patients and caregivers, reducing frustration, and always focusing counseling on making positive progress in treatment. The overwhelming sense of loss that patients or caregivers feel often manifests itself in the stages of grief.

Counseling and the Patient

Tellis and Barone (in press) developed the Counseling-Integration (CI) Matrix. This matrix has four quadrants and pairs the patients' perceived negative impact of their disorder on their quality of life with the patients' willingness to change. Quadrant 1 (Q1), High-High, depicts patients who are experiencing a high negative impact on their quality of a life and a high willingness to change. These patients are energized, eager, dissatisfied, or curious. Patients in quadrant 2 (Q2), High-Low, are experiencing a high negative impact on their quality of life and a low willingness to change. These patients are frustrated, unhappy, resistant, or defeated. In quadrant 3

(Q3), Low-Low, are patients who have a low negative impact on their quality of life and a low willingness to change. Patients in this quadrant are complacent, uninvolved, uncooperative, or indifferent. Quadrant 4 (Q4), Low-High, is the last quadrant. Patients in this quadrant are often reaching the maintenance and generalization phase; they are experiencing a low negative impact on their quality of life and a high willingness to change. Some of the emotional reactions of patients within this quadrant are comfortable, agreeable, controlling, and ready.

Speech-language pathologists need to continually assess the patients' place on the CI Matrix. The degree to which speech-language pathologists counsel patients and the counseling strategies employed depend on which quadrants the patients occupy. Q1 patients are experiencing a negative impact on their quality of life. Although these patients are motivated and probably eager to begin therapy, counseling focuses on providing information about the disorder or disease progression, involving patients and caregivers in making goals and designing the treatment plan, and keeping patients' and caregivers' emotional reactions in check.

Counseling strategies become more necessary with Q2 and Q3 patients because their willingness to change begins to lessen. Speech-language pathologists need to be cognizant of changes in patients' motivational balance. Determine which connections have been lost—purpose, growth, ownership—and counsel patients to reestablish those connections. As patients move into quadrant 4, counseling strategies focus on minimizing the role of speech-language pathologists in the therapy process. Patients recovering from a brain injury who are in quadrant 4 are ready to continue the recovery process alone. They have an established support system and have reached their potential in therapy. Patients with a diagnosis of a progressive disease such as Alzheimer's disease or Huntington's disease might never fully reach quadrant 4. The job of speech-language pathologists is to counsel the patients' caregivers and support system to maintain the patients' quality of life as they deal with end-of-life issues.

Although patients often begin in quadrant 1 and progress through the CI Matrix in numeric order, progression through the matrix is not always a linear process. Patients and caregivers can assume a place in any of the quadrants at any point in therapy. They can start in one quadrant, revert back to an earlier quadrant, and then jump to another quadrant. The patient and caregiver also might not assume the same quadrant at the same time. When there is a conflict with caregivers' and patients' place in the matrix, counseling becomes more important. Take for example a Q1 caregiver, high negative impact on quality of life and high willingness to change, with a Q3 patient, low negative impact on quality of life and a low willingness to change. The caregiver's desire for the patient to participate in therapy is in direct conflict with the patient's unwillingness to participate. Counseling both the patient and caregiver in this example is vitally important.

Many different counseling options are available to speech-language pathologists, and it is the clinician's job to find a method that best suits patients' needs and coincides with the clinician's strengths. No matter which counseling method speech-language pathologists employ, several universal themes enhance any counseling approach and facilitate relationship building between patient and clinician.

- *Build a good rapport with patients.* The cornerstone of all productive therapy and counseling is creating a positive rapport with patients. Rapport comes more quickly when patients feel that they can trust speech-language pathologists. Their relationship with their speech-language pathologist is based on mutual respect. A house can be built only from the foundation up. Rapport is the foundation on which all treatment and counseling approaches are built. If rapport is the foundation of productive therapy, then trust and mutual respect are the mortar and bricks. If rapport has not been established, patients might not trust and respect the treatment methods and recommendations posed by speech-language pathologists. Patients' mistrust of speech-language pathologists creates a barrier to progress in therapy along with potential risks to patient well-being and health.

Rapport can begin before the patient is even met, but it surely is defined by the initial interactions therapists have with patients. Speech-language pathologists need to be sure to make a good first impression. They must introduce themselves appropriately, make good eye contact, and smile. They should take some time to get to know patients before delving right into the evaluation or therapy. The time invested in getting to know patients can help when struggles arise in therapy. At that point, speech-language pathologists will know that they can relate to patients on a personal level.

- *Help patients voice their concerns and have them assist in creating a plan of care to achieve their goals.* Many people with neurogenic communication disorders are not given the opportunity to voice their concerns because of the communication deficits they have acquired. Often speech-language pathologists are the catalyst for advocating communication by patients to caregivers, doctors, and therapists. Speech-language pathologists hold the distinction of being the person many patients turn to when they have concerns about recovery, treatment, and communication deficits. By allowing patients to play an integral part in the creation of goals and always listening to their concerns, speech-language pathologists give their patients a sense of control and a connection to the therapy they are receiving.
- *Avoid contributing to patient frustration.* Creating a positive atmosphere where progress and accomplishments are highlighted, while

negative reactions and errors are diminished, generates an environment which facilitates success. As stated previously, patients who deem certain tasks too difficult or too easy often become frustrated. Frustration is one of the most common demotivators and often results in negative reactions (Tanner, 2003). Speech-language pathologists must carefully walk the line when increasing task difficulty to promote progress in therapy. They might push patients too hard and bring about an increase in errors on task, leading to a feeling of failure by patients. A good rule of thumb for decreasing frustration is to begin with a task that has a very high success rate, and then slowly increase the difficulty level as patients achieve their goals. Adopting this order of treatment can offset the negative feelings of failure with the positive encouragement of success.

- *Acknowledge and allow patients to experience the grieving process and help them through it.* The grieving process is a well-established healthy reaction patients experience after sustaining a loss of any kind (Tanner, 2003). By acknowledging and allowing patients to progress through the grieving process, speech-language pathologists create a safe place where patients are encouraged to explore their feelings of loss and regain their sense of self. Speech-language pathologists can play a central role in continuing the progress of the grieving process through to acceptance, but must also be aware that certain actions and statements can have a negative effect on patients (Tanner, 2003). Therapists must always keep in mind that they are guests that have been invited by the patient to share in a very personal journey. Ultimately, the foundation of trust and respect, hearing the concerns of patients, avoiding frustration, and acknowledging the grieving process enable speech-language pathologists to steer patients down a road that helps them quickly adjust to the new challenges in their life.

Speech-language pathology services focus on the treatment of communication deficits; however, progress in therapy can hinge on the emotional reactions of the patients and, more important, how well they are counseled to deal with those reactions. The emotional reactions of caregivers, family, and friends are also important to the recovery process. Finding creative ways to keep caregivers involved encourages carry-over from the therapy room to the home environment. Caregivers and family members can be a blessing, but they can also become a hindrance to recovery. The ability to counsel them effectively ensures patients' continued success in therapy.

Counseling and the Caregiver

Patients' caregivers, family, and friends can be both helpful and potentially harmful to the therapeutic process. The type of caregivers patients have can be a determining factor in how successful patients are in therapy. For some people, the family dynamic shifts dramatically when the primary provider and caregiver is the one who is experiencing a neurogenic communication disorder. This shift of roles can create obstacles for both patients and new primary caregivers. Upon meeting caregivers and family of patients, the speech-language pathologist should quickly assess them and figure out what role, if any, they will play in aiding in patients' therapy.

Different Types of Caregivers

Ideal caregivers are supportive, motivating, helpful, and empathetic of patients' situations. These caregivers can put aside their own feelings of loss to better facilitate recovery of their loved ones. Conversely, caregivers who are detracting, demotivating, enabling, or sympathizing can cause an interruption of progress toward goals and an increase in patients' negative reactions. Most caregivers are helpful to therapy but can at times possess characteristics that can negatively affect the therapeutic process.

Speech-language pathologists should always be aware that caregivers might not be able to be 100% supportive; they too are coping with a significant loss in their lives. Most negative traits in caregivers can be transferred to positive traits by educating caregivers on the communication deficits their loved ones are experiencing, communicating to them the needs of patients, as well as listening to what they have to say and how their loved ones' communication deficits have affected them. The following are descriptions of some of the more common types of caregivers.

- *Supporter versus detractor.* Supportive caregivers have a positive impact on the motivation of patients and the progress that patients make in therapy, while detractors can have a decidedly less positive impact. Where supporters encourage patients and do not take time away from therapy, detractors diminish the importance and value of the therapy, often causing negative reactions by patients and lost time during the treatment sessions. Speech-language pathologists can turn detractors into supporters by empathizing with their situation, listening to their concerns, and encouraging them to show more supportive behavior.

- *Motivator versus demotivator.* Similar to supporters, motivators aid patients in staying positive and persevering throughout therapy. Demotivators do just the opposite: They cause stress in patients and can sometimes cause catastrophic negative responses, including avoidance, regression, and projection. Without motivation and a desire to improve, patients usually have a much less successful experience in therapy. Turning demotivators into motivators is sometimes a difficult task. Speech-language pathologists should plan a meeting with the caregiver to encourage the person to be a helpful partner in the therapy process. Sometimes caregivers need to be given a role with specific responsibilities. Once they understand their role, they might be more inclined to participate more productively in the therapy process. If the meeting is not successful, then sometimes the best recourse in dealing with demotivators is to adjust therapy schedules to see patients when caregivers are not present.

- *Helper versus enabler.* Helpers do not have trained speech-language pathology skills, but they are caregivers who have the ability to grasp the concepts taught by speech-language pathologists and generalize those concepts to environments outside the clinical experience. Within each therapy session, helpers will try to absorb what speech-language pathologists are doing so that they can continue providing some level of support after the session has ended. Helpers are invaluable to the therapeutic process.

  Enablers think they are helping patients; however, their words and actions usually encourage unproductive behaviors rather than positive ones. Enablers often show no interest in therapy and their actions often counter speech-language pathologists' recommendations or suggestions. These caregivers are usually feeling a tremendous sense of loss and a need to be needed. Speech-language pathologists should provide an open, safe environment for these individuals to discuss their feelings. They should be honest with them about the impact of their actions, educate them on the patients' deficits, and involve them in the process. Speech-language pathologists also need to strive to empower patients to be responsible for their lives and choices and to self advocate.

- *Empathizer versus sympathizer.* The difference between empathy and sympathy is sometimes difficult to discern, but it is an important distinction to make. Empathy is identifying with, sharing in, and understanding patients' circumstances (Shipley & Roseberry-McKibbin, 2006). **Empathizers** are attuned to patients. They seek to learn about the disorder and the related deficits. They are involved in therapy and encourage recovery. **Sympathizers**, however, feel sorry for patients. They often show little understanding of the patients' emotions. Their deep sorrow for their loved one's situation often obstructs any help they can offer in therapy. Caregivers cannot seek a better understanding of their loved ones' circumstance when sympathizing.

> **Empathizer** Caregivers who are attuned to patient needs. They seek to learn about the disorder and related deficits.
>
> **Sympathizer** Caregivers who feel sorry for patients and show little understanding of the patients' emotions.

Speech-language pathologists need to encourage empathizers and reinforce their behavior as helpful. Dealing with sympathizers is more difficult. Speech-language pathologists should provide opportunities for sympathizers to discuss their feelings with their loved ones. They should be open to questions sympathizers have. Sometimes these caregivers benefit just from knowing more about the process. Therapists can show sympathizers when progress is made in therapy. When they see that patients are improving, or that patients are accepting their deficits, they might be more inclined to accept the situation themselves.

Examples of Different Types of Caregivers

The following scenarios are a thought exercise depicting different types of patients and caregivers you, the speech-language pathologist in these scenes, might encounter.

Scenario 1: A young woman sustained a severe TBI from a car accident. She exhibits severe cognitive, orientation, attention, and language deficits. She has a large, supportive family and is never alone in her room. They are very friendly and eager to know how you will be able to help the patient. When you try to conduct your evaluation, everyone stays in the room and the television remains on. You express to the family that the patient needs reduced stimulation and noise during the evaluation. They do not seem to understand, remarking that everyone is there to provide love and support. The family will not leave the room or quiet down. As you continue the evaluation, the patient's parents listen intently and ask questions about what they can to do to help aid in her recovery.

Scenario 2: An elderly man shows signs of dementia and swallowing deficits. He was recently hospitalized following respiratory failure resulting from pneumonia and a urinary tract infection with sepsis. He is on a puréed diet with thickened liquids. His daughter is the primary caregiver. She constantly feeds him french fries and soda from his favorite fast-food restaurant. She refuses to acknowledge that there is anything wrong with her father. She emphasizes that he is only in the hospital for his respiratory issues, and that speech therapy is unnecessary. You notice during your discussions with her that her father coughs on nearly every sip of soda, and there is half-chewed food on the table in front of him. You convince her to allow you to do the evaluation, but throughout the whole assessment she talks loudly on the phone discussing her weekend plans.

Scenario 3: A middle-aged man recently had a left hemisphere stroke. He has moderate expressive language deficits, apraxia of speech, and right hemiparesis. He is entering your hospital for further rehabilitation services. As you begin the assessment, you realize quickly that he is well into the depression stage of grief and is exhibiting negative reactions such as avoidance, projection, and a lack of motivation for therapy and the evaluation. Halfway through the assessment, his wife enters the room and introduces herself. She kisses her husband on the forehead and he scoffs at her, to which she says that she will have none of that. She tells you to continue with the evaluation and sits next to him, holds his hand, and listens quietly with a smile. When you finish, she speaks to you about how upset her husband is. He had been the sole provider for their family and now they are faced with losing their home. She says he is unmotivated to get better, no matter what she does

to motivate him. She has done a lot of research on her husband's condition and has educated herself on what he is going through. She brings him crossword puzzles, something he loved to do before the stroke, and sits with him every day to work on one. Today, she brought a chessboard and stated that she is going to reteach him chess.

In scenario 1, the parents are motivators, helpers, and empathizers, but they exhibit some detractor qualities because of their lack of understanding of how multiple stimuli can be overwhelming to a person with neurogenic communication disorders caused by a TBI. With education, you can easily turn them into supporters and with their help create an environment best suited for successful treatment.

Author's Note

Conclusion

At the conclusion of this chapter, you should be able to answer the following questions: What role do speech-language pathologists play in counseling patients and caregivers and where is the line drawn between counselor and clinician? As you may have noticed, the line is not always clear. Be aware of what issues are within and outside your scope of practice. Make sure to counsel patients and caregivers only on emotions and negative reactions that are directly related to the communication disorders being addressed. Refer to a trained medical professional when necessary. Counseling should be employed to enhance treatment and ensure that your patients achieve their highest level of success. Sometimes counseling might even be the focus of treatment. Once you have a better awareness of the impact negative reactions and negative emotions can have on the therapy process, you can learn to minimize their impact and help patients proceed on a positive course toward achieving their therapy goals. You play an integral part in your patients' ultimate goals—restoring lost abilities, reestablishing a sense of self, overcoming loss, enhancing quality of life, and creating a new, stronger identity.

The daughter in scenario 2 is a detractor, demotivator, enabler, and sympathizer. She feels sorry for her father and enables his bad eating behaviors by providing him food and drink that he is unable to eat safely. She does not motivate him to get better and detracts from his recovery by saying he does not need speech and swallowing therapy. She is in denial about his deficits. When she could have learned more by paying attention during the evaluation, she chose to talk on the phone with her friend instead. This type of caregiver needs to be informed. You will spend time educating her about her father's conditions, the risks associated with his swallowing difficulties, and the impact her actions can have on his health and well-being. Remember to assess the stage of grief she is in as well as her place on the CI Matrix. With a little attention and information, she can be easily persuaded to be a team member in the therapy process.

Finally, scenario 3 depicts a caregiver who is a supporter, motivator, helper, and empathizer. She is a supporter because she agrees with the plan of care and supports the therapy. She motivates her husband by continually finding ways to keep him occupied and happy. She is a helper because she does not accept his bad attitude; she provides stimuli to aid in his recovery. She continually makes attempts to motivate him. She is also an empathizer because she researched his deficits and understands his loss. You need to nurture and preserve the drive of caregivers such as this.

Many negative reactions and actions by caregivers arise out of ignorance about communication disorders and a lack of understanding of how important therapy is in the recovery process. By educating caregivers, counseling them, as well as encouraging their positive traits, speech-language pathologists can transform caregivers' negative characteristics into positive ones, making allies out of even the most obstructive caregivers.

Finally, speech-language pathologists must take a hard look at themselves. Many times speech-language pathologists, other therapists, nurses, and doctors forget that they themselves are caregivers and should be held to the same standards as the family caregivers. Speech-language pathologists should assess their place on the CI Matrix as well as the caregiver traits they have adopted. If necessary, they should be open to changing their attitudes and approaches to treatment and counseling. Speech-language pathologists should strive to always be a model for caregivers and patients by exhibiting the traits of a positive caregiver.

Main Points

- Counseling is important to the therapeutic process.
- To counsel is to provide information, guidance, and assistance.
- The main purpose of counseling patients and caregivers is to reduce the impact that negative reactions have on the therapeutic process and to promote positive progress in therapy.
- Speech-language pathologists should focus on the emotions, thoughts, and behaviors of patients and caregivers that are directly related to the communication disorder.
- Diagnosed or undiagnosed mental health issues and emotions, thoughts, and behaviors of patients and caregivers that are not related to the communication disorder are not within the scope of practice of a speech-language pathologist.
- It is important to consider the location of the brain injury and any known psychoemotional signs associated with damage to that area.
- Speech-language pathologists must recognize emotions, consider their cause, and refer to a professional trained in the medical management of the psychological issues encountered.

- The five stages of the grieving process are as follows:
  - *Denial:* Patients believe that nothing is wrong and that there will never be anything wrong with their speech, language, cognition, or affected abilities. Individuals might confabulate and fabricate reasons for the change in their communication, blame others for communication difficulties, and dismiss evidence of a communication disorder. Speech-language pathologists must be clear, straightforward, and use objective data such as charts or standardized testing results to make it easier for the individual to see the reality of their problems.
  - *Anger:* Patients often feel lack of ownership and frustration because they feel out of control. Speech-language pathologists should remain calm, not become defensive, and validate patients' feelings.
  - *Bargaining:* Patients are searching for hope by looking to a higher being to make a deal.
  - *Depression:* Patients have lost their sense of purpose and can appear apathetic, unmotivated, and discouraged. Speech-language pathologists must help encourage and refer to a medical professional if clinical depression is suspected.
  - *Acceptance:* This stage is where acceptance of deficits and disorders occur, which enables an individual to move forward to progress in therapy. Speech-language pathologists must set appropriate goals and make a plan to achieve those goals while keeping the patients' quality of life in mind.
- Patients can experience the onset of negative attitudes and emotions at any time after the acquisition of a neurogenic communication disorder. Caregivers, family members, and friends of the patient also have reactions of their own.
- Depression: This negative reaction can be evident in patients and caregivers with any etiology that results in neurogenic communication disorders. It is important to recognize the symptoms of clinical depression because appropriate treatment of any psychological problems increases the likelihood that the patient will achieve the therapeutic goals.
- Demotivation: This is the inability to feel connected to goals by purpose, growth, and ownership. Therapy progress suffers if any of the connections is faulty or missing. Individuals feel apathetic, bored, and frustrated. Speech-language pathologists must determine the right balance between tasks that are challenging though not too challenging and find ways to balance the connections between purpose, growth, and ownership.
- Anxiety: This is when frustration becomes extreme and an ownership disconnection is present. Anxiety could lead to irritability, crying, anger, striking out, withdrawal, fainting, and/or depression. Speech-language pathologists must try to restore ownership within the individual or refer to a psychologist or psychiatrist.
- Avoidance or escape behaviors: These behaviors are negative reactions people use to remove themselves from unpleasant, stressful, or feared situations or tasks. Speech-language pathologists must make tasks more achievable, assess why individuals are resisting therapy, and discuss any fears the person might have.
- Displacement and projection: This is when individuals transfer their own feelings of anxiety, fear, loss, or stress onto another person to reduce those feelings within themselves. Speech-language pathologists must remain calm, not become defensive, encourage talking about emotions, and validate the feelings the person is experiencing.
- Disassociation: This is when patients or caregivers unconsciously remove themselves emotionally from painful, stressful, or upsetting situations to alleviate the emotional stress.

Speech-language pathologists must stay attuned to patients' and caregivers' reactions during interactions, encourage the discussion or expression of their feelings, and keep the patient company to help the patient to feel comforted.

- Passive aggression: This is an indirect negative reaction expressed toward others that is masked by timidity and passivity. Passive aggression can present as hostility to the speech-language pathologist in the form of procrastination, delaying, or lack of interest or motivation. Speech-language pathologists must provide an open, nonthreatening environment for patients to discuss their feelings and emotions.

- Repression: This is when a patient consciously suppresses the negative experiences that are the result of their deficits. Speech-language pathologists must build rapport and develop professional relationships with patients by providing opportunities for small successes. Patients need to experience independence from the speech-language pathologist to believe in their own abilities.

- Learned helplessness: When individuals feel a lack of ownership and control they can resort to owning the sick or helpless role. This might be the only part of their life they feel they have control over. Speech-language pathologists must counsel caregivers how to keep their loved ones motivated yet independent to encourage the connection between purpose, growth, and ownership of goals.

- Loss: This is one of the most common reactions of people with neurogenic communication disorders. Loss can be evident in the form of loss of communicative abilities, loss of independence, and loss of the life patients once had.

- The Counseling-Integration Matrix (CI Matrix) pairs the patients' perceived negative impact of their disorder on their quality of life with the patients' willingness to change. Speech-language pathologists must continually assess patients' place on the CI Matrix.
  - Quadrant 1 (Q1), High-High, depicts patients with a high negative impact on their quality of life and a high willingness to change.
  - Quadrant 2 (Q2), High-Low, depicts patients with a high negative impact on their quality of life and a low willingness to change.
  - Quadrant 3 (Q3), Low-Low, depicts patients with a low negative impact on their quality of life and a low willingness to change.
  - Quadrant 4 (Q4), Low-High, depicts patients with a low negative impact on their quality of life and a high willingness to change.

- Counseling the patient includes the following activities:
  - Building positive rapport, helping patients voice their concerns and having them assist in creating a plan of care to achieve their goals, avoiding contributions to patient frustrations, and acknowledging and allowing the patient to experience the grieving process and helping them through it

- The ideal caregiver is one who is supportive, motivating, helpful, and empathetic of patients' situations. There are other types of caregivers, including the following:
  - Supporters versus detractors: Supporters encourage therapy, while detractors diminish the importance and value of therapy.
  - Motivators versus demotivators: Motivators aid patients in staying positive and motivated, while demotivators cause stress and negative responses such as avoidance, regression, and projection.
  - Helpers versus enablers: Helpers understand what speech-language pathologists teach and generalize those ideas outside of the therapy session, while enablers believe they are helping the patient though their words and actions go against the

speech-language pathologists' recommendations or suggestions.

- Empathizers versus sympathizers: Empathizers are attuned to patients and want to learn about the disorder, while sympathizers feel sorry for patients with little understanding of the patients' emotions.

Review Questions

1. What does it mean to counsel?
2. What is the role of the speech-language pathologist in counseling?
3. Name and describe the five stages of the grieving process.
4. What are some signs and symptoms of depression?
5. How might depression and demotivation affect the therapeutic process?
6. How might anxiety and disassociation affect the therapeutic process?
7. How might the speech-language pathologist tailor therapy sessions to a patient with avoidance or escape behaviors?
8. How might the speech-language pathologist tailor therapy sessions to a patient with displacement or projection behaviors?
9. Describe how you would counsel a patient that is passive aggressive.
10. Describe how you would counsel a caregiver that is passive aggressive.
11. Why might the Counseling-Integration Matrix (CI Matrix) be useful?
12. Give an example of an individual who would be placed in quadrant 1 of the CI Matrix and a way in which counseling would be helpful.
13. Give an example of an individual who would be placed in quadrant 2 of the CI Matrix and a way in which counseling would be helpful.
14. How might an individual feel if he is in quadrant 3 of the CI Matrix?
15. How might an individual feel if she is in quadrant 4 of the CI Matrix?
16. In your own opinion, what characteristics would the ideal patient display?
17. In your own opinion, what characteristics would the ideal caregiver display?
18. How are supporters and detractors different?
19. How are helpers and enablers different?
20. Why might sympathizers be detrimental to the therapeutic process?

References

1. Absher, J. R., & Cummings, J. L. (1995). Neurobehavioural examination of frontal lobe functions. *Aphasiology, 9*, 181–192.
2. Ballard, C., Bannister, C., Solis, M., Oyebode, F., & Wilcock, G. (1996). The prevalence, associations, and symptoms of depression amongst dementia sufferers. *Journal of Affective Disorders, 36*, 135–144.
3. Barone, O. R. (1986). *Achieving peak motivation*. Presentation and workshop for the Blue Cross Blue Shield Association, Lafayette, IN.
4. Binder, L. M., Robling, M. L., & Larrabee, G. J. (1997). A review of mild head trauma. Part I: Meta-analytic review of neuropsychological studies. *Journal of Clinical and Experimental Neuropsychology, 19*, 421–431.

5. Burgess, A., & Clements, P. (1998). Stress, coping, and defensive functioning. In A. Burgess (Ed.), *Psychiatric nursing* (pp. 77–90). Stamford, CT: Appleton & Lange.

6. Carlat, D. (1999). *The psychiatric interview*. Philadelphia, PA: Lippincott Williams & Wilkins.

7. Carson, R., Butcher, J., & Coleman, J. (1988). *Abnormal psychology and modern life*. Glenview, IL: Foresman.

8. Craig, A., & Cummings, J. (1995). Neuropsychiatric aspects of aphasia. In H. Kirshner (Ed.), *Handbook of neurological speech and language disorders* (pp. 483–498). New York, NY: Marcel Dekker.

9. Hackett, M. L., Yapa, C., Parag, V., & Anderson, C. S. (2005). Frequency of depression after stroke: A systematic review of observational studies. *Stroke, 36*, 1330–1340.

10. King, N. S. (1996). Emotional, neuropsychological, and organic factors: Their use in the prediction of postconcussion symptoms after moderate and mild head injuries. *Journal of Neurology, Neurosurgery, and Psychiatry, 53*, 293–296.

11. Kolb, L. (1977). *Modern clinical psychiatry*. Philadelphia, PA: Saunders.

12. Korczyn, A. D., & Halperin, I. (2009). Depression and dementia. *Journal of the Neurological Sciences, 283*, 139–142.

13. Kübler-Ross, E. (1969). *On death and dying*. New York, NY: Macmillan.

14. Lishman, W. A. (1988). Physiogenesis and psychogenesis in the "post-concussional syndrome." *British Journal of Psychiatry, 153*, 460–469.

15. Malia, K., Powell, G., & Torode, S. (1995). Personality and psychosocial function after brain injury. *Brain Injury, 9*, 697–712.

16. Masand, P., & Chaudhary, P. (1994). Methylphenidate treatment of poststroke depression in a patient with global aphasia. *Annals of Clinical Psychiatry, 6*, 271–274.

17. Mathias, J. L., & Coats, J. L. (1999). Emotional and cognitive sequelae to mild traumatic brain injury. *Journal of Clinical and Experimental Neuropsychology, 21*(2), 200–215.

18. Mattson, A. J., & Levin, H. S. (1990). Frontal lobe dysfunction following closed-head injury. *Journal of Nervous and Mental Disease, 178*, 282–291.

19. Merriam, A. E., Aronson, M. K., Gaston, P., Wey, S. L., & Katz, K. (1988). The psychiatric symptoms of Alzheimer's disease. *Journal of the American Geriatric Society, 36*, 7–12.

20. National Institute of Mental Health. (2011). *Depression*. U.S. Department of Health and Human Resources. Retrieved from http://www.nimh.nih.gov/health/topics/depression/index.shtml

21. Panza, F., Frisardi, V., Capurso, C., D'Introno, A., Colacicco, A., Imbimbo, B. . . . Solfrizzi, V. (2010). Late-life depression, mild cognitive impairment, and dementia: Possible continuum? *American Journal of Geriatric Psychiatry, 18*(2), 98–116.

22. Servaty-Seib, H. L. (Ed.). (2004). Perspectives on counseling the bereaved. *Journal of Mental Health Counseling, 26*(2), 95–97.

23. Shipley, K. G., & Roseberry-McKibbin, C. (2006). *Interviewing and counseling in communicative disorders: Principles and procedures* (3rd ed.). Austin, TX: Pro-Ed.

24. Stuart, G. (2001a). Anxiety responses and anxiety disorders. In G. Stuart & M. Laraia (Eds.), *Principles and practice of psychiatric nursing* (7th ed., pp. 274–298). St. Louis, MO: Mosby.

25. Stuart, G. (2001b). Self-concept responses and dissociative disorders. In G. Stuart & M. Laraia (Eds.), *Principles and practice of psychiatric nursing* (7th ed., pp. 317–344). St. Louis, MO: Mosby.

26. Stuss, D. T., & Benson, D. F. (1984). Neuropsychological studies of the frontal lobes. *Psychological Bulletin, 95*, 3–28.

27. Stuss, D. T., & Benson, D. F. (1986). *The frontal lobes*. New York, NY: Raven Press.

28. Stuss, D. T., Gow, C. A., & Hetherington, C. R. (1992). "No longer Gage": Frontal lobe dysfunction and emotional changes. *Journal of Consulting and Clinical Psychology, 60*, 349–359.

29. Tanner, D. C. (1980). Loss and grief: Implications for the speech-language pathologist and audiologist. *ASHA, 22*, 916–928.

30. Tanner, D. C. (1999). *The family guide to surviving stroke and communication disorders*. Boston, MA: Allyn & Bacon.

31. Tanner, D. C. (2003). *The psychology of neurogenic communication disorders: A primer for healthcare professionals*. Boston, MA: Allyn & Bacon.

32. Tanner, D. C. (2010). *Exploring the psychology, diagnosis, and treatment of neurogenic communication disorders*. Bloomington, IN: iUniverse.

33. Tanner, D. C., & Gerstenberger, D. (1988). The grief response in neuropathologies of speech and language. *Aphasiology, 1*(6), 79–84.

34. Tellis, C. M., & Barone, O. R. (unpublished manuscript). Interviewing and Counseling in Speech-Language Pathology and Audiology.

Glossary

Acceleration–deceleration closed head injury Damage to the brain created by the external forces that act on the brain when it is moving through space very quickly or coming to an abrupt halt.

Achromatopsia Color blindness, also known as color agnosia.

Acquired immune deficiency syndrome (AIDS) The final stage of HIV disease characterized by severe damage and impairment of the immune system.

Agrammatism The lack of appropriate grammatical construction of language displayed by individuals with aphasia.

Agraphia An acquired impairment in the ability to form letters or form words using letters.

Alexia An acquired impairment of reading.

Alternating attention The ability to move or alternate attention back and forth from one stimulus to another.

Amusia An acquired deficit in the ability to interpret and recognize music.

Anastomosis A connection between blood vessels. (Plural: anastomoses.)

Aneurysm An abnormal stretching and ballooning of the wall of a blood vessel.

Anomia A deficit in word retrieval for expression.

Anomic aphasia An aphasia characterized by fluent speech and intact receptive language but a disproportionately severe deficit in naming abilities.

Anosognosia The pathologic condition of having a deficit and not knowing the deficit exists or denying that the deficit exists despite evidence indicating otherwise.

Anoxia A condition of being completely without oxygen; an extreme lack of oxygen to brain tissue.

Anterior cerebral artery One of a set of paired arteries that originate from the internal carotid arteries at the circle of Willis and course anteriorly to supply blood to the frontal and parietal lobes, basal ganglia, and corpus callosum.

Anterior communicating artery An unpaired anastomosis between the right and left anterior cerebral arteries that forms the anterior portion of the circle of Willis.

Anterograde amnesia An inability to create new memories.

Anxiety A generalized mood with primary emotional components of apprehensiveness and unease.

Aphasia An acquired deficit in language abilities resulting from damage to the brain.

Apraxia of speech An acquired disorder of speech originating from an inability to create and sequence motor plans for speech.

Arachnoid mater A layer of the cerebral meninges that exists between the dura mater and the pia mater that plays a large role in supplying blood to the surface of the brain through the many blood vessels it contains.

Arbor vitae The distinctive plantlike shape of the fibers of the cerebellar hemispheres evident upon dissection and some imaging studies.

Arousal The level of wakefulness and the ability to respond to stimuli.

Association fibers White matter pathways that connect different structures and areas of the brain within a single hemisphere.

Ataxia A set of deficits in the timing and coordination of body movements caused by pathology of the cerebellum.

Ataxic dysarthria The dysarthria produced by the incoordination of the movements of the articulators, which produces a slushy or drunken-like speech quality.

Ataxic gait A type of gait characterized by the feet spread more broadly apart than usual accompanied by irregular footsteps and a greater likelihood of falls; associated with cerebellar pathology.

Atherosclerosis A condition in which a person has a buildup of fatty materials such as cholesterol in the blood and this material accumulates slowly on the walls of the arteries, narrowing the arteries and possibly restricting blood flow.

Athetosis An involuntary slow, writhing movement.

Attention The ability to hold focus on a stimulus when aroused enough to know that the stimulus is there and using orienting skills to direct attention to the stimulus.

Aura The period of time immediately preceding the full onset of a seizure in which a person might experience some warning signs that a seizure is imminent.

Avoidance The act of refusing engagement in a task that is deemed undesirable.

Ballism Bilateral, involuntary, irregular, possibly wild or violent flinging of extremities. A hyperkinesia.

Barotrauma Trauma induced by exposure to intense levels of pressure changes following an explosion.

Basal ganglia A group of subcortical structures located deep within the cerebral hemispheres on either side of the thalamus that works to regulate body movement.

Basilar artery A single unpaired artery that joins the circle of Willis posteriorly and branches into the paired posterior cerebral arteries.

Benign brain tumor A tumor within the brain that cannot spread to other parts of the body.

Bilateral innervation An innervation pattern that occurs when one side of a paired nerve (the right or the left) receives motor plans from both the right and left cerebral hemispheres.

Bilateral On both sides.

Biopsy Surgery to remove a piece of tissue for diagnostic purposes.

Body neglect A deficit in the ability to attend to one side of the body. Also known as personal neglect.

Brain cancer A malignant tumor of the brain or one located centrally within the spinal cord.

Brain tumor An abnormal growth of cells in the brain.

Brain stem A subcortical structure that connects the spinal cord to the rest of the brain and houses many structures involved in autonomic functions.

Broca's area The inferior, posterior region of the frontal lobe of the left hemisphere that is a specialized area of the cerebrum responsible for finding and assembling words for the appropriate expression of thought.

Bulbar polio Poliomyelitis that affects the cranial nerves and the muscles innervated by the cranial nerves.

Bulbospinal polio Poliomyelitis that affects both spinal and cranial nerves and the muscles they innervate.

Capgras delusion A neuropsychiatric deficit characterized by a belief that loved ones, significant others, or family members have been replaced by imposters.

Cauda equina The loose strands of spinal nerves that separate from the inferior termination of the spinal cord.

Central nervous system The brain and spinal cord.

Central sulcus A deep groove that runs down the middle lateral surface of each cerebral hemisphere.

Cerebellum A subcortical structure hanging off the back of the pons and under the occipital lobes that is known as an error control device for body movement and ensures that body movements are smoothly coordinated and as error free as possible.

Cerebral cortex The most superficial layer of the cerebrum.

Cerebral edema The swelling of brain tissue.

Cerebral meninges Three layers of tissues with various functions that encase and envelope the brain and spinal cord.

Cerebrovascular accident A stroke. An interruption of blood flow to or within the brain that permanently destroys brain tissue or causes a temporary cessation of function.

Cerebrum The rounded gray section of the brain with gyri and sulci.

Chorea Involuntary and quick dance-like movements of the feet, hands, extremities, and head and neck. *Chorea* is derived from *choros*, the Greek word for dance.

Chronic traumatic encephalopathy A degenerative disease of the brain caused by repeated head trauma such as repeated concussions in sports or repeated exposure to IED blasts in soldiers that manifests within months or years of brain damage as dementia, confusion, memory loss, headache, depression, and excessive aggression.

Circle of Willis A series of anastomoses that connects the internal carotid and vertebral/basilar system, acts to ensure equal blood flow to all areas of the brain, and acts as a safety valve if an occlusion occurs within the circle of Willis or below the circle of Willis.

Clonic phase The second phase of a tonic clonic seizure characterized by a shaking, jerking, extraneous body movement.

Closed head injury A subcategory of traumatic brain injury in which an individual's skull is not broken open.

Cognition The ability to acquire and process knowledge about the world.

Coma A period of unconsciousness lasting more than 6 hours during which the unconscious individual cannot be awakened and is unresponsive to sensory stimuli.

Commissural fibers White matter pathways that connect analogous areas between the two cerebral hemispheres.

Compensatory strategy A therapy strategy that has the goal of restoring lost function by compensating for underlying deficits.

Complex partial seizure A seizure that occurs over a large section of a single cerebral hemisphere and that creates an altered state of consciousness.

Concussion A pathologic and traumatic event affecting the brain that creates a state of confusion, often with no loss of consciousness.

Conduit d'approche A zeroing-in behavior in which a person with aphasia correctly produces a target word after several repeated and unsuccessful attempts where each failed attempt is closer to the correct production of the target word than the last.

Content words The words that carry the majority of meaning in a sentence.

Contralateral On the opposite side.

Conus medullaris Conical point of inferior termination of the spinal cord in the lumbar region of the lower back.

Copralalia The compulsive and repetitive production of swear words.

Corpus callosum A mass of white matter tracts located at the base of the longitudinal fissure that connects the analogous areas between the two hemispheres.

Cortical aphasia Aphasia that arises as a result of damage to the cortex.

Cortical multi-infarct dementia A form of vascular dementia that is caused by small recurrent ischemic strokes within the cortex.

Counsel To provide information, guidance, and assistance.

Coup–contrecoup A pattern of brain damage that occurs when, due to external forces, the brain bounces back and forth inside the skull causing damage at the sites of impact.

Cranial nerves Nerves that course between the brain stem and the head/neck/face and are either motor/efferent, sensory/afferent, or mixed sensory-motor in function.

Craniotomy A surgery to remove part of the skull to allow the brain to swell without the brain incurring damage from increased pressure within the skull.

Crossed aphasia The condition of having a nonfluent aphasia that, despite the contralateral hemiplegia or hemiparesis, leaves the dominant writing hand ipsilateral to the brain lesion motorically intact (i.e., the damaged language-dominant hemisphere does not control the dominant writing hand).

Declarative memory The ability to remember facts.

Delirium A sudden disturbance in consciousness or a change in cognitive ability that fluctuates through the course of a day with an onset that is a result of a general medical condition.

Dementia A condition of memory loss plus deficits in at least one other of the following areas: verbal expression or auditory and written receptive language skills, recognition and identification of objects, ability to execute motor activities, abstract thinking, judgment, and execution of complex tasks.

Demotivation The lack of a balance between ownership of goals and the therapy process.

Depression A disorder characterized by abnormally low mood that affects individuals' daily lives.

Diaphragm The primary muscle of inspiration.

Diffuse axonal shearing The breaking of neuronal connections that occurs across large areas of the brain and is seen commonly in closed head traumatic brain injury.

Disassociation When patients or caregivers unconsciously remove themselves emotionally from painful, stressful, or upsetting situations to alleviate emotional stress.

Discourse The exchange of communicative information between a speaker and a listener or the back and forth among individuals participating in conversation.

Displacement and projection When patients transfer their own feelings of anxiety, fear, loss, or stress onto another person for the sake of reducing those feelings within themselves.

Divided attention The ability to attend to one stimulus while simultaneously attending to another stimulus. Also known as multitasking.

Dura mater A dense, fibrous protective layer of tissue that envelopes the brain and spinal cord. This is the superficial-most layer of the cerebral meninges.

Dysarthria A group of disorders of speech caused by damage to the central or peripheral nervous system that creates weakness, slowness, incoordination, or abnormal muscle tone in musculature used to produce speech.

Dysmetria The over- or undershooting of a body part while performing a volitional movement such as reaching for an object.

Dystonia An involuntary slow, irregular, often painful twisting of extremities and body parts that often manifests as abnormal and involuntary posturing of the body. A hyperkinesia.

Echolalia The compulsive repetition of someone else's utterances.

Embolic stroke When an embolus lodges within a blood vessel and restricts or cuts off blood circulation to the brain.

Embolus A mass within the blood stream that is carried through the vascular system by the forces of circulation.

Empathizer Caregivers who are attuned to patient needs. They seek to learn about the disorder and related deficits.

Empty speech Speech often produced by those with fluent aphasia that is abundant yet lacking in meaning.

Encephalitis A general term that refers to an acute infection and/or inflammation of the brain or spinal cord.

Epidural hematoma A hematoma that occurs when a blood vessel bursts between the dura mater and the skull.

Epidural hemorrhage A hemorrhage that occurs between the dura mater and the skull, usually of traumatic origin.

Episodic memory The recall of specific, recently experienced events or episodes.

Errorful learning Learning in a way that produces some level of failure. Learning by trial and error.

Etiology The underlying cause of a symptom or deficit.

Evidence-based practice The notion that therapy and evaluation procedures must be determined to be effective based on clinical opinion and/or valid and reliable research.

Executive functions High-level cognitive abilities used to employ other lower-level cognitive functions appropriately to meet high-level goals.

Expressive language deficit Difficulty in formulation and production of language to communicate an intended meaning.

Extinction A mild case of hemispatial neglect in which the affected individual can attend to stimuli within the neglected field of attention but only with prompting.

Festination A progressive speeding up of a repetitive movement often displayed in various forms by individuals with Parkinson's disease.

Fissure A deep groove that creates major divisions in the anatomy of the brain.

Flaccid dysarthria A motor speech disorder resulting from flaccid weakness or paralysis of musculature used to produce speech.

Frontal lobe One of two of the most anterior sections of the cerebral hemisphere that is delineated posteriorly by the central sulcus and inferiorly by the lateral sulcus and that houses expressive language and deals heavily in motor movement.

Frontal lobotomy A procedure of damaging or removing tissue from the prefrontal area of the frontal lobes for the supposed remediation of psychological problems.

Function words The in-between words used to frame the major content words in a sentence.

Generalized seizure A seizure that affects the entire brain and is associated with a total loss of consciousness.

G-force The amount of stress being applied to a body by acceleration forces.

Gray matter Unmyelinated neurons responsible for the processing and regulating of information within the nervous system.

Gyrus Ridges forming the visible portion of the cerebral cortex.

Hematoma The gathering of blood outside a blood vessel following a hemorrhage.

Hemiballism Unilateral, involuntary, irregular, possibly wild or violent flinging of extremities. A hyperkinesia.

Hemiparesis A unilateral spastic weakness of the body.

Hemiplegia A unilateral spastic paralysis of the body.

Hemispatial neglect A deficit in the ability to attend to one side of the environment.

Hemorrhage Bleeding of an open blood vessel.

Hemorrhagic stroke A cerebrovascular accident that occurs when a blood vessel within the brain ruptures.

Hippocampus A region of the temporal lobe responsible for storing and creating memories. (Plural: hippocampi.)

HIV/AIDS dementia Cognitive changes as a result of HIV/AIDS which are severe enough to affect an individual's activities of daily living.

Human immunodeficiency virus (HIV) The virus that leads to AIDS (acquired immune deficiency syndrome).

Hyperkinesia Extra and involuntary movement of the body or body parts. Also known as dyskinesia.

Hyperkinetic An excess of movement, too much movement to be appropriate.

Hyperkinetic dysarthria The dysarthria created by the presence of hyperkinesias that interfere with speech production.

Hyperreflexia An excess of reflexes, overactive reflexes.

Hypertension High blood pressure.

Hypertonic An excess of muscle tone, an excessively tight muscle tone.

Hypokinetic A lack of appropriate level of movement. Too little movement.

Hypokinetic dysarthria The dysarthria that results from pathology at the basal ganglia or its connections to other structures in the central nervous system.

Hyporeflexia A lack of appropriate reflexes.

Hypotonic A lack of appropriate muscle tone. A loose muscle tone.

Hypoxia A condition in which the body lacks appropriate oxygen supply.

Ictus The main stage of the seizure during which the primary symptoms are experienced.

Idiopathic To be of unknown origin.

Impact-based TBI A form of closed head injury in which a moving object impacts the head forcing the skull inward on the brain producing focal damage to the area of the brain compressed.

Increased intracranial pressure A raised level of pressure within the skull above the normal and healthy level.

Inferencing The ability to take previous knowledge and experience and apply it to the interpretation of the present situation. The ability to make a leap in judgment to a correct interpretation of the overall meaning.

Interictal period The time between the end of one seizure and the beginning of the next seizure.

Internal carotid artery One of a set of paired arteries that course superiorly from the thorax within the anterior portion of the neck to the base of the brain to link with the circle of Willis.

Intracerebral hemorrhage A hemorrhage that occurs within the brain, often of traumatic origin.

Intracranial pressure The level of pressure within the skull and therefore the amount of pressure that is exerted on the brain.

Ipsilateral To be on the same side.

Ischemia Blockage of or restriction in a blood vessel.

Ischemic core The location of the focal damage of tissue within the brain following ischemia. Also known as the infarct.

Ischemic penumbra An area of tissue within the brain surrounding the ischemic core that has lost the appropriate level of blood supply to function but that is still receiving enough collateral blood flow from other vessels to stay alive.

Ischemic stroke A cerebrovascular accident that occurs as a result of a blood vessel becoming occluded or blocked.

Lacunar state A form of vascular dementia that is the result of multiple subcortical thrombotic ischemic strokes occurring in small and deep blood vessels that supply circulation to the brain stem, basal ganglia, and other subcortical structures.

Language A set of symbols used to communicate meaning.

Lateral sulcus A deep groove that begins at the lower frontal aspect of each of the two cerebral hemispheres and travels at an upward angle, passes the central sulcus, and then terminates.

Learned helplessness A condition in which a person behaves in a helpless manner even though he or she has opportunities to improve their situation.

Learned nonuse When an individual learns to compensate for a deficit by employing other intact abilities and, in doing so, ceases to exercise the physical or intellectual ability in which the deficit is present.

Leptomeninges The thin layers of the meninges including the arachnoid mater and the pia mater.

Lesion An abnormal change in body tissue usually as a result of disease or trauma.

Lesion localization The practice of identifying the location of pathology in the brain based on the profile of deficits the individual displays.

Lissencephaly A group of congenital malformations that create a lack of appropriate gyri and sulci of the cortex and a consequent reduction in cortical tissue.

Logorrhea A near nonstop, usually meaningless and tangential, output of speech.

Longitudinal fissure A deep groove running front to back along the brain that divides the brain into the right and left cerebral hemispheres.

Long-term memory The ability to retain information successfully for months or years.

Lower motor neuron (LMN) The efferent component of a cranial or spinal nerve. Also known as the final common pathway.

Macrostructure The bigger picture composed of many details. Also known as the gestalt.

Macrostructure processing The ability to generate a correct perception of macrostructure.

Malignant brain tumor Brain cancer.

Mandibular branch A branch of the trigeminal nerve with both sensory and motor functions. The afferent portion of this nerve carries sensory information from the lower teeth, lower gums, bottom lip, as well as somatic information from portions of the tongue. The efferent component innervates muscles of mastication.

Mass effect The displacement effect or crushing force on nearby tissues that a tumor exerts.

Maxillary branch A branch of the trigeminal nerve that is sensory in nature and is responsible for transmitting sensory information from the teeth, upper lip, buccal and nasal cavities, as well as the sides of the face to the central nervous system.

Maximum performance tasks Tasks used to test an individual's maximum limit of ability and to compare the individual's greatest effort on a task with the known average performance rate of unimpaired individuals.

Medulla The superior-most section of the spinal cord that connects the spinal cord to the pons and is the site of decussation of a large portion of the motor tracts descending through the brain stem.

Metastatic tumor A cancerous tumor that spread from a primary tumor to grow in another part of the body. Also known as a secondary tumor.

Midbrain The superior-most section of the brain stem that houses the substantia nigra.

Middle cerebral artery One of a set of paired arteries that originate from the internal carotid arteries at the circle of Willis and course laterally to supply blood flow to Broca's area, Wernicke's area, the temporal lobes, and the primary motor cortex.

Mild cognitive impairment Subtle cognitive changes that are often prediagnostic signs of dementia and usually manifest as decreased ability to concentrate, decreased word finding abilities, decreased short-term memory, and difficulty following detail-heavy conversations or writings.

Mixed aphasia A nonspecific form of fluent or non-fluent aphasia that combines attributes of more distinctive forms of aphasia.

Mixed dysarthria A simultaneous manifestation of more than one type of dysarthria.

Motivation The achievement of a balanced state among an individual's sense of purpose, perception of growth or improvement, and ownership of his or her goals, therapy, and the therapy process.

Motor homunculus A visual illustration of the amount of cortical tissue dedicated to the movement of each body part within the primary motor cortex.

Motor neglect A condition of displaying diminished use of a neglected limb, despite the limb being motorically intact.

Motor speech programmer A network of neural structures that contribute to the function of creating appropriate motor plans for speech.

Multi-infarct dementia A form of vascular dementia caused by many small infarcts usually to various areas of the brain.

Myelin An insulating layer of protein and fatty substances that forms a layer around the axons of certain neurons, which allows for the fast and effective transmission of neural impulses.

Myoclonus An involuntary rapid twitching of a muscle or group of muscles.

Neglect A general term used to describe a deficit in the ability to attend to sensory stimuli from one side of the body or the environment.

Neologism An error in speech that occurs when an individual produces a word that is entirely different from the intended word and is mostly unintelligible.

Neoplasm A brain tumor. An abnormal growth of cells in the brain that serves no purpose to the body.

NeuroAIDS Neurological changes as a result of HIV/AIDS that create cognitive deficits and dementia. Also known as HIV/AIDS dementia and HIV-associated neurocognitive disorder (HAND).

Neurogenic communication disorder A disorder of communication arising from damage to the nervous system.

Neuroplasticity The ability of a part of the brain to change its previous function and to take on and learn a new and previously unknown role.

Neurosyphilis A variation of syphilis that infects the nervous system.

Nonspeech compensatory strategy A compensatory strategy that entirely bypasses speech production to focus on improving overall communication.

Nystagmus Involuntary and rapid back-and-forth motion of the eyes.

Occipital lobe The most posterior section of the cerebrum that is dedicated to receiving and processing neural impulses related to vision.

Oligodendroglioma A brain tumor arising from oligodendrocytes, which are myelin-producing cells within the brain.

Open head TBI A form of TBI in which the skull is broken open and the brain is penetrated.

Ophthalmic branch A branch of the trigeminal nerve that is sensory in nature and transmits afferent information from the upper face, forehead, and scalp to the central nervous system.

Oral motor evaluation An evaluation of the oral structures and functions used in speech.

Orientation The ability of individuals to know who they are, where they are, and when they are.

Orienting The ability to direct attention toward a stimulus.

Paralysis A total loss of movement.

Paraphasia An error in expressive language that is not related to motor deficits but that is linked to higher-level language deficits associated with aphasia.

Paresis A partial or incomplete loss of movement (weakness).

Paresthesia A sensory abnormality usually characterized by the sensation of pins and needles, or tingling, or burning on the skin as well as general body aches.

Parietal lobe A section of the cerebrum located posterior to the frontal lobes and anterior to the occipital lobes that is largely responsible for receiving and processing sensory information concerning the body.

Partial seizure A seizure in which pathologic levels of electricity in the brain remain confined to a particular region of the brain.

Passive aggression An indirect negative reaction expressed toward others that is masked by timidity and passivity.

Peduncles Attachments between the cerebellum and the pons.

Peripheral nervous system The nerve tracts outside of the central nervous system that work to connect the central nervous system to the rest of the body.

Perseverate To do something repeatedly, redundantly, and, more often than not, inappropriately.

Perseveration A word that is said repeatedly and inappropriately.

Perseverative paraphasia A word that is produced repeatedly and inadvertently by an individual with aphasia instead of the intended word.

Persistent vegetative state A vegetative state lasting longer than 4 weeks.

Petit mal seizure A generalized seizure in which an individual loses awareness for a few seconds and might seem simply to stare off into space before coming to.

Phonemic paraphasia An error in speech in which the word produced is discernable, mostly correct, and yet there are phoneme-level mistakes.

Phrenic nerve A spinal nerve that provides innervation to the diaphragm.

Pia mater The innermost and most delicate layer of the cerebral meninges that hugs the surface of the brain and spinal cord closely as it rises and falls along the gyri, sulci, and fissures of the brain.

Poliomyelitis A virus that attacks the peripheral nervous system and causes paralysis and absent reflexes. Also known as polio.

Polypharmacy The unexpected and unknown side effects of taking many prescription drugs at once.

Polytrauma A profile of traumatic injury resulting from many different types of trauma.

Pons The middle and slightly bulbous portion of the brain stem that provides an attachment between the cerebellum (not cerebrum) and the rest of the central nervous system.

Post ictus The stage of seizure that follows the ictus and that can last for minutes or hours and during which people might display lethargy and confusion and experience memory loss, weakness, and depression.

Post polio syndrome Symptoms of muscle weakness, muscle pain, and fatigue within those limbs that were affected by a previous polio infection.

Posterior cerebral artery One of a set of paired arteries that branch off the basilar artery at the circle of Willis to course posteriorly and deliver blood to the occipital lobes, cerebellum, and the inferior temporal lobes.

Posterior communicating artery Paired anastomoses coursing from the left posterior cerebral artery to the left middle cerebral artery and also coursing from the right posterior cerebral artery to the right middle cerebral artery.

Post-ictal confusion The short-lived cognitive deficits following the ictus stage of a seizure.

Post-traumatic amnesia Memory loss following trauma to the brain that is usually a combination of retrograde and anterograde amnesia.

Post-traumatic epilepsy Seizures that occur as a result of a traumatic brain injury.

Primary auditory cortex A region of cortex located within the temporal lobes responsible for receiving and processing neural impulses related to sound.

Primary motor cortex A strip of tissue oriented vertically along the last gyrus of each frontal lobe that plays a large role in voluntary motor movement.

Primary sensory cortex A section of cortex along the first gyrus of the parietal lobe dedicated to receiving and processing sensory information.

Primary tumor A tumor that originates at its location within the body.

Primary visual cortex The posterior-most section of the occipital lobes dedicated to receiving neural impulses of vision from the eyes.

Prion A small infectious protein with its own genetic coding that attacks structures within the central or peripheral nervous system.

Problem solving The ability to find an appropriate solution to a problem.

Procedural memory Memory of sequences of individual actions used to achieve larger objectives.

Projection fibers White matter pathways that project from the brain to the spinal cord and transmit motor (movement) signals from the central nervous system out to the peripheral nervous system and also transmit sensory signals from the peripheral nervous system back up through the lower central nervous system to be processed in the brain.

Proprioception An individual's sense of where their extremeties and their body is in space.

Prosody The changes in pitch, stress, timbre, cadence, and tempo a person uses to infuse utterances with emotional content.

Prosopagnosia A neurologic deficit in the specific ability to cognitively process sensory information regarding the faces of others for the purposes of recognition.

Protective redundancy When the body duplicates systems to protect proper functioning.

Pseudodementia An outdated term once used to indicate cognitive changes and deficits brought on by depression.

Receptive language deficit A deficit in the ability to derive meaning from language.

Reflex The production of a physical movement that occurs automatically in response to a stimulus and is initiated below the level of awareness.

Repression Occurs when an individual suppresses acknowledgment of the negative experiences that are the result of his or her deficits.

Resistance to passive movement The body resisting movement of a body part by an outside force.

Restorative strategy A therapy strategy that has the goal of restoring lost function by reducing the severity of the underlying deficits.

Reticular formation A series of nuclei stretching among the midbrain, pons, and medulla that regulates arousal, respiration, and blood pressure.

Secondary tumor A cancerous tumor that spread from another part of the body. Also known as a metastatic tumor.

Seizure A sudden, often periodic, abnormal level of electrical discharge occurring within the brain.

Selective attention The ability to hold attention on a stimulus while ignoring the presence of competing stimuli.

Self-repair When a speaker restates or revises a word or phrase in an attempt to produce it in an error-free fashion or refine it to better reflect the intended meaning.

Semantic paraphasia An error in speech in which one word is substituted for another word that is similar in meaning.

Sensory homunculus A visual illustration of the amount of cortical tissue within the primary sensory cortex dedicated to processing sensory information from each body part.

Shaken baby syndrome A profile of traumatic brain injury seen in infants and small children most often caused by physical abuse, usually a shaking of the child, by the caregiver.

Short-term memory The retention of information for longer than 30 seconds to a few hours.

Simple partial seizure A partial seizure during which the seizure activity within the brain is limited to a small area within one cerebral hemisphere and the individual experiencing the seizure remains conscious.

Simultagnosia A neurologic disorder that produces the inability to visually perceive many details at once.

Somatophrenia A deficit in the ability to perceive parts of one's own body as belonging to oneself.

Spasm An involuntary and sudden muscle contraction.

Spastic dysarthria A motor speech disorder resulting from spasticity of musculature used to produce speech.

Spasticity A combination of hypertonia and the resistance to passive movement caused by a hyperactive stretch reflex that makes movement of a body part difficult.

Speech The sounds made with the vocal and articulatory structures of the body to produce verbal language.

Speech compensatory strategy A compensatory technique that increases intelligibility of the speaker and reduces the impact of dysarthria on speech while not directly targeting the pathologic neuromotor condition producing the dysarthria.

Speech systems Systems that support the production of speech, including the articulatory system, the resonatory system, the phonatory system, and the respiratory system.

Spinal cord A bundle of white matter tracts and gray matter housed within the bony vertebral column that enables afferent (sensory) impulses coming from the body to be transmitted to brain and efferent (motor) impulses from the brain to be transmitted to the body.

Spinal nerves Nerves that course between the spinal cord and the body.

Spinal polio Poliomyelitis that affects the spinal nerves and the muscles innervated by the spinal nerves.

Status epilepticus A state of constant seizure. When an individual experiences one seizure that leads right into another seizure with no interictal period.

Stretch reflex A contraction of a muscle in response to a passive stretching of a muscle spindle within a muscle. This reflex enables the body to correct any unintended changes in body position in a timely manner without waiting for input from the cerebral cortex as well as keep appropriate tone in the muscles.

Striatocapsular aphasia Language deficits associated with lesion at the striatum that occur as a result of a lack of blood flow to the cortical language areas.

Stroke A lesion in the brain that occurs when brain tissue is either permanently destroyed or temporarily ceases to function as a result of a lack of blood flow or a disturbance of blood supply to the affected area.

Subarachnoid hemorrhage A hemorrhagic stroke that occurs when a blood vessel between the arachnoid mater and the pia mater ruptures.

Subcortex The portion of the brain located beneath the cortex that deals less in reasoning abilities and higher-level cognition and more in autonomic, life-sustaining functions.

Subcortical aphasia Aphasia that arises as a result of damage to subcortical structures.

Subdural hematoma A hematoma that occurs when veins between the dura mater and the brain are broken and bleed out between the dura mater and brain.

Subdural hemorrhage A hemorrhage that occurs between the dura mater and the arachnoid mater, usually of traumatic origin.

Substantia nigra A structure located within the midbrain responsible for the production of the neurotransmitter dopamine.

Sulcus An inward fold of the cerebral cortex.

Surgical trauma The collateral damage to the tissues of the body that occurs during the process of surgery.

Sustained attention The ability to hold attention on a single stimulus.

Sympathizer Caregivers who feel sorry for patients and show little understanding of patients' emotions.

Syphilis A sexually transmitted disease that is caused by corkscrew-shaped bacterium called spirochetes. Syphilis is highly treatable and curable with the antibiotic penicillin.

Temporal lobe A section of the cerebrum located inferior to the parietal lobes that is largely responsible for memory and processing of auditory stimuli.

Thalamus A subcortical structure that rests on top of the brain stem beneath the cerebrum and functions as a relay station for neural impulses of sensation (excluding olfaction).

Thalamic aphasia Language deficits as a result of lesion at the thalamus that is characterized by almost fluent speech, significant anomia in spontaneous speech but less so in confrontational naming tasks, impaired receptive language, perseverative semantic paraphasias, normal articulation, hypophonic voice, intact repetition, and intact grammar.

Thrombo-embolus When a piece of a thrombus breaks off and travels through the circulatory system, thereby becoming an embolus.

Thrombotic stroke A cerebrovascular accident that occurs when a thrombus forms and interrupts blood flow to the brain.

Thrombus A site of occlusion of a blood vessel usually the result of slow accumulation of fatty materials such as cholesterol on the walls of the artery.

Tic An involuntary, quick, repetitive, and stereotyped movement. A hyperkinesia.

Tissue necrosis The death of body tissue.

Titubation Involuntary, rapid, and small back–and-forth rhythmic movements of a body part.

Tonic clonic seizure A seizure in which an individual passes through a stage of muscle contraction and loss of consciousness (tonic phase) followed by a stage of abnormal motor activity (clonic phase).

Tonic phase The initial phase of a tonic clonic seizure characterized by a sudden stiffening of the body and limbs due to muscle contractions and a loss of consciousness.

Transient ischemic attack A small ischemia within the brain that resolves itself within 24 hours.

Trauma Serious and potentially life-threatening levels of physical injury.

Traumatic brain injury Damage to the brain that is the result of an external and forceful event.

Traumatic hemorrhage Bleeding as a result of trauma.

Traumatic hydrocephalus A disruption of the brain's ability to reabsorb excess cerebrospinal fluid that is caused by a traumatic event and leads to a life-threatening increase in intracranial pressure.

Tremor An involuntary, rhythmic, and quick movement usually occurring three to five times per second.

Unilateral To be on one side.

Unilateral innervation An innervation pattern that occurs when a nerve receives motor plans from only the contralateral cerebral hemisphere.

Unilateral upper motor neuron (UUMN) dysarthria The dysarthria that results from unilateral UMN damage.

Unrelated verbal paraphasia A verbal substitution of a word that is unrelated in meaning to the intended word.

Upper motor neurons (UMNs) Descending (efferent) tracts of axons that originate in the cerebral cortex and travel in the central nervous system to synapse with the lower motor neurons of the peripheral nervous system at the cranial and spinal nerve nuclei.

Vegetative state A condition in which a person is minimally responsive to stimuli but lacking consciousness and cognition.

Verbal comprehension deficit An inability to comprehend the verbal language produced by others.

Vermis The midline gray matter that connects the two cerebellar hemispheres and receives somatosensory information about the body through projections coursing through the pons.

Vertebral artery One of a set of paired arteries that course superiorly through the cervical vertebrae of the spinal column in the posterior aspect of the neck and come together to form the basilar artery at the pons.

Vigilance The ability to stay alert to the occurrence of a possible stimulus.

Visual agnosia An inability to appropriately perceive visual stimuli resulting from damage to the central nervous system, not peripheral damage to the eyes or optic nerve.

Visual association cortex A section of cortex within the occipital-parietal region responsible for processing and interpreting visual information received from the primary visual cortex.

Visuospatial processing The ability to understand visual information, visual representations, and spatial relationships among objects.

Wernicke's aphasia A fluent aphasia with receptive deficits, repetition deficits, verbal output void of meaning, and a usual lack of awareness of the presence of these deficits.

Wernicke's area A specialized portion of the cerebrum located at the superior marginal gyrus of the left hemisphere's temporal lobe that is responsible for interpreting and deriving meaning from the speech of others.

White matter Myelinated neurons responsible for transmission of impulses from one area of the brain to another.

Working memory The ability to hold a finite amount of information in the mind for immediate processing and manipulating.

Zone of language The anatomic area within the language-dominant hemisphere that houses Broca's and Wernicke's areas as well as the arcuate fasciculus.

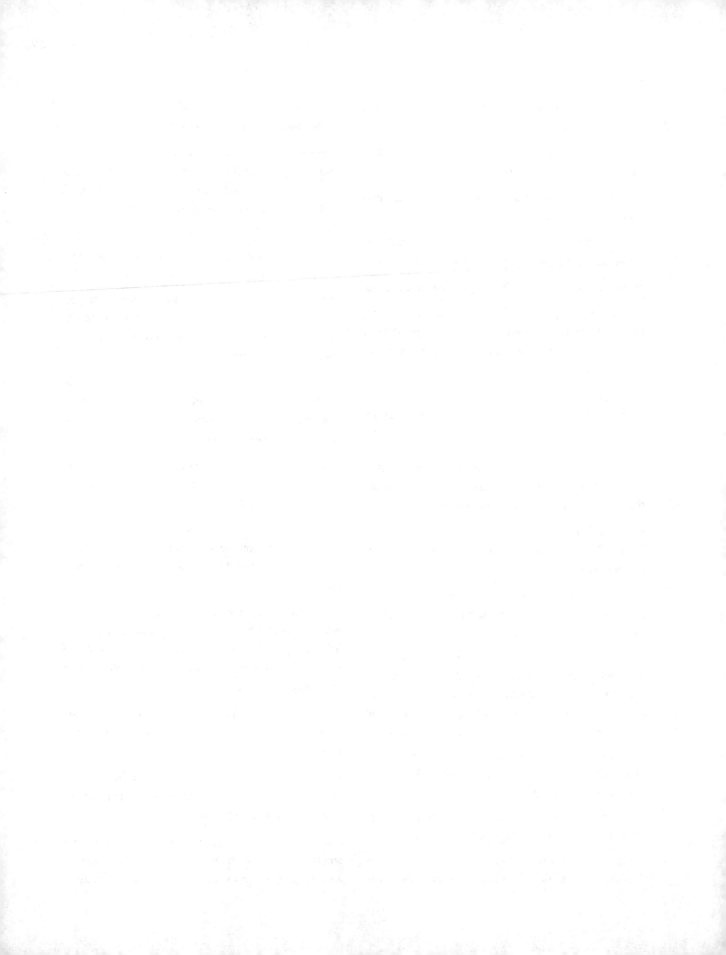

Index

NOTE: page numbers followed by *f* indicate figures and *t*, tables.